Multiple Sclerosis: Diagnosis and Treatment

Multiple Sclerosis: Diagnosis and Treatment

Edited by Floyd Freemont

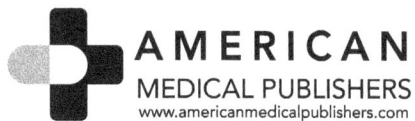

AMERICAN
MEDICAL PUBLISHERS
www.americanmedicalpublishers.com

American Medical Publishers,
41 Flatbush Avenue,
1st Floor, New York,
NY 11217, USA

Visit us on the World Wide Web at:
www.americanmedicalpublishers.com

ISBN: 978-1-63927-306-5

Cataloging-in-Publication Data

Multiple sclerosis : diagnosis and treatment / edited by Floyd Freemont.
p. cm.
Includes bibliographical references and index.
ISBN 978-1-63927-306-5
1. Multiple sclerosis. 2. Multiple sclerosis--Diagnosis. 3. Multiple sclerosis--Treatment.
4. Neurology. I. Freemont, Floyd.
RC377 .M85 2022
616.834--dc23

Table of Contents

Permissions

List of Contributors

Index

Preface

This book has been a concerted effort by a group of academicians, researchers and scientists, who have contributed their research works for the realization of the book. This book has materialized in the wake of emerging advancements and innovations in this field. Therefore, the need of the hour was to compile all the required researches and disseminate the knowledge to a broad spectrum of people comprising of students, researchers and specialists of the field.

Multiple sclerosis is a neurological disease in which the insulating covers of nerve cells of the brain and spinal cord are damaged. This obstructs the ability of the parts of the nervous system to communicate. It causes certain physical, mental as well as psychiatric problems such as double vision, blindness in one eye, muscle weakness, and trouble with sensation and coordination. The causes of multiple sclerosis include destruction by the immune system or failing of the myelin-producing cells. It can also occur due to genetic and environmental factors such as viral infection. It is diagnosed on the basis of signs and symptoms along with medical tests. The most commonly used method of diagnosis is McDonald criteria, which focuses on clinical, radiologic and laboratory evidence of lesions in different areas and times. This book presents researches and studies performed by experts across the globe. Some of the diverse topics covered herein address the varied diagnostic techniques and treatment strategies of this disease. It is appropriate for students seeking detailed information in this area as well as for experts.

At the end of the preface, I would like to thank the authors for their brilliant chapters and the publisher for guiding us all-through the making of the book till its final stage. Also, I would like to thank my family for providing the support and encouragement throughout my academic career and research projects.

Editor

Exercise prescription for patients with multiple sclerosis; potential benefits and practical recommendations

Farzin Halabchi[1], Zahra Alizadeh[1], Mohammad Ali Sahraian[2] and Maryam Abolhasani[3,4]*

Abstract

Background: Multiple sclerosis (MS) can result in significant mental and physical symptoms, specially muscle weakness, abnormal walking mechanics, balance problems, spasticity, fatigue, cognitive impairment and depression. Patients with MS frequently decrease physical activity due to the fear from worsening the symptoms and this can result in reconditioning.
Physicians now believe that regular exercise training is a potential solution for limiting the reconditioning process and achieving an optimal level of patient activities, functions and many physical and mental symptoms without any concern about triggering the onset or exacerbation of disease symptoms or relapse.

Main body: Appropriate exercise can cause noteworthy and important improvements in different areas of cardio respiratory fitness (Aerobic fitness), muscle strength, flexibility, balance, fatigue, cognition, quality of life and respiratory function in MS patients.
Aerobic exercise training with low to moderate intensity can result in the improvement of aerobic fitness and reduction of fatigue in MS patients affected by mild or moderate disability.
MS patients can positively adapt to resistance training which may result in improved fatigue and ambulation. Flexibility exercises such as stretching the muscles may diminish spasticity and prevent future painful contractions. Balance exercises have beneficial effects on fall rates and better balance.
Some general guidelines exist for exercise recommendation in the MS population.
The individualized exercise program should be designed to address a patient's chief complaint, improve strength, endurance, balance, coordination, fatigue and so on.
An exercise staircase model has been proposed for exercise prescription and progression for a broad spectrum of MS patients.

Conclusion: Exercise should be considered as a safe and effective means of rehabilitation in MS patients. Existing evidence shows that a supervised and individualized exercise program may improve fitness, functional capacity and quality of life as well as modifiable impairments in MS patients.

Keywords: Multiple sclerosis, Exercise, Fitness, Balance, Fatigue

* Correspondence: m_abolhasani@tums.ac.ir
[3]Sports and Exercise Medicine, MS Research Center, Neuroscience Institute,
Tehran University of Medical Sciences, Tehran, Iran
[4]Sports and Exercise medicine, Sina MS Research Center, Department of
Sports Medicine, Sina Hospital, Hassan Abad Square, Tehran, Iran
Full list of author information is available at the end of the article

Background

MS or demyelinating disease of central nervous system is characterized with neurodegeneration, inflammation, axonal demyelination and transaction [1–3].

This disease has a chronic nature and affects young people, especially women [3]. However, it can be identified in childhood or late adulthood, although this is rare [4–6].

The chronic course of multiple sclerosis can result in significant mental and physical symptoms and irreversible neurologic deficits, including muscle weakness, ataxia, tremor, spasticity, paralysis, balance disorder, cognitive impairment, loss of vision, double vision, vertigo, impaired swallowing and speech, sensory deficits, bladder and bowel dysfunction, pain, fatigue, and depression [3–5, 7].

Motor dysfunctions in MS patients are frequently due to muscle weakness, abnormal walking mechanics, balance problems, spasticity and fatigue [6, 8, 9].

MS has an unpredictable progressive nature and defects and restrictions of activities may suddenly occur and proceed further than the expected time [10].

It is reported that nearly 50% of multiple sclerosis patients use a an accessory device for moving following 15 years from the beginning of disease [11, 12]. Patients frequently reduce their activities due to their fear of symptoms exacerbation [13]. Limited activities increase disability,unfitness, mobility, quality of life (QOL),gait abnormalitiesand lack of stability and muscle strenght [14, 15].

Impairments related to the disease process itself are irreversible by exercise, but impairments resulting from deconditioning are often reversible with exercise [16]. Furthermore, inactivity places MS patients in raised possibility of comorbid health dependent conditions.

Hypercholesterolemia, hypertension, obesity, type 2 diabetes, cancer, arthritis, osteoporosis, depression, fatigue and death from cardiovascular diseases are the most frequently reported comorbid health -related conditions [13, 16].

These comorbidities in MS have further been connected with a raised possibility of inability development because of reduced aerobic capacity, decreased muscle strength, increased muscle atrophyas well as further neurologic risks (e.g., stroke, etc) [16].

For many years, physicians advised newly diagnosed persons with MS to avoid anyphysical activity and exercise. But now, we believe that regular exercise and training is a possible solution during disease period by limiting the deconditioning process and achieving an optimal level of patient activity, functions and many physical and mental health benefits without any concern about a triggering onset or exacerbation of disease symptoms or relapse [13, 16].

We review in this paper, therapeutic function of physical training in multiple sclerosis. The aim of this narrative review is to emphasize the current documents in exercise recommendation including aerobic, resistance, balance or combined trainingin MS patients, and to provide instructions for the sensible use of the physical modalities. Another aim is to outline the impacts of exercise on MS patients by summarizing the physiologic and health view of multiple sclerosis disease.

Part I

Physiological profile of MS patients

MS patients, especially with more severe impairments, may exhibit some differences in their physiological characteristics in comparison tohealthy age-matched people in terms of cardiovascular and muscle physiology [16].

Decreased aerobic capacity and cardiorespiratory fitness, in expression of VO_2max or maximal oxygen consumption, among MS patients has been about 30% lower than the healthy controls. Respiratory dysfunction due to respiratory muscle weakness and external causes like muscle defect and tiredness are contributing factors in reducing aerobic fitness [14, 16–18].

Another cardiac factors such as basic heart rate and minimum blood pressure are noted to be increased in multiplesclerosis because of impairments in the autonomic control of cardiovascular function that has been estimated about 7% to 60% among MS patients [13, 19].

Also, decreased muscle force calculated by isokinetic and isometric muscle contractions and endurance,muscle mass in total body and increased muscle atrophy are seen in MS patients [13, 16, 20, 21].

It must be shown that muscle strength defect appears particularly clear in the lower extrimities in comparison to the upper extrimities [8, 13].

Flexibility is another physiological characteristic that has diminished in MS patients specially in those with spasticity [16].

About 80% of MS patients feel high temperature intolerance that may be correlated with temporary exacerbation of clinical manifestations of the MS [22]. This is an important concern about MS and exercise. Physical activity is beneficialand important for people with MS, but it should not causeoverheating symptoms [22, 23].

Benefits of exercise for MS patients

Appropriate exercise can lead to significant and important improvements in different areas of cardiorespiratory fitness (Aerobic fitness), muscle strength, flexibility, stability, tiredness, cognition, quality of life and respiratory function. At this section, the details of benefits are described [3].

Cardiorespiratory fitness

Aerobic training in MS patients is more extensively studied than resistance training. During aerobic training, the patients use multiple muscle acts opposite a low burdon with aim of increasing cardiovascular fitness [16].

In summary, aerobic training of low to moderate intensity is effective on cardiovascular fitness, mood and QOL(quality of life) in multiple sclerosis patients with EDSS < 7. This type of exercise is safe and tolerable in many individuals with MS. multiple sclerosis patients are shown to make favorable gains in cardiorespiratory fitness within a short term of exercise (for example, 4 weeks) [18, 24].

Cardiorespiratory exercise training in MS is associated with increased VO_2 Max or VO_2peak and working capacity, respiratory function and reduction of fatigue [18, 25].

A number of studies have made better in cardiorespiratory fitness and aerobic capacity in response to exercise interventions. For instance, Rampello et al. (2007) showed that cardiorespiratory training is better than neurorehabilitation in improvement of functional and moving capacity in multiple sclerosis patients with EDSS < 7 [26].

In another study, Swank et al. (2013) showed that structural cardiorespiratory training can cause improvement in quality of life and emotion of multiple sclerosis patients [2].

In addition cardiorespiratory training can can increase aerobic fitness and reduce tiredness in MS patients some degrees of disability [27]. However, it is not clear whether MS patients with sever impairments have similar adaptations to the cardiorespiratory training benefits or not [13].

Muscle strength and endurance

During strength training, the patients use muscle contractions against a load for increasing muscle strength. Some studies have demonstrated the benefits strenght exercises in MS patients [16, 28].

Increased muscular strength and endurance have also been shown following other exercise interventions in multiple sclerosis patients [18]. Increased strength in lower limbs, could be an important benefit of strnght training in MS. Strength of the lower limb is affected by the disease often previously and to a more range than arms and hands [29, 30].

White et al. (2004) revealed the effects of the strenght exercise on leg strength, moving ability and self-reported fatigue and disability and showed significant improvements in knee extensor and plantar flexor muscle forces and thenwalking performance [8].

MS patients can make good adjustments to strenght trainings in accompanying by improvement in moving capacity and tiredness [30]. Gutierrez.et al. (2005) revealed that strenght training is a good intervention to improve moving and functional capacity in MS patients having moderate disabilities [9]. Surakka et al. (2004) reported that cardiorespiratory and strength training improves tiredness in MS patients with some degree of disabilities and the training type was more achievable in women patients with less disability in comparison to men patients with more disabilities [27]. In general, resistance training with moderate intensity can induce improvements in muscle strength and function among moderately impaired persons with MS. Thistype of exercise is safe and well tolerated in multiple sclerosis [8, 9, 16, 25, 29].

Bone health

The use of therapeutic corticosteroids and inactivity may both lead to osteoporosis and pathologic fractures in MS patients. Furthermore, the chronic process of disease and inactivity in multiple sclerosis patients can cause loss of muscle and bone mass. Shabas et al. (2000) showed that among 220 women with MS, 82% had corticosteroid's history of use and 53% had loss of mobility and bone mass [31].

Weight - bearing exercise can slow the loss of muscle and bone mass in MS. For this reason, the resistance training program is recommended for maintaining and developing the muscle and bone mass in the whole of body [18].

Flexibility

People with multiple sclerosis frequently have limitation in joint motion because of spasticity and prolonged inactivity. Goals of flexibility exercises are to lengthen the muscles, enhance joint range of motion, reduce spasticity, and maintain good posture and balance [16, 18].

Avoidance of spasticity in early stages of disease is very noted. Lenghening the muscles can delay coming aching muscle contractions and spasms. Studies regarding the effects of flexibility exercise on MS are limited, but this type of exercise are recommended. These exercises must be performed by using proprioceptive facilitation techniques and stretching tight muscles in pelvis, chest, leg and hip flexores. For preventing spasticity aggravation, activities like for example indicating the toes during traing must be prevented [6, 13, 16, 18].

Balance

Impairments of balance, such as difficulty in maintenance of upright posture, are common in MS patients. Swing during silent standing, moving slowly following postural disturnances and inability to maintain the balance are common in multiple sclerosis and may be related to falling [5, 32, 33].

Some articles showed the effects of balance training in stability of MS patients. Improvements in balance assessed by Berg Balance Scale (BBS), are shown following group aquatic and stability training [34, 35].

Cattaneo et al. (2007) studied the effects of stability training on multiplesclerosis patients and demonstrated that stability training is effective to reduce the falling and improve stability [36].

Generally, balance training has small, but statistically significant effect on improving stability and reducing falling risk in MS patients with some degrees of disabilities. There was limited data on patients with severe MS who are not ambulatory [33, 37].

Tiredness
Tiredness is greatly seen in MS patients and leads to exacerbation of the neurological and other symptoms of MS such as depression, pain, anxiety and cognitive dysfunction [18, 37]. The underlying mechanisms of fatigue are unknown.

Physical inactivity and mental disorders because of MS or comorbidities have been suggested to cause tiredness.

Exercise can cause some changes such as neuroprotection and neuroplasticity, reduction of long-term inactivityand deregulation of hypothalamus-pituitary-adrenal (HPA) axis and then reduction of tiredness in patients [38].

Evidence has revealed that exercise can manage energy and tierdness levels in healthy peoples. Results are much less conclusive with relation to the exercise and tiedness management in MS patients, although several studies provide support for the potential benefits of exercise in these patients [25, 37, 39].

Cardiorespiratory training and neurorehabilitation, energy storage programs and cooling devices and plans have also been shown as good and effective interventions [24, 40, 41]. Petajan et al. showed that regular aerobic exercisecan reduce fatigue in MS patients, and improve both mood and the QOL(quality of life) [42].

Kargarfard et al. (2012), revealed that aquatic training is effective on tierdness and QOL of women with MS [34].

Establishing a safe and effective exercise program may be considered as an important option while planning for treatment of fatigue and should be encouraged [37].

Quality of life
HRQOL(Health-related quality of life) has diminished in MS patients. The reduced QOL may be related with deterioration of symptoms, walking and cognition in patients [14].

Stuifbergen (2006) studied the positive effects of regular exercises in general health, liveliness and function of patients [43]. The results of several studies on patients with MS confirm the effectiveness of exercise on long period improvement in physical and social function and quality of life [25, 42, 44].

In summary, exercise training can cause prominent and positive effects in QOL of persons with MS [3].

CNS morphology and imaging findings
Until now, no evidence has been foundabout the effects of exercise training on brain structure in multiple sclerosis disease. Any way, some studies revealed the effects of cardiorespiratory training on volume of brain grey matter volume and unity of white matter tract as well as functional connectivity of the hippocampus and cortex in people with MS [5, 45]. Despite the limited data on exercise performance on the brain structureon, some studies revealed regular cardiorespiratory training work against brain degeneration in relapsing-remitting type of MS and probably is a protective strategy.

Some studies proposed detection of morphological changes with exercise in the CNS of MS patients by imaging techniques. Although, evidence is still not enoughto demonstrate effects of exercise on brain structure in multiple sclerosis [46].

Implications for practice
The evidence confirms that individuals with MS are less active than healthy individuals [28]. This is important when designing effective exercise programs for both increasing the tendency and adherence to exercise and createing potential beneficial effects.

Despite all the limitations, exercise has beneficial effects on individuals with multiple sclerosis. Furthermore, no side effects from exercise have been seen in most studies [14, 23, 46–48].

Part II: Exercise recommendations
Growing evidence exists in favour of exercise as an effective treatment for MS patients, and therefore it should be recommended in the rehabilitation process [7, 49].

Some general guidelines exist for exercise prescription in the MS population. In this part, we will discuss the practical points for exercise prescription in MS patients.

Pre-exercise evaluation
A comprehensive pre-exercise screening should be considered before designing an individualized exercise program. This should be preferably performed by sports medicine physician, physical medicine and rehabilitation physician, exercise physiologist or physical therapist with proper expertise on MS patients [13, 16, 18, 23, 50].

The evaluation should include a thorough physical examination and history, including MS, functional, and exercise histories. A cardiopulmonary function review should also be done [6, 49]. Patients should also be screened for risk factors or presence of cardiovascular, respiratory or metabolic disorders [51].

Some authors have recommended a baseline ECG or submaximal stress test for this review [52]. However, some others do not always find these tests necessary unless individual cardiovascular risk factors and cardiac history mandate further evaluations [23]. In these cases, MS patients, stratified as "high risk" for medical problems during exercise should undergo a supervised exercise test before participating in an exercise routine [51].

Also, some authors recommend fitness evaluations to be used as a baseline for exercise prescription in MS patients. Using these assessments, the physician can formulate an appropriate initial exercise program [53].

After medical clearance was obtained by physician, exercise professionals should use proper fitness tests to estimate the patient's cardiorespiratory, musculoskeletal fitness, as well as neuromuscular/functional competence [53]. These tests should be selected according to the patient's tolerance and goals [18, 54, 55]. Fitness tests should be performed according to the guidelines of American College of Sports Medicine [51]. The six minute walk test

(6MWT) requiring minimal apparatus, is a valid tool for MS patients, and is applicable for patients who use walkers, canes, and assistive devices [56, 57]. Other proper tests consist of arm, leg, or combined leg and arm cycle ergometry and recumbent stepping.

Table 1 describes suggestions for testing cardiorespiratory and musculoskeletal fitness, as well as neuromuscular/functional competence.

Exercise program

The individualized exercise program should be designed to address a patient's chief complaint or goal—to improve strength, endurance, balance, coordination, fatigue, etc. It should consider a patient's baseline impairments and capabilities [18, 50]. The prescription should include all the necessary components, such as frequency, duration,

Table 1 Recommendations for exercise testing in MS patients [53–55]

Fitness Parameter	Measures	Comments
Aerobic fitness		
6-min walk test. It is used to measure improvements and differences in Pre and Post program performances but not to compare them to "healthy individuals."	Total distance walked, heart rate, RPE[a], BP. The HR response to exercise may be decreased due to autonomic dysfunction. Therefore, the use of the RPE scale is preferred in these patients.	Using air conditioner for all aerobic testing. Spasticity, lower limb weakness, and paralysis will preclude walking tests in some patients.
Submaximal, upright, or recumbent leg cycle ergometry. Intermittent instead of continuous protocol may be indicated. Increase work rate by 12–25 W per stage.	Workload and steady-state heart rate to predict VO$_2$peak; RPE.	Toe clips and foot straps may be necessary in persons with tremors, spasticity, or weakness in the lower extremities. Begin with a warm-up of unloaded pedaling or cranking.
Combination arm/leg cycle ergometry.	Workload and steady-state heart rate to predict VO$_2$peak; RPE.	May reduce difficulty in individuals with lower extremity uncoordination Experience.
Arm ergometry—increase work rate 8–12 W per stage.	Workload and steady-state heart rate to predict VO$_2$peak;RPE.	Alternative for persons with lower extremity weakness or paralysis.
Muscular Strength/Endurance		
30-s sit-to-stand test These tests are used to measure improvements and differences in pre- and postprogram performance but not to compare them to "healthy individuals."	Number of times patient comes to a full stand with arms crossing a standard size chair.	A functional measure of lower extremity strength, power, and muscle endurance.
10RM Testing.	Maximal weight lifted for 10 repetitions (reps).	Machines provide test reliability, support, and joint stability. Remind patients to exhale on concentric action and avoid breath holding.
Flexibility		
Modified bench sit and reach test (1 ft on floor and other straight).	Distance reached in hip/trunk flexion.	Administer test with client seated on a table.
Goniometry.	Range of motion.	Focus on flexibility of hamstrings, hip flexors, ankle plantar flexors, shoulder adductors, and internal rotators.
Power/functional		
Timed up and go test.	Time to stand from a chair, walk a 3-m round trip, and sit back down on the same chair.	Results correlate with gait speed, balance, functional level, the ability to go out.
Five-times sit-to-stand test.	Time to stand and sit 5 consecutive times on a standard size chair.	Most useful in patients ≤60 y.

BP blood pressure, RPE ratings of perceived exertion, HR heart rate, MS multiple sclerosis; RM, repetition maximum
[a]RPE is a subjective rating scale ranging from six to 20 that gives an indication of the workout intensity level

intensity, modalities to be used, and precautions to be observed [50].

Exercise staircase model

An exercise staircase model has been proposed for exercise prescription and progression for a broad spectrum of MS patients [23].

At the base of the staircase is the passive range of motion exercises. This serves as the foundation and is suitable for the most physically and cognitively disabled. These exercises should be done no less than once daily.

The next step up the staircase is the active range of motion exercises. These are proper for less disabled MS individuals and may be carried out with or without gravity eliminationas strength allows. Even when diffused weakness exists, resistance exercises of cautiously chosen muscles, perhaps not more than 2 per limb, may still permit efficient strengthening. In motivated patients with mild MS, focused muscle strengthening with progressive resistive exercises may be effective.

The third and highest step in the staircase is integrated exercises. Integrated exercises use a combination of strength, endurance, flexibility, balance, and coordination exercises [16, 23]. Recent studies have also shown that combined exercisetraining may have advantages, especiallyin reducing fatigue perception, and improving someaspects of QOL [58, 59]. The exact combination of exercises should be individualized according to patient needs and capabilities. Aquatic exercise is a good example of an integrated exercise, simultaneously incorporating endurance, resistance, flexibility and balance components [16, 23].

Aerobic exercises

In general, aerobic training of low to moderate intensity produced improvements in aerobic capacity and in measures of HRQL, mood, and depression in patients with mild to moderate MS (EDSS < 7). Aerobic training is generally safe and well tolerated in these patients [13, 16]. Individuals with MS have been shown to make favorable gains in cardiorespiratory fitness within a short span of 4 weeks [18, 60].

Bicycle ergometry, arm ergometry, arm-leg ergometry, aquatic exercise, and treadmill walking may all be suggested, although rowing and running are only recommended for MS patients with proper functioning [13, 54, 55, 60–67]. Currently, the use of robot assisted weight supported treadmills has shown promising results in MS patients [68–71]. Exercise frequency of 2–5 weekly sessions is recommended according to the patient's toleration. It is preferred to set these sessions in non-resistance training days [13, 53–55]. Starting with intensity of 40%–70% of VO$_2$max, 60%–80% of maximal heart rate or 40%–60% heart rate reserve is recommended [13, 18, 53, 63, 64]. A rating of percieved exertion (RPE) scale of 11–13 (fairly light to somewhat hard) is another valuable alternative for exercise intensity. As autonomic dysfunction (a common finding in MS patients) may attenuate the HR response to exercise in MS patients, the use of the RPE scale is advised throughout the exercise [13, 53–55].

Depending on the level of patient's disability, the initial training duration of 10–40 min is suggested. At first, it may be splitted to three 10-min bouts [13, 53–55]. During the first 2–6 months, progression should be attained by increasing the duration or frequency of exercise sessions. After this time, it should be checked to find out whether a higher intensity is tolerable. In this condition, one training session may be replaced with interval training (up to 90% of VO$_2$max) [13, 18, 53–55].

Resistance exercises

It is important that resistance training should be supervized for safety by an experienced staff until the MS patient is contented with the program [13]. Other than safety concern, it has been shown that supervised is more effective than nonsupervised resistance training [13, 72].

In terms of resistance training modalities, the use of weight machines (i.e., closed kinetic chains) is preferred to free weights (i.e., open kinetic chains) for safety, especially in the initial training phase [13]. If weight machines are not practicable, a home based exercise program using elastic bands and/or body weight as resistance should be considered as a substitute. However, it is not easy to achieve the same benefit from this type of exercises, as it can be achieved using weight machines [13, 18].

Training frequency of 2–3 weekly sessions is well tolerated and gives rise to significant progress in patients. Training intensity should be set in the range of 8 to 15 repetition maximum (RM) with 60%–80% of 1RM. Initial starting intensities of approximately 15 RM is suitable [53–55]. This should be gradually increased over several months toward intensities of approximately 8 to 10 RM [8, 18]. Resistance can be securely added by 2% to 5% when 15 repetitions are properly carried out in successive training sessions [8, 18]. However, day-to-day variability in fatigue will likely justify flexibility in the resistance program. The rate of progression should permit for full recovery between exercise sessions to prevent overuse musculoskeletal injuries [13, 18].

The patient should begin with 1 to 3 sets, which can be gradually increased over a few months to 3 to 4 sets of each exercise. Allow rest breaks of 2 to 4 min between sets and exercises [16].

Regarding the number of exercises, a whole-body program including 4 to 10 exercises is suitable. As a general rule regarding the exercise order, large muscle group exercises should be performed before small muscle group exercises, and multiple-joint exercises before single-joint exercises [13, 53, 73]. Prioritize lower extremity over upper extremity exercises. In MS patients, the lower extremity strength deficit is greater than that of the upper extremity [13, 74].

Balance training of agonist/antagonist muscle groups is also necessary. Particular emphasis should be placed on the posterior shoulder girdle, spine, hip and knee extensors, and dorsiflexor muscles [4–6, 9]. However, any contraindications based on individual impairments should be addressed [16, 18].

Sample exercises include shoulder press, seated scapular row, latissimus pull-downs, chest press, knee extensions, seated leg press, seated hamstring curls, biceps curls, seated triceps extensions, seated back extensions and abdominal crunches, and chair sit to stands [53–55].

In terms of precautions, weight lifting in a seated position (as in most weight machines) is preferred to minimize the risk of falling with free weights. If an individual has impaired proprioception or coordination, the exercise should be done under supervision [16, 18]. Also, compared to the endurance exercise, resistance training in heat sensitive patients less frequently cause symptom exacerbations due to increased body temperature [18].

Flexibility and stretching exercises

Individuals with MS usually have limited range of motion as a result of spasticity and prolonged immobility. Flexibility exercises are recommended to lengthen muscles, offset the effects of spasticity, enhance joint mobility, and improve balance and posture [18]. These exercises should be performed at least daily for 10 to 15 min [18, 75, 76]. Stretching should be done before and after exercise sessions and must involve both upper and lower body muscle groups used in the program. The neck extensors, anterior shoulder girdle, hip flexors, hamstring, hip adductors and plantar flexors should be especially emphasized [53–55]. Spastic muscles must be particularly targeted. Stretches should be slow, gentle, and prolonged. The stretch should be up to the end of the comfort range and held there for 20 to 60 s. Ballistic stretch or bouncing with the stretch is not recommended. Furthermore, stretching should not be painful. Individuals who need assistance with stretching may use a towel, rope, or partner. For immobilized patients with spasticity, passive stretching may be done by an expert therapist. Passive range of motion above the joint of a paralysed area is recommended. Complementary techniques such as deep breathing, light massage and progressive muscle relaxation techniques may also be beneficial. Supervised yoga or tai chi classes may be suitable for doing stretching exercises in higher-functioning MS patients [16, 18, 62].

Balance and coordination exercises

Particular attention should be paid to include activities for improvement of balance and coordination. In these activities, the MS patient should shift the centre of gravity and respond to external signals. Swiss ball exercise with coordinated movements and bilateral muscle actions may increase coordination and balance, as well. This type of exercise is extremely helpful to increase strength and flexibility, as well. Tai Chi exercises with slow eccentric movements may also be beneficial to maintain balance, strength and range of motion. For patients with insufficient stability or strength to take part in the mentioned activities, coordination and balance drills may be done in shallow pools. In this milieu, the risk of falling or injury due to balance loss is minimised and support of the water will permit the accomplishment of challenging movements, when it is not possible on land. Improvement of posture, flexibility, coordination and muscle tone are potential advantages of water exercise [6].

Respiratory muscle training

Adaptation of respiratory muscles to training programs can occur similar to skeletal muscles [18].

In a study, Foglio et al. (1994) examined respiratory muscle function and exercise capacity in MS patients. They concluded that in patients, reduction in exercise tolerance may be associated, at least partially, to diminished respiratory muscle strength [77].

O'Kroy et al. (1993) showed that respiratory muscle training enhanced maximal inspiratory and expiratory pressures, controlled breathing exercises and increased respiratory muscle endurance in MS patients. The use of ventilatory resistance training devices may be helpful and increase respiratory muscle strength [78].

Special precautions

MS patients are especially susceptible to exercise-related fatigue, heat intolerance, and falling [53–55]. Furthermore, some problems such as spasticity, neurologic or cognitive deficits, and urinary incontinence may influence the exercise program. So, special measures should be considered in these cases. A summary of these precautions and safety recommendations are listed in Table 2.

Fatigue

There are some concerns about the potential effect of exercise on exacerbation of fatigue in MS patients. However, the existing evidence supports the fact that regular exercise training is linked with a small but important reduction in fatigue among persons with MS [39, 63, 79].

Exercise on elliptical machine may result in significant reduction of fatigue among MS patients. So, this type of exercise may be a useful part of MS rehabilitation

Table 2 Special considerations and precautions for exercise prescription in MS patients

Special considerations	Precautions
Fatigue	Schedule resistance training on non-endurance training days [13, 53, 54].
Spasticity	Consider foot and/or hand straps for ergometers. Use machines instead of free weights [53–55].
Heat intolerance and reduced sweating response	Encourage adequate hydration, keep room temperature between 20 and 22° C. Using of cooling fans and precooling before aerobic exercise might have positive effects on performance. It is better to plan exercise in the morning when body temperature is at the lowest [53, 54, 93].
Cognitive deficits	Provide written instructions, diagrams, frequent instructions, and verbal cues [53–55, 94]. Exercise tasks should be initially performed with minimal resistance. Individuals with cognitive impairments may require additional supervision during exercise to ensure their safety [18].
Lack of coordination in extremities	Consider using a synchronized upright or recumbent arm/leg ergometer to ensure balance and safety [53–55, 94].
Sensory loss and balance problems	Perform all exercises preferably in a seated position; use machines or elastic bands instead of free weights [53–55, 94].
Higher energy cost of walking (2–3 times greater than age-matched healthy persons)	Adjust workloads to maintain target heart rate and check heart rate regularly [13, 53–55, 94].
Daily variations in symptoms	Provide close exercise supervision and make daily modifications to exercise variables [13, 53–55, 94].
Urinary incontinence /urgency	Ensure adequate hydration, and schedule exercise in close proximity to restrooms [53–55, 94].
Symptom exacerbation	Discontinue exercises and refer the patient to a physician. Resume exercise program. Once symptoms are stable and the patient is medically ready to continue [13, 53–56, 94].

programs [80]. Aquatic exercise may also successfully improve fatigue of MS patients and may be considered in the rehabilitation of these patients [34].

Heat intolerance

A common concern with exercise in MS patients is potentially prompting Uhthoff phenomenon. Uhthoff phenomenon is defined as developing transient symptoms such as amblyopia or blurred vision triggered by overheating from exercise [6, 23]. The exact mechanism of Uhthoff phenomenon is not determined. It may be the result of heat-worsened conduction across partially demyelinated axons, fatigue of damaged neuronal pathways with repetitive nerve transmission, [23, 81] or a hormonal factor produced by cooling [16]. Exercise-induced Uhthoff phenomenon should not be considered as a contraindication for exercise [23]. Fortunately, temporary and mild heat stress causes only transient exacerbation of symptoms without apparent remaining impairment after normothermia is achieved [18]. It often settles within an hour or even sooner with rapid cooling [23]. Moreover, it is still more common in MS patients to respond to exercise in heat conditions with just general fatigue rather than Uhthoff phenomenon with focal neurologic deficits [23, 82]. Studies have demonstrated that usual exercise does not considerably increase core body temperature. A study reported a

mean rectal temperature change of 0.1 C during land-based exercise and - 0.1C during water-based exercise [83]. Alternatively, normal thermoregulatory responses (e.g., sweating and peripheral vasodilatation) that preserve a stable core temperature during usual exercise may be impaired in MS patients. In such cases, an increase in core temperature of even less than 1 C may trigger heat-related symptoms [16, 23]. The use of cooling devices such as head-vest liquid cooling garment may provide some modest benefits for MS patients [84, 85]. Another study showed the reduced fatigue and improved ambulation for up to 3 h postcooling with the use of either the liquid cooling system or an icepack suit [23, 85, 86]. When engaging in pool-based aquatic exercises, the ideal water temperature for heat sensitive MS patients seems to be between 27 and 29 C [18, 23, 87, 88]. Temperatures below 27 C can paradoxically enhance spasticity [23, 89].

MS patients, especially those who are heat-sensitive, should avoid scheduling exercise sessions in the hottest times of the day or times when they experience greater fatigue. Exercise sessions in the early morning, when there is cooler temperature and lower body temperature, may be more endurable than in the afternoon [18, 90]. Moreover, resistance exercise is more tolerable than endurance exercise for heat sensitive MS patients and should be encouraged to incorporate resistance exercises in their routines [91].

Particularly for individuals with heat sensitivity, several investigators have recommended pre-exercise cooling strategies, such as the use of cooling devices, [6, 18, 50, 92] cold water lower body immersion, [18] or taking a tepid bath 20 to 30 min before (and after) exercise [23]. Individuals should wear light exercise clothing or may even try exercising with a cooling vest. The exercise area temperature should be kept cool through the use of fans or air conditioning [16, 23].

Risk of falling

Special attention is needed for patients at high risk of falling due to the balance and coordination problems as well as sensory and proprioceptive deficits. These issues should be particularly considered when planning and supervising exercise sessions in MS patients [13, 16].

Conclusion

Exercise should be considered as a safe and effective means of rehabilitation in MS patients. Existing evidence has shown that a supervised and individualized exercise program can improve physical fitness, functional capacity, quality of life and modifiable impairments in MS patients. There are general guidelines that may be followed for exercise prescription for the MS population. These guidelines should be adapted according to the patient's needs, abilities and preferences.

Abbreviations
BP: blood pressure; EDSS: Expanded Disability Status Scale; HR: heart rate; HRQOL: Health related quality of life; MS: Multiple sclerosis; QOL: Quality of life; RM: repetition maximum; RPE: Rate of precieved exhaustion; RPE: ratings of perceived exertion; VO$_2$max: maximal oxygen consumption; VO$_2$peak: peak oxygen consumption

Acknowledgements
The authors would like to thank Development and Research center of Sina Hospital and Mrs. Pourmand (Urology Research Center, Tehran University of Medical Sciences) for editing the manuscript.

Funding
We did not have any sources of funding.

Authors' contributions
HF and AM Wrote the primary draft. SMA Proposed the idea and revised the primary draft. AZ reviewed the literature and approved the primary draft. All authors read and approved the final manuscript.

Competing interests
None of the authors had any financial or personal conflicts of interest.

Author details
[1]Sports and Exercise Medicine, Sports Medicine Research Center, Neuroscience Institute, Tehran University of Medical Sciences, Tehran, Iran. [2]Neurology, MS fellowship, MS Research Center, Neuroscience Institute, Tehran University of Medical Sciences, Tehran, Iran. [3]Sports and Exercise Medicine, MS Research Center, Neuroscience Institute, Tehran University of Medical Sciences, Tehran, Iran. [4]Sports and Exercise medicine, Sina MS Research Center, Department of Sports Medicine, Sina Hospital, Hassan Abad Square, Tehran, Iran.

References
1. Pilutti LA, Platta ME, Motl R, Latimer-Cheung AE. The safety of exercise training in multiple sclerosis: a systematic review. J Neurol Sci [review]. 2014;343:3–7.
2. Swank C, Thompson M, Medley A. Aerobic exercise in people with multiple sclerosis: its feasibility and secondary benefits. Int J MS Care. 2013;15(3):138–45.
3. Motl RW, Sandroff BM. Benefits of exercise training in multiple sclerosis. Curr Neurol Neurosci Rep. 2015;15(9):62.
4. Romberg A, Virtanen A, Aunola S, Karppi SL, Karanko H, Ruutiainen J. Exercise capacity, disability and leisure physical activity of subjects with multiple sclerosis. Mult Scler. 2004;10(2):212–8.
5. Motl RW, Pilutti LA. The benefits of exercise training in multiple sclerosis. Nat Rev Neurol. 2012;8(9):487–97.
6. Petajan JH, White AT. Recommendations for physical activity in patients with multiple sclerosis. Sports Med. 1999;27(3):179–91.
7. Sa MJ. Exercise therapy and multiple sclerosis: a systematic review. J Neurol. 2014;261(9):1651–61.
8. White L, McCoy S, Castellano V, Gutierrez G, Stevens J, Walter G, et al. Resistance training improves strength and functional capacity in persons with multiple sclerosis. Mult Scler. 2004;10(6):668–74.
9. Gutierrez GM, Chow JW, Tillman MD, McCoy SC, Castellano V, White LJ. Resistance training improves gait kinematics in persons with multiple sclerosis. Arch Phys Med Rehabil. 2005;86(9):1824–9.
10. Asano M, Dawes DJ, Arafah A, Moriello C, Mayo NE. What does a structured review of the effectiveness of exercise interventions for persons with multiple sclerosis tell us about the challenges of designing trials? Mult Scler. 2009;15(4):412–21.
11. O'Connor P. Key issues in the diagnosis and treatment of multiple sclerosis. An overview Neurology. 2002;59(6 Suppl 3):S1–33.
12. Grima DT, Torrance GW, Francis G, Rice G, Rosner AJ, Lafortune L. Cost and health related quality of life consequences of multiple sclerosis. Mult Scler. 2000;6(2):91–8.
13. Dalgas U, Stenager E, Ingemann-Hansen T. Multiple sclerosis and physical exercise: recommendations for the application of resistance-, endurance- and combined training. Mult Scler. 2008;14(1):35–53.
14. Gallien P, Nicolas B, Robineau S, Petrilli S, Houedakor J, Durufle A. Physical training and multiple sclerosis. Ann Readapt Med Phys. 2007;50(6):373–6. 69-72
15. Pilutti LA, Platta ME, Motl RW, Latimer-Cheung AE. The safety of exercise training in multiple sclerosis: a systematic review. J Neurol Sci. 2014;343(1):3–7.
16. Sandoval AE. Exercise in multiple sclerosis. Phys Med Rehabil Clin N Am. 2013;24(4):605–18.
17. Feltham MG, Collett J, Izadi H, Wade DT, Morris MG, Meaney AJ, et al. Cardiovascular adaptation in people with multiple sclerosis following a twelve week exercise programme suggest deconditioning rather than autonomic dysfunction caused by the disease Results from a randomized controlled trial. Eur J Phys Rehabil Med. 2013;49(6):765–74.
18. White LJ, Dressendorfer RH. Exercise and multiple sclerosis. Sports Med. 2004;34(15):1077–100.
19. Huang M, Jay O, Davis SL. Autonomic dysfunction in multiple sclerosis: implications for exercise. Auton Neurosci. 2015;188:82–5.
20. Formica CA, Cosman F, Nieves J, Herbert J, Lindsay R. Reduced bone mass and fat-free mass in women with multiple sclerosis: effects of ambulatory status and glucocorticoid use. Calcif Tissue Int. 1997;61(2):129–33.

21. Lambert CP, Lee Archer R, Evans WJ. Body composition in ambulatory women with multiplesclerosis. Arch Phys Med Rehabil. 2002;83(11):1559–61.
22. White AT, Wilson TE, Davis SL, Petajan JH. Effect of precooling on physical performance in multiple sclerosis. Mult Scler. 2000;6(3):176–80.
23. Brown TR, Kraft GH. Exercise and rehabilitation for individuals with multiple sclerosis. Phys Med Rehabil Clin N Am. 2005;16(2):513–55.
24. Mostert S, Kesselring J. Effects of a short term exercise training programme on aerobic fitness, fatigue, health perception and activity level of subjects with multiple sclerosis. multiple sclerosis. 2002;8(2):161–8.
25. Latimer-Cheung AE, Pilutti LA, Hicks AL, Martin Ginis KA, Fenuta AM, MacKibbon KA, et al. Effects of exercise training on fitness, mobility, fatigue, and health-related quality of life among adults with multiple sclerosis: a systematic review to inform guideline development. Arch Phys Med Rehabil. 2013;94(9):1800–28. e3
26. Rampello A, Franceschini M, Piepoli M, Antenucci R, Lenti G, Olivieri D, et al. Effect of aerobic training on walking capacity and maximal exercise tolerance in patients with multiple sclerosis: a randomized crossover controlled study. Phys Ther. 2007;87(5):545–55.
27. Surakka J, Romberg A, Ruutiainen J, Aunola S, Virtanen A, Karppi SL, et al. Effects of aerobic and strength exercise on motor fatigue in men and women with multiple sclerosis: a randomized controlled trial. Clin Rehabil. 2004;18(7):737–46.
28. Motl RW, McAuley E, Snook EM. Physical activity and multiple sclerosis: a meta-analysis. Mult Scler. 2005;11(4):459–63.
29. DeBolt LS, McCubbin JA. The effects of home-based resistance exercise on balance, power, and mobility in adults with multiple sclerosis. Arch Phys Med Rehabil. 2004;85(2):290–7.
30. Kjølhede T, Vissing K, Dalgas U. Multiple sclerosis and progressive resistance training: a systematic review. Mult Scler J. 2012;18(9):1215–28.
31. Shabas D, Weinreb H. Preventive healthcare in women with interferon beta-1b in MS: results of an open label trial. Neurol- multiple sclerosis. J Womens Health Gend Based Med. 2000;9(4):389–95.
32. Motl RW, Learmonth YC, Pilutti LA, Gappmaier E, Coote S. Top 10 research questions related to physical activity and multiple sclerosis. Res Q Exerc Sport. 2015;86(2):117–29.
33. Cameron MH, Lord S. Postural Control in Multiple Sclerosis: Implications for Fall Prevention. Curr Neurol Neurosci Rep. 2010;10:407–12.
34. Kargarfard M, Etemadifar M, Baker P, Mehrabi M, Hayatbakhsh R. Effect of aquatic exercise training on fatigue and health-related quality of life in patients with multiple sclerosis. Arch Phys Med Rehabil. 2012; 93(10):1701–8.
35. Rafeeyan Z, Azarbarzin M, Moosa FM, Hasanzadeh A. Effect of aquatic exercise on the multiple sclerosis patients' quality of life. Iran J Nurs Midwifery Res. 2010;15(1):43–7.
36. Cattaneo D, Jonsdottir J, Zocchi M, Regola A. Effects of balance exercises on people with multiple sclerosis: a pilot study. Clin Rehabil. 2007;21(9):771–81.
37. Motl RW. Benefits, safety, and prescription of exercise in persons with multiple sclerosis. Expert Rev Neurother. 2014;14(12):1429–36.
38. Heine M, van de Port I, Rietberg MB, van Wegen EE, Kwakkel G. Exercise therapy for fatigue in multiple sclerosis. Cochrane Database Syst Rev. 2015; 11(9):CD009956.
39. Andreasen AK, Stenager E, Dalgas U. The effect of exercise therapy on fatigue in multiple sclerosis. Mult Scler. 2011;17(9):1041–54.
40. Karpatkin HI. Multiple sclerosis and exercise: a review of the evidence. Int J MS Care. 2005;7(2):36–41.
41. Braley TJ, Chervin RD. Fatigue in multiple sclerosis: mechanisms, evaluation, and treatment. Sleep. 2010;33(8):1061–7.
42. Petajan JH, Gappmaier E, White AT, Spencer MK, Mino L, Hicks RW. Impact of aerobictraining on fitness and quality of life in multiple sclerosis. Ann Neurol. 1996;39:432–41.
43. Stuifbergen AK, Blozis SA, Harrison TC, Becker HA. Exercise, functional limitations, and quality of life: a longitudinal study of persons with multiple sclerosis. Arch Phys Med Rehabil. 2006;87(7):935–43.
44. Dalgas U, Stenager E, Jakobsen J, Petersen T, Hansen HJ, Knudsen C, et al. Fatigue, mood and quality of life improve in MS patients after progressive resistance training. Mult Scler. 2010;16(4):480–90.
45. Prakash RS, Snook EM, Motl RW, Kramer AF. Aerobic fitness is associated with gray matter volume and white matter integrity in multiple sclerosis. Brain Res. 2010;1341:41–51.
46. Doring A, Pfueller CF, Paul F, Dorr J. Exercise in multiple sclerosis – an integral component of disease management. EPMA J. 2011;3(1):2.

47. Dalgas U, Stenager E. Multiple sclerosis and physical training. Ugeskr Laeger. 2005;167(14):1495–9.
48. Dalgas U, Stenager E. Exercise and disease progression in multiple sclerosis: can exercise slow down the progression of multiple sclerosis? Ther Adv Neurol Disord. 2012 Mar;5(2):81–95.
49. Rietberg MB, Brooks D, Uitdehaag BM, Kwakkel G. Exercise therapy for multiple sclerosis. Cochrane Database Syst Rev. 2005;1:CD003980.
50. Vollmer T, Benedict R, Bennett S. Exercise as prescriptive therapy in multiple sclerosis. Int J MS Care. 2012;14:2–14.
51. Medicine ACoS. ACSM's Guidelines for exercise testing and prescription: Lippincott Williams & Wilkins; 2013.
52. Taylor R. Rehabilitation of persons with multiple sclerosis. Phys Med Rehabil Phila: WB Saunders. 1996:1105–7.
53. Ronai P, LaFontaine T, Bollinger L. Exercise guidelines for persons with multiple sclerosis. Strength & Conditioning Journal. 2011;33(1) 30–3
54. Jackson K, Mulcare J. Multiple sclerosis. In: Myers J, Nieman D, editors. ACSM's Resources for clinical exercise physiology. 2nd ed. Baltimore: Lippincott Williams & Wilkins; 2009. p. 34–43.
55. Jackson K, Mulchare J. Multiple sclerosis. In: Durstine JL, Moore GE, Painter PL, Roberts SO, editors. ACSM's Exercise Management for Persons with chronic diseases and disabilities. 3rd ed. Champaign, IL: Human kinetics; 2009. p. 321–6.
56. Goldman MD, Marrie RA, Cohen JA. Evaluation of the six-minute walk in multiple sclerosis subjects and healthy controls. Mult Scler. 2008;14(3):383–90.
57. Savci S, Inal-Ince D, Arikan H, Guclu-Gunduz A, Cetisli-Korkmaz N, Armutlu K, et al. Six-minute walk distance as a measure of functional exercise capacity in multiple sclerosis. Disabil Rehabil. 2005;27(22):1365–71.
58. Gobbi E, Carraro A. Effects of a combined aerobic and resistance exercise program in people with multiple sclerosis: a pilot study. Sport Sciences for Health. 2016;12(3):437–42.
59. Latimer-Cheung AE, Pilutti LA, Hicks AL, Ginis KAM, Fenuta AM, MacKibbon KA, et al. Effects of exercise training on fitness, mobility, fatigue, and health-related quality of life among adults with multiple sclerosis: a systematic review to inform guideline development. Arch of Phys Med Rehabil. 2013;94(9) 1800–28. e3
60. Mostert S, Kesselring J. Effects of a short-term exercise training program on aerobic fitness, fatigue, health perception and activity level of subjects with multiple sclerosis. Mult Scler. 2002;8(2):161–8.
61. Kileff J, Ashburn A. A pilot study of the effect of aerobic exercise on people with moderate disability multiple sclerosis. Clin Rehabil. 2005;19(2):165–9.
62. Oken BS, Kishiyama S, Zajdel D, Bourdette D, Carlsen J, Haas M, et al. Randomized controlled trial of yoga and exercise in multiple sclerosis. Neurology. 2004;62(11):2058–64.
63. Petajan JH, Gappmaier E, White AT, Spencer MK, Mino L, Hicks RW. Impact of aerobic training on fitness and quality of life in multiple sclerosis. Ann Neurol. 1996;39(4):432–41.
64. Ponichtera-Mulcare JA, Mathews T, Barrett PJ, Gupta SC. Change in aerobic fitness of patients with multiple sclerosis during a 6-month training program. Res Sports Med: An Int J. 1997;7(3–4):265–72.
65. Schulz K-H, Gold SM, Witte J, Bartsch K, Lang UE, Hellweg R, et al. Impact of aerobic training on immune-endocrine parameters, neurotrophic factors, quality of life and coordinative function in multiple sclerosis. J Neurol Sci. 2004;225(1):11–8.
66. Van den Berg M, Dawes H, Wade D, Newman M, Burridge J, Izadi H, et al. Treadmill training for individuals with multiple sclerosis: a pilot randomised trial. J Neurol Neurosurg Psychiatry. 2006;77(4):531–3.
67. Newman M, Dawes H, Van den Berg M, Wade D, Burridge J, Izadi H. Can aerobic treadmill training reduce the effort of walking and fatigue in people with multiple sclerosis: a pilot study. Mult Scler. 2007;13(1):113–9.
68. Lo AC, Triche EW. Improving gait in multiple sclerosis using robot-assisted, body weight supported treadmill training. Neurorehabil Neural Repair. 2008; 22(6):661–71.
69. Giesser B, Beres-Jones J, Budovitch A, Herlihy E, Harkema S. Locomotor training using body weight support on a treadmill improves mobility in persons with multiple sclerosis: a pilot study. Mult Scler. 2007;13(2):224–31.
70. Pilutti LA, Lelli DA, Paulseth JE, Crome M, Jiang S, Rathbone MP, et al. Effects of 12 weeks of supported treadmill training on functional ability and quality of life in progressive multiple sclerosis: a pilot study. Arch Phys Med Rehabil. 2011;92(1):31–6.
71. Wier LM, Hatcher MS, Triche EW, Lo AC. Effect of robot-assisted versus conventional body-weight-supported treadmill training on quality of life for people with multiple sclerosis. J Rehabil Res Dev. 2011;48(4):483–92.

72. Mazzetti SA, Kraemer WJ, Volek JS, Duncan ND, Ratamess NA, Gomez A, et al. The influence of direct supervision of resistance training on strength performance. Med Sci Sports Exerc. 2000;32(6):1175–84.

73. Kraemer WJ, Adams K, Cafarelli E, Dudley GA, Dooly C, Feigenbaum MS, et al. American College of Sports Medicine position stand. Progression models in resistance training for healthy adults. Med Sci Sports Exerc. 2002;34(2):364–80.

74. Schwid S, Thornton C, Pandya S, Manzur K, Sanjak M, Petrie M, et al. Quantitative assessment of motor fatigue and strength in MS. Neurology. 1999;53(4):743.

75. Durstine JL. American college of sports medicine's exercise management for persons with chronic diseases and disabilities: human kinetics 10%; 2009.

76. Burks JS, Johnson KP. Multiple sclerosis: diagnosis, medical management, and rehabilitation: diagnosis, medical management, and rehabilitation: demos medical; 2000.

77. Foglio K, Clini E, Facchetti D, Vitacca M, Marangoni S, Bonomelli M, et al. Respiratory muscle function and exercise capacity in multiple sclerosis. Eur Respir J. 1994;7(1):23–8.

78. O'Kroy JA, Coast JR. Effects of flow and resistive training on respiratory muscle endurance and strength. Respiration. 1993;60(5):279–83.

79. Pilutti LA, Greenlee TA, Motl RW, Nickrent MS, Petruzzello SJ. Effects of exercise training on fatigue in multiple sclerosis: a meta-analysis. Psychosom Med. 2013;75(6):575–80.

80. Huisinga JM, Filipi ML, Stergiou N. Elliptical exercise improves fatigue ratings and quality of life in patients with multiple sclerosis. J Rehabil Res Dev. 2011;48(7):881–90.

81. Van Diemen H, Van Dongen M, Dammers J, Polman C. Increased visual impairment after exercise (Uthhoff's phenomenon) in multiple sclerosis: therapeutic possibilities. Eur Neurol. 1992;32(4):231–4.

82. Ponichtera-Mulcare JA. Exercise and multiple sclerosis. Med Sci Sports Exerc. 1993;25(4):451–65.

83. Ponichtera-Mulcare J, Glaser R, Mathews T, Camaione D. In the Field-Maximal aerobic exercise in persons with multiple sclerosis. Clinical Kinesiology. 1993;46:14.

84. Capello E, Gardella M, Leandri M, Abbruzzese G, Minatel C, Tartaglione A, et al. Lowering body temperature with a cooling suit as symptomatic treatment for thermosensitive multiple sclerosis patients. Ital J Neurol Sci. 1995;16(7):533–9.

85. Kraft GH, Alquist AD. Effect of microclimate cooling on physical function in multiple sclerosis (MS). J Rehabil Res Dev. 1997;34:198.

86. Syndulko K, Woldanski A, Baumhefner RW, Tourtellotte WW. Preliminary evaluation of lowering tympanic temperature for the symptomatic treatment of multiple sclerosis. Neurorehabil Neural Repair. 1995;9(4):205–15.

87. Peterson C. Exercise in 94 degrees F water for a patient with multiple sclerosis. Phys Ther. 2001;81(4):1049–58.

88. Peterson J, Bell G. Aquatic exercise for individuals with multiple sclerosis. Clinical Kinesiology. 1995;49:69.

89. Chiara T, Carlos J, Martin D, Miller R, Nadeau S. Cold effect on oxygen uptake, perceived exertion, and spasticity in patients with multiple sclerosis. Arch Phys Med Rehabil. 1998;79(5):523–8.

90. Noronha M, Vas C, Aziz H. Autonomic dysfunction (sweating responses) in multiple sclerosis. J Neurol Neurosurg Psychiatry. 1968;31(1):19.

91. Skjerbaek AG, Moller AB, Jensen E, Vissing K, Sorensen H, Nybo L, et al. Heat sensitive persons with multiple sclerosis are more tolerant to resistance exercise than to endurance exercise. Mult Scler. 2013;19(7):932–40.

92. Grahn DA, Murray JL, Heller HC. Cooling via one hand improves physical performance in heat-sensitive individuals with multiple sclerosis: a preliminary study. BMC Neurol. 2008;8(1):14.

93. Mulchare J, Webb P, Mathews T, Gupta S. Sweat response in persons with multiple sclerosis during submaximal aerobic exercise. Int J Mult Scler Care. 2001;3:26–33.

94. LaFontaine T. Clients with spinal cord injury, multiple sclerosis, epilepsy, and cerebral palsy. NSCA's Essentials of Personal Training Earle RW and Baechle TR, eds Champaign, IL: Human Kinetics. 2004:565–8.

2

Comprehensive catwalk gait analysis in a chronic model of multiple sclerosis subjected to treadmill exercise training

Danielle Bernardes and Alexandre Leite Rodrigues Oliveira[*]

Abstract

Background: Multiple sclerosis (MS) is a demyelinating disease with a wide range of symptoms including walking impairment and neuropathic pain mainly represented by mechanical allodynia. Noteworthy, exercise preconditioning may affect both walking impairment and mechanical allodynia. Most of MS symptoms can be reproduced in the animal model named experimental autoimmune encephalomyelitis (EAE). Usually, neurological deficits of EAE are recorded using a clinical scale based on the development of disease severity that characterizes tail and limb paralysis. Following paralysis recovery, subtle motor alterations and even mechanical allodynia investigation are difficult to record, representing sequels of peak disease. The aim of the present study was to investigate the walking dysfunction by the catwalk system (CT) in exercised and non-exercised C57BL/6 mice submitted to EAE with MOG_{35-55} up to 42 days post-induction (dpi).

Methods: Twenty-four C57BL/6 female mice were randomly assigned to unexercised ($n = 12$) or exercised ($n = 12$) groups. The MOG_{35-55} induced EAE model has been performed at the beginning of the fifth week of the physical exercise training protocol. In order to characterize the gait parameters, we used the CT system software version XT 10.1 (Noldus Inc., The Netherlands) from a basal time point (before induction) to 42 days post induction (dpi). Statistical analyses were performed with GraphPad Prisma 4.0 software.

Results: Data show dynamic gait changes in EAE mice including differential front (FP) and hind paw (HP) contact latency. Such findings are hypothesized as related to an attempt to maintain balance and posture similar to what has been observed in patients with MS. Importantly, pre-exercised mice show differences in the mentioned gait compensation, particularly at the propulsion sub-phase of HP stand. Besides, we observed reduced intensity of the paw prints as well as reduced print area in EAE subjects, suggestive of a development of chronic mechanical allodynia in spite of being previously exercised.

Conclusions: Our data suggest that Catwalk system is a useful tool to investigate subtle motor impairment and mechanical allodynia at chronic time points of the EAE model, improving the functional investigation of gait abnormalities and demyelination sequelae.

Keywords: Experimental autoimmune encephalomyelitis (EAE), Walking impairment, Treadmill exercise, Catwalk (CT), Neuropathic pain

* Correspondence: alroliv@unicamp.br
Department of Structural and Functional Biology, Institute of Biology, University of Campinas, Rua Monteiro Lobato, 255, Campinas, Sao Paulo 13.083-862, Brazil

Background

Multiple sclerosis (MS) is the most frequent demyelinating disease worldwide, affecting around 2.3 million people. The majority of the patients (80–85%) present the remitting-recurrent clinical form with transient symptoms that are associated with inflammatory infiltrates followed by demyelination that progress chronically to permanent neurological damage [1]. As it is a disease with disseminated lesions in time and space in the central nervous system (CNS), clinical signs and symptoms of MS can be variable between patients and include mostly motor and sensory dysfunctions [2, 3].

Indeed, motor and balance disorders contribute to the progressive gait weakness, so that about 50% of patients may require ambulation support in approximately 10–20 years from diagnosis [4]. Noteworthy, the walking instability is associated with falls that lead to essential approaches aiming its prevention [5]. Also, pain affects around 63% of MS patients, and it is composed of a variety of pain syndrome, including neuropathic pain, which is present in 26% of the cases [6]. Of note, a characteristic symptom of neuropathic pain is mechanical allodynia in which an exaggerated response to non-noxious stimuli is observed, constituting a significant clinical problem [7, 8].

Some of MS symptoms as well as the histopathological hallmarks of the disease can be deeply investigated in the so-called experimental autoimmune encephalomyelitis (EAE) animal model [9]. Such studies have helped to understand the mechanisms of the disease along with the detection of some therapeutic approaches. Accordingly, the EAE model induced by myelin oligodendrocyte glycoprotein (MOG)$_{35-55}$ peptide offers the possibility to study chronic disease, and it is a well-accepted model for testing neuroprotective strategies since it presents pronounced axonal/neuronal damage [10].

Remarkably, neurological deficits in mice subjected to EAE are classically recorded using a clinical scale with several levels of disease severity representing a broad-spectrum ranging from walking impairment to paralysis [11, 12]. However, subtle gait alterations are hard to detect after disease score stabilization in the chronic periods. Besides, neuropathic pain investigation is biased by this approach as it depends on the subjective observation of the investigator. Thus, mechanical allodynia has usually been evaluated by the von Frey filaments test in rodents [13, 14].

The catwalk automated quantitative gait analysis (CT) is a computer-assisted method for locomotor analysis in which is possible to quantify several and refined gait parameters and detect innumerous motor abnormalities [15]. In addition, different parameters investigated by CT method show a high degree of correlation with mechanical allodynia measured by von-Frey filaments test [7, 16, 17].

Quantitative gait analysis by CT method has been performed in the EAE model using Lewis rats [18] or Brown Norway rats [19]. However, von-Frey filaments method studies show hyper nociception mostly before the onset of motor dysfunction [8, 13, 14]. Also, gait analysis showed no preclinical abnormalities in EAE animals [18, 19].

Regarding strategies to prevent mechanical allodynia, exercise-preconditioning protocols aim developing neuroprotective mechanisms [20], which may have a positive impact on walking impairment [21, 22]. In this sense, a significant clinical score attenuation of EAE after specific programs of regular exercise in mice was previously reported [23, 24]. To our knowledge, specific investigation of subtle walking impairment and neuropathic pain has never been performed in exercised mice. Such approach may provide useful information regarding functional recovery and neuroprotection. Therefore, the CT system has been used in the present study aiming to investigate the walking dysfunction in exercised and non-exercised C57BL/6 mice induced to EAE with MOG$_{35-55}$ in a chronic approach from immunization to 42 days post-induction (dpi).

Methods
Animals

The Multidisciplinary Center for Biological Research (CEMIB/UNICAMP, Campinas, SP, Brazil) supplied the female C57BL/6 mice (4–6 weeks old) used herein. The animals were maintained on a 12/12 h light/dark cycle and were provided with food and water ad libitum. Efforts were made to avoid any unnecessary distress to the animals, and all experiments were carried out in accordance with international guidelines and principles regulated by the National Council of Animal Experimentation (CONCEA, Brazil) for the care and use of animals. The Ethics Committee on Animal Experimentation of University of Campinas (CEUA/UNICAMP, protocol n° 3844–1) approved the protocols, and the animals were randomly assigned to unexercised (EAE; $n = 12$) or exercised (EAE-Ex; $n = 12$) groups.

Physical exercise protocol

Based on previous work that promoted significant attenuation of EAE clinical score [24–26], we investigated whether a similar volume and duration of exercise executed in a treadmill equipment would have the same effect. For that, mice were familiarized to the motorized treadmill for five consecutive days with a progressive increase of time (5 to 25 min), a speed of 6 m/min and 11° of inclination. Next, the exercise protocol consisted of five more weeks (5 days/week) of forced running at 11 m/min, one session/day for 30 min. To account the stress associated with the environment, the unexercised mice were placed on a bench on the side of the treadmill.

With this approach, the animals performed 6 weeks of pre-conditioning exercise before the onset of the EAE clinical scale.

EAE induction and clinical assessment

The MOG_{35-55} peptide injection has been performed at the beginning of the fifth week of the physical exercise training protocol, as it has been previously standardized [25]. Accordingly, EAE was induced by subcutaneous immunization (in the tail base) with an emulsion containing 100 μg of MOG_{35-55} peptide in complete Freund's adjuvant (CFA), supplemented with 4 mg/ml *Mycobacterium tuberculosis* H37Ra (Difco Laboratories, Detroit, MI, USA). *Bordetella pertussis* toxin (300 ng/animal; Sigma-Aldrich, St. Louis, MO, USA) was injected i.p. on the day of immunization and after 48 h. This protocol promoted the development of EAE clinical signs from 11 to 12 dpi and peaked at around 16–17 dpi, according to the clinical score assessment. To that end, animal weight and clinical score were monitored daily. The scores were defined as follows: 0 no clinical signs, 1 tail paralysis (or loss of tail tone), 2 tail paralysis and hind-limb weakness (visible paresis) and 3 one or two hind-limb paralysis.

Gait analysis

The CatWalk system (CT) consists in an objective test to detect relevant functional changes in studies regarding regenerative strategies using the EAE model [19]. Therefore, in a first attempt to characterize the gait parameters in a chronic approach in this model, we used the CT system software version XT 10.1 (Noldus Inc., The Netherlands). The system was used to analyze gait profile in female C57BL6/J mice induced to EAE model by MOG_{35-55} peptide injection from a basal time point (before induction) to 42 days post induction (dpi). Therefore, the data were normalized against basal values, which were settled as 100% in each parameter. Of note, the study was initiated with 12 animals per group (sedentary and exercised). In the CT system method, animals must cross an illuminated walkway with a glass floor to the collection of the paw prints. However, with the disease progression, some animals were not able to cross the walkway in some of the time points. Therefore, the number of animals analyzed at each time point is described in Table 1.

For the analysis, each animal was placed into the walkway and was allowed to move freely in both directions with a run duration between 0.50 and 5.00 s and a maximum allowed speed variation of 60%. A high-speed camera carried out data acquisition and the software automatically classified the paw prints. The camera gain was set to 25.01 and the detection threshold to 0.25, for the detection of all parameters used in the experiments.

Table 1 Animals analyzed at each time point

Time point of analysis	EAE mice	EAE-Exercised mice
Basal	12 (100%)	12 (100%)
5 dpi	12 (100%)	12 (100%)
12 dpi	12 (100%)	12 (100%)
19 dpi	07 (58%)	04 (33%)
22 dpi	10 (83%)	08 (67%)
25 dpi	08 (67%)	05 (42%)
28 dpi	10 (83%)	07 (58%)
31 dpi	06 (75%)	05 (63%)
36 dpi	07 (88%)	04 (50%)
42 dpi	07 (88%)	04 (50%)

Data are presented as absolute number (percentage)

Four compliant runs were acquired per trial and no food restriction or reward was used.

Rotarod

Before collection of the data, animals were familiarized with the equipment for three consecutive days. Every session, each mouse was placed 3 times on the turning wheel for 5 min with 20–30 min of rest between the trials. The velocities (rotations per minute, rpm) were 5 rpm, 10 rpm and 16 rpm on the first, second and third day, respectively. On the fourth day, the basal time point test consisted on the acceleration from 5 to 25 rpm for 6 min (360 s), being finalized when the animal did not maintain itself on the turning wheel voluntarily, losing the balance. Two to three attempts were recorded and the average calculated for each animal. On days 5, 12, 19, 22, 25, 28, 31, 36 and 42 post induction (the same for catwalk evaluation), the animals were retested. In turn, rotarod data collections occurred always before catwalk session in the morning. As it is possible to observe in Fig. 1, almost all animals can keep walking on the turning wheel by the whole period of acceleration from 5 to 25 rpm on basal and 5 dpi time points.

Statistical analysis

Statistical analyses were performed with GraphPad Prisma 4.0 software and data are shown as mean ± standard error. The differences between groups were considered significant when P-values were minor than 0.05. All data were subject to a two-way analysis of variance (ANOVA) with *Bonferroni* post-test in order to investigate the percentage of variation caused by the exercise, by the disease per se or by the interaction between these two factors. When applicable, a one-way ANOVA with *Newman-Keuls* multiple comparison tests was performed in order to investigate the effect of the disease progression, which can be observed on the figure legends (comparisons between time points). Additionally, a

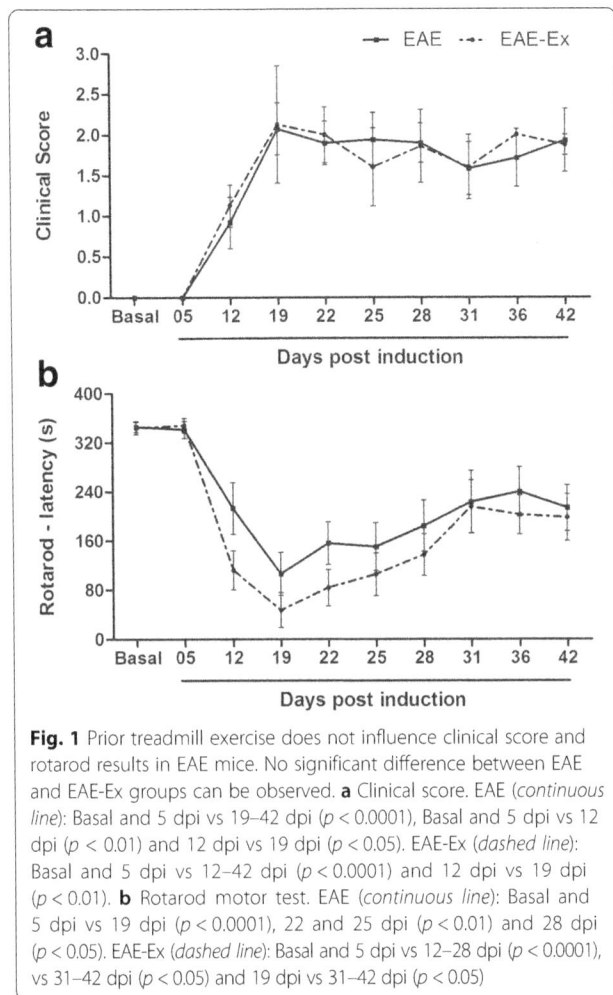

Fig. 1 Prior treadmill exercise does not influence clinical score and rotarod results in EAE mice. No significant difference between EAE and EAE-Ex groups can be observed. **a** Clinical score. EAE (*continuous line*): Basal and 5 dpi vs 19–42 dpi ($p < 0.0001$), Basal and 5 dpi vs 12 dpi ($p < 0.01$) and 12 dpi vs 19 dpi ($p < 0.05$). EAE-Ex (*dashed line*): Basal and 5 dpi vs 12–42 dpi ($p < 0.0001$) and 12 dpi vs 19 dpi ($p < 0.01$). **b** Rotarod motor test. EAE (*continuous line*): Basal and 5 dpi vs 19 dpi ($p < 0.0001$), 22 and 25 dpi ($p < 0.01$) and 28 dpi ($p < 0.05$). EAE-Ex (*dashed line*): Basal and 5 dpi vs 12–28 dpi ($p < 0.0001$), vs 31–42 dpi ($p < 0.05$) and 19 dpi vs 31–42 dpi ($p < 0.05$)

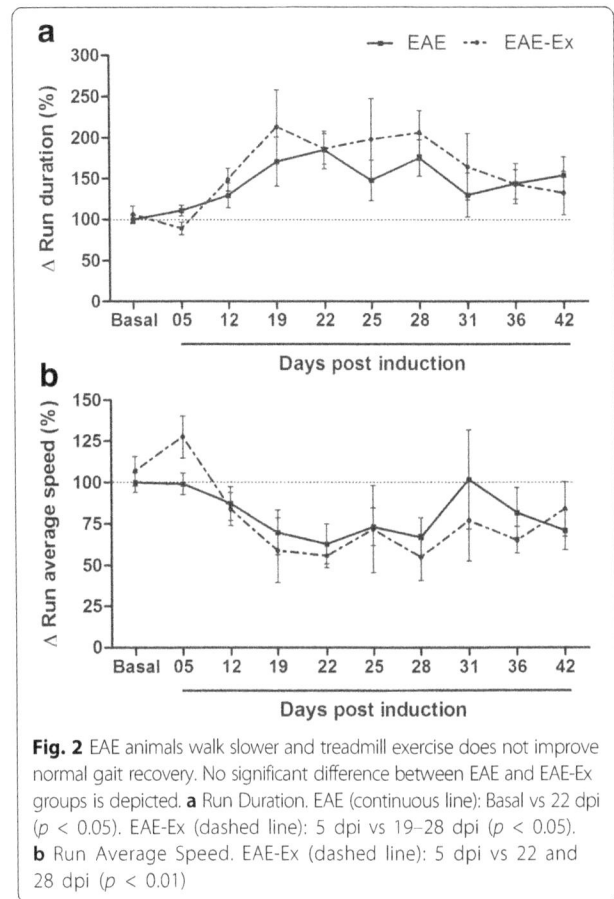

Fig. 2 EAE animals walk slower and treadmill exercise does not improve normal gait recovery. No significant difference between EAE and EAE-Ex groups is depicted. **a** Run Duration. EAE (continuous line): Basal vs 22 dpi ($p < 0.05$). EAE-Ex (dashed line): 5 dpi vs 19–28 dpi ($p < 0.05$). **b** Run Average Speed. EAE-Ex (dashed line): 5 dpi vs 22 and 28 dpi ($p < 0.01$)

correlation analysis between clinical score and run duration with all the other parameters was also performed using the Pearson test.

Results

Regular treadmill exercise previously to EAE onset does not influence clinical score, rotarod data, and speed of the walking in EAE mice

Figures 1 and 2 (and Additional file 1: raw data) demonstrate that there is no effect of the exercise approach used in the present study on the clinical score, rotarod data and speed of the walking on CT apparatus in EAE mice. For rotarod motor test data, the two-way ANOVA revealed an isolated effect of exercise ($p < 0.05$). However, there was a higher impact of the disease ($p < 0.0001$) and no interaction between exercise and EAE ($p > 0.05$) and no *Bonferroni* post hoc differences between these two groups. Similar to what has occurred to clinical score, the one-way ANOVA of rotarod data revealed some differences between time points for EAE (continuous line) and EAE-Ex (dashed line) groups (Fig 1).

Figure 2 shows the data about the gait speed and the two-way ANOVA revealed only a pronounced effect of the disease ($p < 0.0001$). On the same way, the one-way ANOVA showed some differences between time points for the two groups. Interestingly, the statistical differences were more evident in the exercised group although the correlation data presented in Table 2 are statistically similar for the two groups (EAE and EAE-Ex). Observe the values of correlation between clinical score (CS) and run duration (RD) and between rotarod (R) and CS and RD. Taken together, these data suggest that EAE animals walk slower especially around 19–28 dpi.

EAE animals present decreased inter-paw coordination, and prior exercise seems to modify the style of support during the progression of the disease

Table 2 demonstrates, along with Fig. 3 (and Additional file 1: raw data), the inter-paw coordination such as cadence, regularity index, phase dispersions, couplings and styles of support. The two-way ANOVA revealed that there was no interaction between exercise and disease for any of these variables ($p > 0.05$). However, the correlation data in Table 2 and some distinction of the one-way ANOVA between the time points suggest a

Table 2 Correlation of clinical score, run duration and rotarod with some of CT parameters

Parameters	EAE			EAE-Ex		
	CS	RD	R	CS	RD	R
Clinical score	–	0.73#	−0.73#	–	0.72#	−0.77#
Run Duration (s)	0.73#	–	−0.65#	0.72#	–	−0.64#
Rotarod (s)	−0.73#	−0.65#	–	−0.77#	−0.64#	–
Run Average Speed (cm/s)	−0.65#	−0.87#	0.60#	−0.73#	−0.95#	0.59#
Cadence (steps/s)	−0.67#	−0.88#	0.61#	−0.66#	−0.93#	0.60#
Regularity Index (%)	−0.65#	−0.67#	0.59#	−0.75#	−0.69#	0.58#
Phase Dispersions RF → LH	0.35+	0.38+	−0.34+	0.64#	0.51#	−0.34+
Phase Dispersions LF → RH	0.32+	0.29+	−0.22*	0.61#	0.55#	−0.38+
Couplings RF → LH	−0.69#	−0.67#	0.62#	−0.54#	−0.45+	0.32+
Couplings LF → RH	−0.63#	−0.50#	0.47#	−0.51#	−0.44+	0.28*
Diagonal Support (%)	−0.62#	−0.73#	0.48#	−0.62#	−0.75#	0.39+
Lateral Support (%)	0.51#	0.33+	−0.42#	0.71#	0.35+	−0.40+
Three Support (%)	0.36+	0.59#	−0.21*	0.38+	0.66#	−0.27*
Girdle Support (%)	0.35+	0.39+	−0.43#	0.30*	0.20	−0.22
Zero Support (%)	0.17	0.01	−0.08	0.41+	−0.01	−0.27*

Legend: #$p < 0.0001$; +$p < 0.01$; *$p < 0.05$; CS: Clinical Score; RD: Run Duration and; R: Rotarod. Data are demonstrated per group (EAE: non-exercised mice and EAE-Ex: exercised mice)

differential exercise and non-exercise modulation of the inter-paw coordination after EAE induction. An isolated effect of the disease was observed with $p < 0.01$ for cadence (steps/s) and $p < 0.0001$ for regularity index and the correlation values of these parameters with CS, RD, and R were all high and significant (Table 2). However, although the correlation values were similar for both exercised and non-exercised animals, the statistical differences between time points were more evident for the exercised group (Fig. 3).

Gait alterations may be related to phase dispersion results (Table 2), although these effects were not detected by the one-way ANOVA between time points. Besides, in spite of phase dispersion RF- > LH has been affected by the disease ($p < 0.01$, two-way ANOVA), no other effects were observed and phase dispersion LF- > RH was not affected by any of the variables herein investigated. On the other hand, couplings (both RF- > LH and LF- > RH) were strongly affected by the disease ($p < 0.0001$; two-way ANOVA) and both groups (exercise-trained and untrained) presented significant reduction of this parameter during disease progression in comparison to basal time point (Fig. 3 c, d). Interestingly, couplings LF- > RH presented significant reduction on days 31–42 in comparison to both basal and 5 dpi just for the exercised group while the non-exercised group recovered to values close to the basal line at these time points (Fig 3 d). Taken together, these data suggest that EAE animals in spite of being previously exercised present decreased inter-paw coordination.

The measure of limb support in the present study comprised diagonal, lateral, three, girdle and no support

at all (zero). Of these, the disease affected support diagonal (RF-LH or LF-RH) for both exercised and non-exercised EAE mice (Table 2, $p < 0.01$, two-way ANOVA). That means EAE mice presented reduced proportion of diagonal support, which is the most used in healthy conditions (60–70% of the all types of support). This reduction was slightly more evident in the EAE-Ex (Fig 3e). The reduction of diagonal support was mainly compensated by an increase in the lateral support (RF-RH or LF-LH) that was more evident in the EAE-Ex group. Indeed, two-way ANOVA showed that there was an isolated effect of exercise on lateral support ($p < 0.05$) and, by the data presented in Table 2, we can see that exercised animals increased this type of support with the progression of the disease in a higher magnitude that the non-exercised ones. In fact, 31 dpi shows a statistical difference between the two groups ($p < 0.05$; Fig 3f). Lateral support accounts for 0–1% of the all types of support used in healthy conditions and it was increased to 5% between the non-exercised and to 9–10% between the exercised mice in the chronic phase of EAE. Support three, which represents around 20–30% of all types of support in healthy conditions, was almost unaffected by the disease although a high correlation value was observed with RD for both groups (Table 2). That means how slow the EAE animals walk so that three paws are constantly used as support. Girdle support (RF-LF or RH-LH), which represents 1–2% of all types of support used in healthy conditions, was increased to 8% around 19 dpi for the EAE group and to 7% around 28 dpi for the EAE-Ex group. The two-way ANOVA

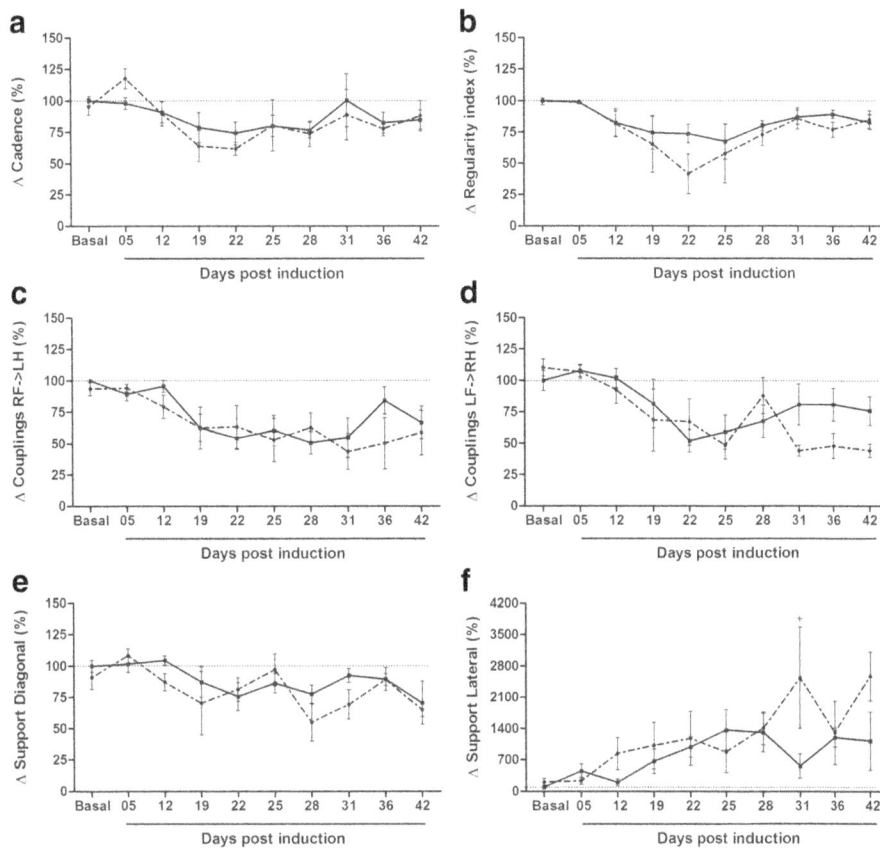

Fig. 3 Exercised and non-exercised EAE animals present decreased inter-paw coordination. **a** Cadence. EAE-Ex (*dashed line*): 5 dpi vs 22 dpi (*p* < 0.01). **b** Regularity Index. EAE-Ex (*dashed line*): 5 dpi vs 22 dpi (*p* < 0.01). **c** Couplings RF- > LH. EAE (*continuous line*): Basal vs 22, 25 and 31 dpi (*p* < 0.05). EAE-Ex (*dashed line*): Basal and 5 dpi vs 31 dpi (*p* < 0.05). **d** Couplings LF- > RH. EAE (*continuous line*): Basal and 12 dpi vs 22 dpi (*p* < 0.05). EAE-Ex (*dashed line*): Basal and 5dpi vs 22–25 and 31–42 dpi (*p* < 0.05). **e** Support diagonal. EAE-Ex (*dashed line*): 5 dpi vs 28 dpi (*p* < 0.01). **f** Support lateral. EAE-Ex (*dashed line*): Basal and 5 dpi vs 31 and 42 dpi (*p* < 0.05). + Represents *p* < 0.05 between EAE and EAE-Ex at 31 dpi

showed an isolated effect of disease (*p* < 0.01) and a moderate correlation is observed in Table 2.

Differential modulation of dynamic and static gait parameters of front (FP) and hind paws (HP) in EAE and exercised EAE (EAE-ex) animals

Overall, the remaining data are related to static and dynamic CT parameters of FP and HP of EAE and EAE-Ex mice. Unless for max contact at, the two-way ANOVA also revealed that there was no significant interaction between exercise and disease (*p* > 0.05). In fact, most of them were just related to the effect of the disease, as seen in Fig. 4 about stride length (*p* < 0.0001 for FP and HP), body speed (*p* < 0.0001 for FP and HP) and swing speed (*p* < 0.01 for FP and *p* < 0.0001 for HP). Although the one-way ANOVA has shown some effect between time points, mostly for the exercised animals, Table 3 demonstrates similar correlation values between these parameters and CS and RD for both groups. Noteworthy, as these results are strongly affected by run duration, the statistical

differences between time points were more evident for the EAE-Ex group.

Table 3 (and Additional file 1: raw data) shows that the disease and the reduced gait speed have increased parameters related to the stance of the FP such as step cycle, stand, duty cycle, initial and terminal dual stance. It is note worth that stand/stance is the duration in seconds of contact while swing is the duration in seconds of no contact of a paw with the glass plate. Therefore, step cycle represents the sum of swing and stand duration while duty cycle represents stand as a percentage of step cycle. Dual stand/stance is the duration in seconds of contact for both limbs simultaneously (hind or forelimbs). Therefore, initial and terminal dual stance are, respectively, the first and the second time in a step cycle of a paw and its contralateral when making contact with the glass plate. All of these parameters for FP were also strongly affected by the disease (two-way ANOVA, *p* < 0.0001; Fig. 5 a and c). These data suggest that EAE animals keep FP more time on the glass while walking. On the other hand, only step cycle for hind paws were

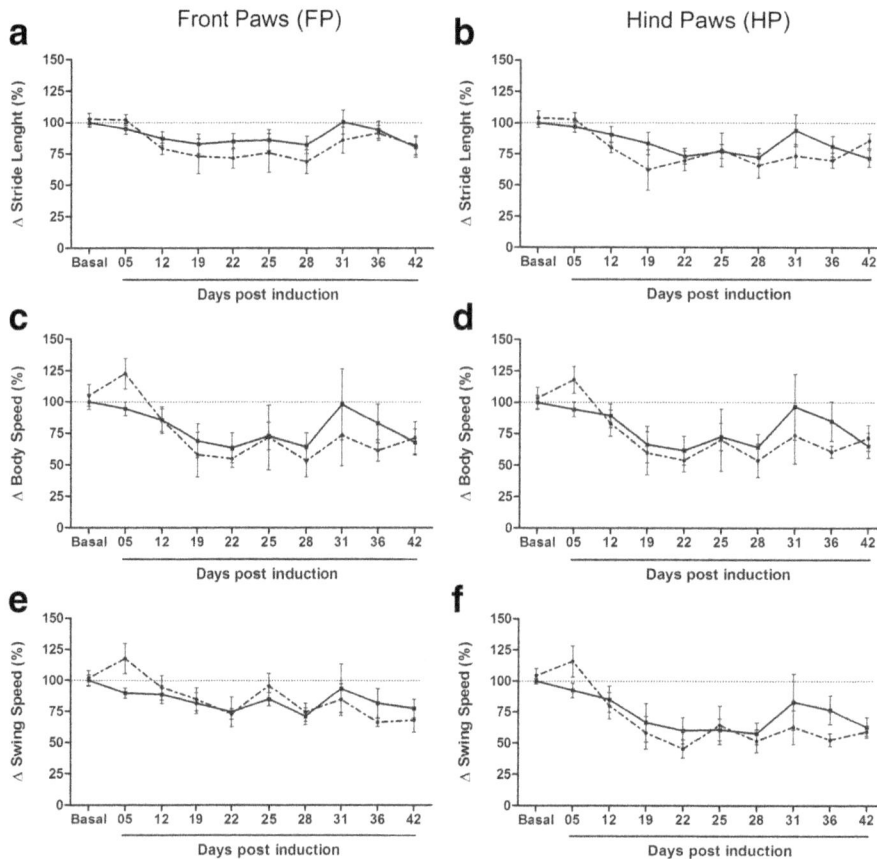

Fig. 4 EAE animals walk slower (body and swing speed) and with short footsteps (stride length). No differences between EAE and EAE-Ex groups at any time point for any of the parameters can be observed. **a** Front paws stride length. EAE-Ex (dashed line): Basal and 5 dpi vs 22 and 28 dpi ($p < 0.05$). **b** Hind paws stride length. EAE-Ex (dashed line): Basal and 5 dpi vs 19, 22 and 28 dpi ($p < 0.05$). **c** Front paws body speed. EAE-Ex (dashed line): 5 dpi vs 22 and 28 dpi ($p < 0.05$). **d** Hind paws body speed. EAE-Ex (dashed line): 5 dpi vs 22 and 28 dpi ($p < 0.05$). **e** Front paws swing speed. No differences detected. **f** Hind paws swing speed. EAE (continuous line): Basal vs 28 dpi ($p < 0.05$). EAE-Ex (dashed line): 5 dpi vs 12–42 dpi ($p < 0.05$) and Basal vs 22 and 28 dpi ($p < 0.05$)

positive and significantly correlated with CS and RD for both groups and the two-way ANOVA shows an isolated effect of disease ($p < 0.05$). The disease also affected duty cycle for hind paws ($p < 0.01$), but the correlation data shows a moderate and negative relationship between them (Table 3). Noteworthy, stand, initial and terminal dual stance for hind paws were not affected by the disease, although some positive correlation with RD can be observed in Table 3. Taken together, this differential FP and HP response may suggest a compensation mechanism in order to maintain gait and balance with a shift of the center of gravity to FP because of the overt dysfunction of HP.

A differential response from the EAE condition between FP and HP was also observed for the base of support (BOS) data (Table 3; Fig. 5 e-f). In this case, highly positive correlations with CS and RD are observed for FP with a strong effect from disease ($p < 0.0001$; two-way ANOVA), starting after 22 dpi (Fig. 5 e). Since this parameter is related to the perpendicular distance of both paws to each other, these analyses demonstrate that

EAE animals walk with a wider distance between the front paws. Curiously, unpaired t-test analysis for basal time point (before induction) demonstrates that 6 weeks of treadmill exercise decreased the distance between the left and the right FP during the walking ($p < 0.05$; sedentary: 1.42 ± 0.03 cm and exercised: 1.26 ± 0.06 cm). However, this basal difference did not influence the development of wider BOS of FP after EAE induction.

Detailed unpaired t-test analysis for basal time point of all parameters revealed several differences, suggesting some effect of exercise on the walking pattern. For example, exercise increased FP print width (Fig. 7 a; $p < 0.01$; sedentary: 0.74 ± 0.006 cm and exercised: 0.78 ± 0.010 cm) but reduced its max intensity at (Fig. 6 e; $p < 0.01$; sedentary: $31.68 \pm 1.91\%$ and exercised: $24.19 \pm 1.42\%$) and its max contact at (Fig. 6 g; $p < 0.05$; sedentary: $37.27 \pm 1.26\%$ and exercised: $33.73 \pm 0.99\%$). In its way, exercise increased HP print area (Fig. 7 F; $p < 0.05$; sedentary: 0.32 ± 0.014 cm and exercised: 0.39 ± 0.018 cm) and its mean intensity of the 15 most intense pixels (Fig. 6 d; $p < 0.05$;

Table 3 Correlation of clinical score and run duration with other CT parameters

Parameters	Front paws (FP)				Hind paws (HP)			
	EAE		EAE-Ex		EAE		EAE-Ex	
	CS	RD	CS	RD	CS	RD	CS	RD
Stride Length (cm)	$-0.60^{\#}$	$-0.84^{\#}$	$-0.74^{\#}$	$-0.80^{\#}$	$-0.72^{\#}$	$-0.85^{\#}$	$-0.68^{\#}$	$-0.78^{\#}$
Body Speed (cm/s)	$-0.67^{\#}$	$-0.89^{\#}$	$-0.74^{\#}$	$-0.95^{\#}$	$-0.69^{\#}$	$-0.89^{\#}$	$-0.75^{\#}$	$-0.95^{\#}$
Swing Speed (cm/s)	$-0.51^{\#}$	$-0.71^{\#}$	-0.42^{+}	$-0.63^{\#}$	$-0.73^{\#}$	$-0.85^{\#}$	$-0.75^{\#}$	$-0.83^{\#}$
Step Cycle (s)	$0.64^{\#}$	$0.82^{\#}$	$0.45^{\#}$	$0.77^{\#}$	$0.58^{\#}$	$0.88^{\#}$	$0.44^{\#}$	$0.73^{\#}$
Stand (s)	$0.70^{\#}$	$0.93^{\#}$	$0.57^{\#}$	$0.88^{\#}$	0.18	$0.43^{\#}$	0.06	$0.45^{\#}$
Duty Cycle (%)	$0.56^{\#}$	$0.81^{\#}$	$0.64^{\#}$	$0.85^{\#}$	-0.30^{+}	-0.14	-0.36^{+}	0.02
Initial Dual Stance (s)	$0.66^{\#}$	$0.90^{\#}$	$0.63^{\#}$	$0.88^{\#}$	0.07	0.37^{+}	0.06	$0.53^{\#}$
Terminal Dual Stance (s)	$0.67^{\#}$	$0.90^{\#}$	$0.64^{\#}$	$0.87^{\#}$	0.16	$0.47^{\#}$	0.11	$0.57^{\#}$
Base of Support (cm)	$0.58^{\#}$	$0.61^{\#}$	$0.72^{\#}$	$0.73^{\#}$	-0.31^{+}	-0.18	-0.44^{+}	-0.20
Max Contact Max Intensity	-0.13	0.15	$-0.46^{\#}$	-0.15	$-0.55^{\#}$	-0.36^{+}	$-0.76^{\#}$	$-0.47^{\#}$
15 Most Intense Pixels	-0.08	0.20	-0.31^{+}	-0.02	$-0.53^{\#}$	-0.28^{+}	$-0.73^{\#}$	$-0.46^{\#}$
Max Intensity At (%)	$0.51^{\#}$	$0.40^{\#}$	$0.52^{\#}$	$0.43^{\#}$	$-0.64^{\#}$	-0.37^{+}	$-0.73^{\#}$	$-0.54^{\#}$
Max Contact At (%)	0.25^{*}	$0.38^{\#}$	$0.44^{\#}$	$0.58^{\#}$	$-0.44^{\#}$	-0.39^{+}	-0.25^{*}	-0.27^{*}
Print Width (cm)	$-0.40^{\#}$	-0.28^{+}	$-0.66^{\#}$	-0.42^{+}	$-0.51^{\#}$	-0.31^{+}	-0.41^{+}	-0.20
Print Length (cm)	-0.16	-0.02	-0.29^{*}	-0.07	-0.18	-0.03	-0.26^{*}	-0.09
Print Area (cm^2)	-0.15	0.11	-0.36^{*}	-0.10	-0.27^{*}	-0.05	$-0.45^{\#}$	-0.22

Legend: $^{\#}p < 0.0001$; $^{+}p < 0.01$; $^{*}p < 0.05$; CS: Clinical Score; RD: Run Duration. Data are demonstrated per group and per pair of paws

sedentary: 221.7 ± 1.98 and exercised: 229.4 ± 2.09 cm). Analogous to BOS of FP, these last basal alterations did not influence the course of each parameter during disease.

Similarly to BOS of FP, hind paws were positioned with a narrower distance after 6 weeks of exercise (basal time point on Fig. 5 f; $p < 0.0001$; sedentary: 2.5 ± 0.06 cm and exercised: 2.2 ± 0.09 cm), meaning that 6 weeks of treadmill exercise decrease the BOS for FP and HP of mice in healthy condition. However, for BOS of the HP, a detached curve of exercised from sedentary mice is visible on the graph and the effect of exercise is quite significant during all the period studied (Fig. 5 f; $p < 0.0001$; two-way ANOVA). No effects from disease were observed either by the two- or one-way ANOVA and a negative correlation were observed (Table 3), suggesting that EAE animals may decrease the distance between the hind paws over the walking dysfunction. Therefore, the overall response of BOS between FP and HP were opposite during disease progression, which, along with data about stance, is suggestive of a compensation mechanism.

Max intensity at (Fig. 6 e-f) and *max contact at* (Fig. 6 g-h) were also altered in an opposite manner with overall positive correlations with CS and RD for FP while negative values were observed for the HP (Table 3). This discrepancy is quite visible on the graphs of *max intensity at*, which was affected by the disease with ($p < 0.0001$) for both FP and HP and had several overt differences between the time points with a noticeable increase for FP after 22 dpi and decrease for HP after 12 dpi. Similar results were

observed with max contact at even though two important dissimilarities are worth mentioning. Firstly, two-way ANOVA revealed an effect of the disease ($p < 0.01$) for both FP and HP and a significant interaction between exercise and disease for HP ($p < 0.05$). Secondly, this interaction effect caused reduced correlation values with CS and RD and no difference between the time points for the EAE-Ex group. Therefore, it seems that 6 weeks of treadmill exercise has attenuated the variations on max contact at of HP caused by the EAE induction. In other words, our data suggest that EAE mice show some fluctuations on the time spent for the transition of braking into propulsion sub-phase of stand during disease progression and it seems that prior treadmill exercise attenuates that changings for HP.

The present correlation data suggest that exercise may have had a negative synergistic effect with the disease for max contact max intensity and mean intensity of the 15 most intense pixels (Table 3). For FP only the exercised mice showed a significant and negative correlation between clinical score and gait parameters, although the two-way ANOVA revealed a strong effect of the disease ($p < 0.0001$) In turn one-way ANOVA indicated several significant differences between time points for both groups. For HP, both groups demonstrated a significant and negative correlation between these parameters and both CS and RD. However, the disease demonstrated the highest effect ($p < 0.0001$) and, one-way ANOVA presented several significant differences between time points

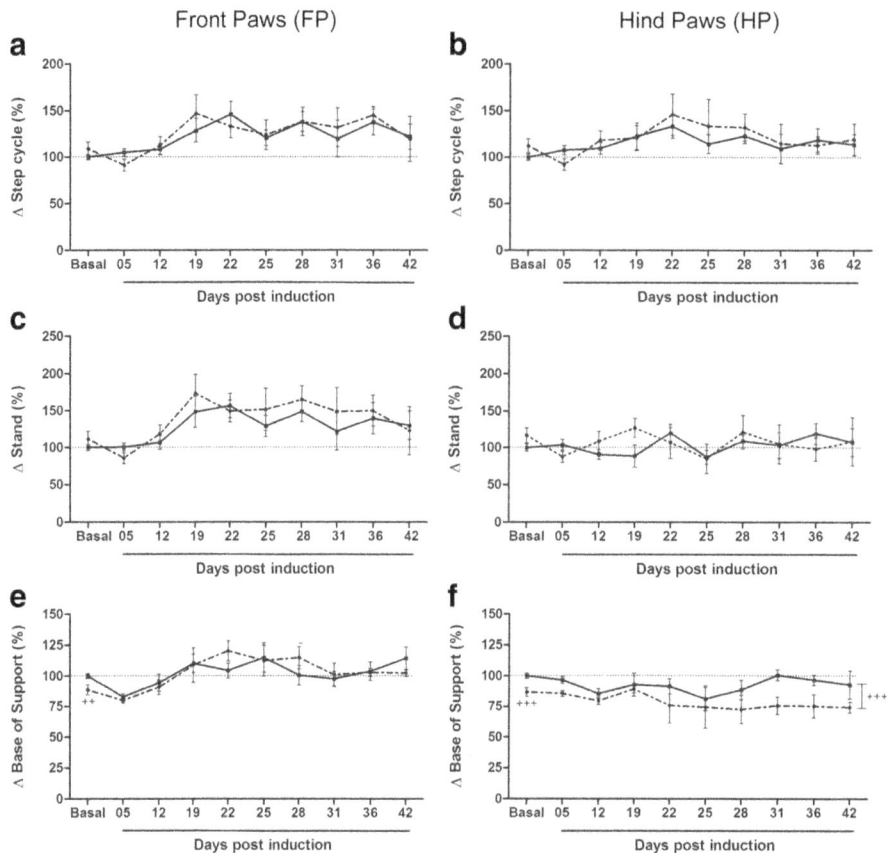

Fig. 5 EAE animals present increased stance phase of step cycle for front paws. **a** Front paws step cycle. EAE (continuous line): Basal and 5 dpi vs 22 dpi ($p < 0.05$). **b** Hind paws step cycle. No differences detected. **c** Front paws stand. EAE-Ex (dashed line): 5 dpi vs 19 and 28 dpi ($p < 0.05$). **d** Hind paws stand. No differences detected. **e** Front paws base of support. EAE (continuous line): 5 dpi vs 25 and 42 dpi ($p < 0.050$). EAE-Ex (dashed line): 5 dpi vs 22–28 dpi ($p < 0.05$) and Basal and 12 dpi vs 22 dpi ($p < 0.05$). ++ Represents $p < 0.01$ between EAE and EAE-Ex at Basal time point. **f** Hind paws base of support. $^{+++}p < 0.0001$ between the curves (EAE vs EAE-Ex) by student T test

for both groups. Taken together, these data suggest that EAE animals present reduced intensity of paw prints from 12 dpi to 42 dpi and that treadmill exercise may have strengthened this result.

In the same way, print width, print length, and print area were decreased with the progression of the disease (Fig. 7). Exercise strengthened such results, since the highest values of negative correlation between these parameters and CS were observed for the EAE-Ex group (Table 3). However, there was no interaction or isolated effect of exercise and FP was strongly affected by the disease from 12 dpi ($p < 0.0001$, one-way ANOVA). The hind paws were also affected but with variable values of P (print width: $p < 0.0001$; print length: $p < 0.05$; print area: $p < 0.01$). These data suggest that EAE animals present decreased contact area of the paw prints at chronic disease, especially for FP.

Discussion

Several studies using treadmill exercise performed during short periods of training (2–25 days) have shown none or undersized effects on development and progression of clinical signs in EAE animals [27–31]. Therefore, we chose to investigate volume and duration of exercise similar to the protocol of swimming we have used previously in which we observed an important clinical score attenuation [24, 25].

We used regular treadmill exercise in this study in order to prepare animals in a similar ability to what they would be evaluated such as the CT system and motor rotarod, in which animals are forced to walk on the apparatus. Indeed, the basal data of the present work show several subtle motor alterations that represent an isolated effect of exercise on gait pattern in healthy condition, before the EAE induction. First, 6 weeks of treadmill exercise significantly decreased the BOS for FP and HP irrespective to the body weight. Based upon some data with animal models of ataxic gait such as cerebral ischemia [32], thyroid system dysfunction [33] and Leigh disease [34], in which an increased BOS was observed, we may suggest that exercised mice presented an increased gait stability before EAE induction.

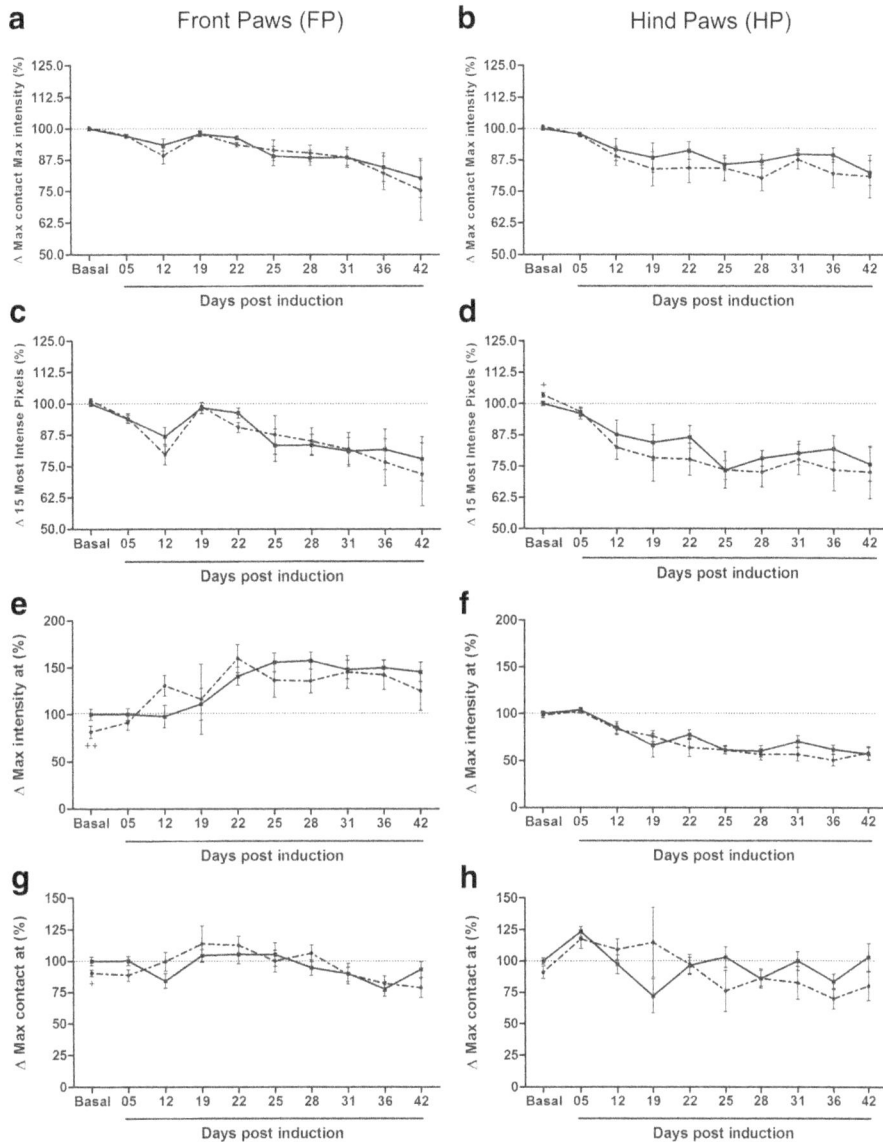

Fig. 6 EAE animals present reduced intensity of paw prints at chronic disease. $^{+}p < 0.05$ and $^{++}p < 0.01$ between EAE and EAE-Ex groups. **a** Front paws max contact max intensity. EAE (continuous line): Basal vs 36 dpi ($p < 0.05$) and Basal to 22 dpi vs 42 dpi ($p < 0.05$). EAE-Ex (dashed line): Basal vs 36 dpi ($p < 0.05$) and Basal, 5, 19 and 22 dpi vs 42 dpi ($p < 0.05$). **b** Hind paws max contact max intensity. EAE (continuous line): Basal vs 25, 28 and 42 dpi ($p < 0.05$) and 5 dpi vs 42 dpi. EAE-Ex (dashed line): Basal vs 28 and 42 dpi ($p < 0.05$) and 5 dpi vs 28 dpi. **c** Front paws mean intensity of the 15 most intense pixels. EAE (continuous line): Basal vs 42dpi ($p < 0.05$). EAE-Ex (dashed line): Basal vs 12, 36 and 42 dpi ($p < 0.05$). **d** Hind paws mean intensity of the 15 most intense pixels. EAE (continuous line): Basal and 5 dpi vs 25, 28 and 42 dpi ($p < 0.05$). EAE-Ex (dashed line): Basal vs 12–42 dpi ($p < 0.05$) and 5 dpi vs 28 dpi ($p < 0.05$). + Represents $p < 0.05$ between EAE and EAE-Ex at Basal time point. **e** Front paws max intensity at. EAE (continuous line): Basal, 5 and 12 dpi vs 22–42 dpi ($p < 0.05$) and 19 dpi vs 28 dpi ($p < 0.05$). EAE-Ex (dashed line): Basal vs 22 and 31 dpi ($p < 0.05$) and 5 dpi vs 31 dpi ($p < 0.01$). ++ Represents $p < 0.01$ between EAE and EAE-Ex at Basal time point. **f** Hind paws max intensity at. EAE (continuous line): Basal and 5 dpi vs 19–42 dpi ($p < 0.01$) and 12 dpi vs Basal, 5, 25, 28, 36 and 42 dpi ($p < 0.05$). EAE-Ex (dashed line): Basal and 5 dpi vs 12–42 dpi ($p < 0.05$) and 12 dpi vs 22–42 dpi ($p < 0.05$). **g** Front paws max contact at. + Represents $p < 0.05$ between EAE and EAE-Ex at Basal time point. **h** Hind paws max contact at. EAE (continuous line): 5 dpi vs 19, 28 and 36 dpi

In addition, exercised mice showed increased FP print width (Fig 7 a) with reduced both max intensity at and max contact at, suggesting that exercised mice anticipate the shifting of brake to propulsion sub-phase of stand for FP. On the other hand, an increased HP print area with increased mean intensity of the 15 most intense pixels at basal time point was observed for the exercised group, suggesting a compensation of the pressure between FP and HP. These subtle and prior adaptations caused by the exercise may have affected some of the gait parameters during the progression of the disease. First, it seems that 6 weeks of treadmill exercise have

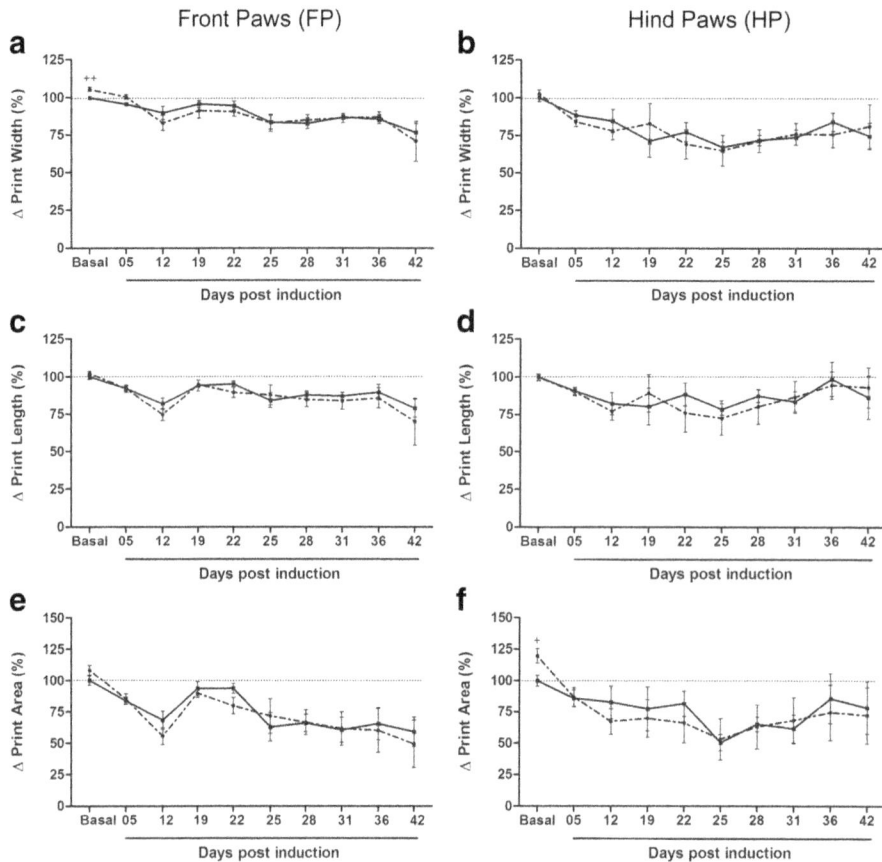

Fig. 7 EAE animals present decreased contact area of the paw prints at the chronic disease. **a** Front paws print width. EAE (continuous line): Basal vs 25, 28, 36 and 42 dpi ($p < 0.05$), 19 dpi vs 12 and 42 dpi ($p < 0.05$) and 5 and 22 dpi vs 42 dpi. EAE-Ex (dashed line): Basal vs 12, 25–31 and 42 dpi ($p < 0.05$) and 5 dpi vs 12 and 42 dpi. ++ Represents $p < 0.01$ between EAE and EAE-Ex at Basal time point. **b** Hind paws print width. EAE (continuous line): Basal vs 19, 25 and 28 dpi ($p < 0.05$). EAE-Ex (dashed line): Basal vs 22–28 dpi ($p < 0.05$). **c** Front paws print length. EAE (continuous line): Basal vs 12, 25 and 42 dpi ($p < 0.05$). EAE-Ex (dashed line): Basal vs 12 and 42 dpi ($p < 0.01$). **d** Hind paws print length. No differences detected. **e** Front paws print area. EAE (continuous line): Basal vs 12 and 25–42 dpi ($p < 0.05$). EAE-Ex (dashed line): Basal vs 05–12 and 22–42 dpi. **f** Hind paws print area. EAE-Ex (dashed line): Basal vs 25–28 dpi ($p < 0.05$). + Represents $p < 0.05$ between EAE and EAE-Ex at Basal time point

attenuated the fluctuations on the time spent for the transition of braking into propulsion sub-phase of the stand of HP. Second, BOS of HP was decreased during the studied period for the EAE-Ex group in comparison to the EAE group. These data are in agreement with evidence showing that repeated treadmill-walking tests increase gait stability in mice that is maybe associated to a habituation response to the dynamic daily feedbacks from proprioceptive, vestibular, and visual inputs [35]. However, unless for some negative effects related to neuropathic pain that will be discussed later, these subtle effects of the protocol of exercise used herein had no significant impact on EAE walking dysfunction.

Literature has shown greater effects of swimming over treadmill running on elevation of serum adrenocorticotropic hormone and corticosterone [36]; activation of sympathetic nervous system [37] increase of cell proliferation in the hippocampal dentate gyrus [38] and even preservation of spinal motoneurons [39]. Perhaps, swimming promotes

specific neuroimmune modulation that counts in favor of a clinical score attenuation of EAE mice that may not be depicted with the forced running approach.

Noteworthy, our results show that EAE animals present decreased inter-paw coordination, a wider distance of perpendicular support between FP and a reduced intensity of the paw prints as well as reduced print area when compared to the basal time point. These alterations were evident until 42 dpi. In a transient way, especially from 19 to 28 dpi, EAE animals walk slower, with shorter footsteps (decreased stride length) and an increased time of FP stand, suggesting the development of a compensation mechanism to maintain gait and balance during periods of more significant walking dysfunction. Reduced velocity of movement has been demonstrated in EAE mice at 4 dpi and it was associated with the stress caused by the injections necessary to the induction procedure [40]. The speed of the walking is an important parameter of debate in walking dysfunctions since it can affect other dynamic gait parameters [16, 41–43]. For example, it is classically recognized that decreased speed of walking leads to increased period of paw contact [44] and that hind paws are much less variable with velocity than the front paws [45].

Accordingly, EAE animals keep FP more time on the glass because of the delayed time to shift brake into propulsion sub-phase of stand and that was accompanied by increased BOS, i.e., wide perpendicular distance between FP. These results were observed especially after 22 dpi with no positive effect of exercise pre-training. Overall, the present evidences that EAE mice try to keep posture and balance, by changing the center of gravity to the FP, as illustrated by positive phase dispersion and the more negative values of couplings during the progression of the disease [43].

Of note, reduction of the regularity index has been observed in the rat model of EAE [18]. In addition, rotarod motor test data presented correlation values with gait parameter similar to the ones observed with the clinical score, illustrating the important walking dysfunction during the course of the disease [46]. EAE animal's shorter footsteps provide additional confirmation of the altered gait pattern observed herein. In this sense, a similar result has been established on 15 and 20 dpi in EAE mice [47]. Besides, reduced stride length was also observed in a mouse model of pyramidotomy [48] and in a model of reduced levels of striatal dopaminergic neurons [49].

In fact, damage to both corticospinal tract [50] and striatum [51], as well as alteration of the dopaminergic system [52], has been observed in EAE animals. In addition, reduced levels of dopamine have been associated with lower velocities of walking [53] as well as dysfunction of locomotor circuits in the lumbar spinal cord [54]. Recently, Fiander and colleagues demonstrated that EAE mice present changed angle and range of motion for hip, knee and ankle joints suggesting that these deficits are caused by reduced corticospinal axon conduction as well as reduced synchronization of the activities from the basal ganglia [12]. In turn, our study suggests that reduced stride length may be also related to a damaged corticospinal tract or even reduced dopaminergic activity caused by the disease.

It is important to highlight that EAE-Ex group presented some worsened gait parameters such as those related to intensity and contact area of the paw prints, especially FP. Such reduction started at 12 dpi and resulted in a decreased print area, what may be associated to mechanical allodynia [7, 15, 17]. Pain enhancement can be associated with demyelinating lesions, axonal damage, and release of pro-inflammatory cytokines, activated glial cells as well as excitatory neurotransmission that are characteristic of EAE development [8]. Exercising may lead to pro-inflammatory responses, especially if performed close to the onset of the disease.

Conclusions

The great magnitude of alterations on gait parameters observed herein, during the course of EAE may be related to the fact that several areas of the CNS are affected in this model as is observed in patients with multiple sclerosis (MS). The present study demonstrates for the first time that walking speed, stride length, inter-paw coordination, intensity and area of the paw prints, base of support as well as stand are relevant parameters for gait monitoring during EAE. Such parameters can in turn be used to evaluate new treatments that result in motor preservation/recovery.

Abbreviations
ANOVA: Analysis of variance; BOS: Base of support; CEMIB/UNICAMP: Multidisciplinary Center for Biological Research of University of Campinas; CEUA/UNICAMP: Ethics Committee on Animal Experimentation of University of Campinas; CFA: Complete Freund's adjuvant; CNS: Central nervous system; CONCEA: National Council of Animal Experimentation; CS: Clinical score; CT: Catwalk; Dpi: Days post induction; EAE: Experimental autoimmune encephalomyelitis; EAE-Ex: EAE animals submitted to prior regular exercise; FP: Front paws; HP: Hind paws; LF- > RH: Left front to right hind; MOG: Myelin oligodendrocyte glycoprotein; MS: Multiple sclerosis; R: Rotarod; RD: Run duration; RF- > LH: Right front to left hind; rpm: Rotations per minute

Acknowledgement
None.

Funding
This work was supported by Fapesp (2014/06892–3). Bernardes D receives a scholarship from FAPESP (2015/04665–2). Oliveira, A.L.R. receives a fellowship from CNPq (Brazil).

Authors' contributions
DB and ALRO contributed to conception and design and wrote the manuscript. DB contributed to acquisition, analysis, and editing of data. ALRO provided the supervision. All authors read and approved the final manuscript.

Competing interests
The authors declare that they have no competing interests.

References
1. Loleit V, Bieberacher V, Hemmer B. Current and future therapies targeting the immune system in multiple sclerosis. Curr Pharm Biotechnol. 2014;15:276–96.
2. Bagnato F, Centonze D, Galgani S, Grasso MG, Haggiag S, Strano S. Painful and involuntary multiple sclerosis. Expert Opin Pharmacother. 2011;12:763–77.
3. Doshi A, Chataway J. Multiple sclerosis, a treatable disease. Clin Med (Northfield II). 2016;16:53–9.
4. Motl RW, Goldman MD, Benedict RHB. Walking impairment in patients with multiple sclerosis: exercise training as a treatment option. Neuropsychiatr Dis Treat. 2010;6:767–74.
5. Comber L, Galvin R, Coote S. Gait deficits in people with multiple sclerosis: a systematic review and meta-analysis. Gait Posture. 2017;51:25–35.
6. Foley PL, Vesterinen HM, Laird BJ, Sena ES, Colvin LA, Chandran S, et al. Prevalence and natural history of pain in adults with multiple sclerosis: systematic review and meta-analysis. Pain. 2013;154:632–42.
7. Vrinten DH, Hamers FFT. "CatWalk" automated quantitative gait analysis as a novel method to assess mechanical allodynia in the rat; a comparison with von Frey testing. Pain. 2003;102:203-9.
8. Khan N, Smith MT. Multiple sclerosis-induced neuropathic pain: pharmacological management and pathophysiological insights from rodent EAE models. Inflammopharmacology. 2014;22:1–22.

9. Lühder F, Gold R, Flügel A, Linker RA. Brain-derived neurotrophic factor in neuroimmunology: lessons learned from multiple sclerosis patients and experimental autoimmune encephalomyelitis models. Arch Immunol Ther Exp. 2013; 61:95–105.

10. Lassmann H, Bradl M. Multiple sclerosis: experimental models and reality. Acta Neuropathol. 2017;133(2):223–44.

11. Recks MS, Addicks K, Kuerten S. Spinal cord histopathology of MOG peptide 35-55-induced experimental autoimmune encephalomyelitis is time- and score-dependent. Neurosci Lett. 2011;494:227–31.

12. Fiander MDJ, Stifani N, Nichols M, Akay T, Robertson GS. Kinematic gait parameters are highly sensitive measures of motor deficits and spinal cord injury in mice subjected to experimental autoimmune encephalomyelitis. Behav Brain Res. 2017;317:95–108.

13. Rodrigues DH, Sachs D, Teixeira AL. Mechanical hypernociception in experimental autoimmune encephalomyelitis. Arq Neuropsiquiatr. 2009; 67:78–81.

14. Rodrigues DH, Leles BP, Costa VV, Miranda AS, Cisalpino D, Gomes DA, et al. IL-1b is involved with the generation of pain in experimental autoimmune encephalomyelitis. Mol Neurobiol. 2016;53:6540–7.

15. Chen Y-J, Cheng F-C, Sheu M-L, Su H-L, Chen C-J, Sheehan J, et al. Detection of subtle neurological alterations by the catwalk XT gait analysis system. J Neuroeng Rehabil. 2014;11:62.

16. Gabriel AF, Marcus MAE, Honig WMM, Walenkamp GHIM, Joosten EAJ. The CatWalk method: a detailed analysis of behavioral changes after acute inflammatory pain in the rat. J Neurosci Methods. 2007;163:9–16.

17. Pitzer C, Kuner R, Tappe-theodor A. Voluntary and evoked behavioral correlates in inflammatory pain conditions under different social housing conditions. Mol Pain. 2016;12:1–15.

18. Silva GAA, Pradella F, Moraes A, Farias A, dos Santos LMB, de Oliveira ALR, et al. Impact of pregabalin treatment on synaptic plasticity and glial reactivity during the course of experimental autoimmune encephalomyelitis. Brain Behav. 2014;4:925–35.

19. Herold S, Kumar P, Jung K, Graf I, Menkhoff H, Schulz X, et al. CatWalk gait analysis in a rat model of multiple sclerosis. BMC Neurosci. BioMed Central; 2016; 17:78.

20. Basso DM, Hansen CN. Biological basis of exercise-based treatments: spinal cord injury. Phys Med Rehabil. 2011;3:S73–7.

21. Pearson M, Dieberg G, Smart N. Exercise as a therapy for improvement of walking ability in adults with multiple sclerosis: a meta-analysis. Arch Phys Med Rehabil. 2015;96:1339–48.

22. Jung SY, Kim DY, Yune TY, Shin DH, Baek S Bin, Kim CJ. Treadmill exercise reduces spinal cord injury-induced apoptosis by activating the PI3K/Akt pathway in rats. Exp Ther Med. 2014; 7:587–93.

23. Rossi S, Furlan R, De Chiara V, Musella A, Lo Giudice T, Mataluni G, et al. Exercise attenuates the clinical, synaptic and dendritic abnormalities of experimental autoimmune encephalomyelitis. Neurobiol Dis. 2009;36:51–9.

24. Bernardes D, Brambilla R, Bracchi-Ricard V, Karmally S, Dellarole A, Carvalho-Tavares J, et al. Prior regular exercise improves clinical outcome and reduces demyelination and axonal injury in experimental autoimmune encephalomyelitis. J Neurochem. 2016;136:63–73.

25. Bernardes D, Oliveira-Lima OC, da Silva TV, Faraco CCF, Leite HR, Juliano MA, et al. Differential brain and spinal cord cytokine and BDNF levels in experimental autoimmune encephalomyelitis are modulated by prior and regular exercise. J Neuroimmunol. 2013;264:24–34.

26. Bernardes D, Oliveira-Lima OC, da Silva TV, Juliano MA, Dos Santos DM, Carvalho-Tavares J. Metabolic alterations in experimental autoimmune encephalomyelitis in mice: effects of prior physical exercise. Neurophysiology. 2016;48:117–21.

27. Le Page C, Ferry A, Rieu M. Effect of muscular exercise on chronic relapsing experimental autoimmune encephalomyelitis. J Appl Physiol. 1994;77(5):2341–7.

28. Le Page C, Bourdoulous S, Béraud E, Couraud PO, Rieu M, Ferry A. Effect of physical exercise on adoptive experimental auto-immune encephalomyelitis in rats. Eur J Appl Occup Physiol. 1996;73(1-2):130–5.

29. Patel DI, White LJ. Effect of 10-day forced treadmill training on neurotrophic factors in experimental autoimmune encephalomyelitis. Appl Physiol Nutr Metab. 2013;38:194–9.

30. Wens I, Dalgas U, Verboven K, Kosten L, Stevens A, Hens N, et al. Impact of high intensity exercise on muscle morphology in EAE rats. Physiol Res. 2015;32:1–37.

31. Patel DI, White LJ, Lira VA, Criswell DS, Physiology A. Forced exercise increases muscle mass in EAE despite early onset of disability. Physiol Res. 2016;65:1013–7.

32. Parkkinen S, Ortega FJ, Kuptsova K, Huttunen J, Tarkka I, Jolkkonen J. Gait impairment in a rat model of focal cerebral ischemia. Stroke Res Treat. 2013; 2013:1–12.

33. Bárez-López S, Bosch-García D, Gómez-Andrés D, Pulido-Valdeolivas I, Montero-Pedrazuela A, Obregon MJ, et al. Abnormal motor phenotype at adult stages in mice lacking type 2 deiodinase. PLoS One. 2014;9:e103857.

34. de Haas R, Russel FG, Smeitink JA. Gait analysis in a mouse model resembling Leigh disease. Behav Brain Res. 2016;296:191–8.

35. Wooley CM, Xing S, Burgess RW, Cox GA, Seburn KL. Age, experience and genetic background influence treadmill walking in mice. Physiol Behav. 2009;96:350–61.

36. Contarteze RVL, Manchado FDB, Gobatto CA, De Mello MAR. Stress biomarkers in rats submitted to swimming and treadmill running exercises. Comp Biochem Physiol - A Mol Integr Physiol. 2008;151:415–22.

37. Baptista S, Piloto N, Reis F, Teixeira-de-Lemos E, Garrido AP, Dias A, et al. Treadmill running and swimming imposes distinct cardiovascular physiological adaptations in the rat: focus on serotonergic and sympathetic nervous systems modulation. Acta Physiol Hung. 2008;95:365–81.

38. Ra S-M, Kim H, Jang M-H, Shin M-C, Shin M-C, Lee T-H, et al. Treadmill running and swimming increase cell proliferation in the hippocampal dentate gyrus of rats. Neurosci Lett. 2002;333:123–6.

39. Deforges S, Branchu J, Biondi O, Grondard C, Pariset C, Lécolle S, et al. Motoneuron survival is promoted by specific exercise in a mouse model of amyotrophic lateral sclerosis. J Physiol. 2009;587:3561–72.

40. Sheridan GK, Dev KK. Targeting S1P receptors in experimental autoimmune encephalomyelitis in mice improves early deficits in locomotor activity and increases ultrasonic vocalisations. Sci Rep. 2014;4:1–6.

41. Deumens R, Jaken RJP, Marcus MAE, Joosten EAJ. The CatWalk gait analysis in assessment of both dynamic and static gait changes after adult rat sciatic nerve resection. J Neurosci Methods. 2007;164:120–30.

42. Herbin M, Hackert R, Gasc JP, Renous S. Gait parameters of treadmill versus overground locomotion in mouse. Behav Brain Res. 2007;181:173–9.

43. Batka RJ, Brown TJ, Mcmillan KP, Meadows RM, Jones KJ, Haulcomb MM. The need for speed in rodent locomotion analyses Richard. Anat Rec. 2014; 297:1839–64.

44. Górska T, Majczyński H, Zmysłowski W. Overground locomotion in intact rats: contact electrode recording. Acta Neurobiol Exp (Wars). 1998;58:227–37.

45. Clarke K, Still J. Gait analysis in the mouse. Physiol Behav. 1999;66:723–9.

46. Moore S, Khalaj AJ, Patel R, Yoon J, Ichwan D, Hayardeny L, et al. Restoration of axon conduction and motor deficits by therapeutic treatment with glatiramer acetate. J Neurosci Res. 2014;92:1621–36.

47. Mitra NK, Bindal U, Hwa WE, Chua CLL, Tan CY. Evaluation of locomotor function and microscopic structure of the spinal cord in a mouse model of experimental autoimmune encephalomyelitis following treatment with syngeneic mesenchymal stem cells. Int J Clin Exp Pathol. 2015;8:12041–52.

48. Starkey ML, Barritt AW, Yip PK, Davies M, Hamers FPT, McMahon SB, et al. Assessing behavioural function following a pyramidotomy lesion of the corticospinal tract in adult mice. Exp Neurol. 2005;195:524–39.

49. Guillot TS, Asress SA, Richardson JR, Glass JD, Miller GW. Treadmill gait analysis does not detect motor deficits in animal models of Parkinson's disease or amyotrophic lateral sclerosis. J Mot Behav. 2008;40:568–77.

50. Liu Z, Li Y, Zhang J, Elias S, Chopp M. Evaluation of corticospinal axon loss by fluorescent dye tracing in mice with experimental autoimmune encephalomyelitis. J Neurosci Methods. 2008;167:191–7.

51. Centonze D, Muzio L, Rossi S, Cavasinni F, De Chiara V, Bergami A, et al. Inflammation triggers synaptic alteration and degeneration in experimental autoimmune encephalomyelitis. J Neurosci. 2009;29:3442–52.

52. Gentile A, Fresegna D, Federici M, Musella A, Rizzo FR, Sepman H, et al. Dopaminergic dysfunction is associated with IL-1b-dependent mood alterations in experimental autoimmune encephalomyelitis. Neurobiol Dis. 2015;74:347–58.

53. Serradj N, Jamon M. The adaptation of limb kinematics to increasing walking speeds in freely moving mice 129/Sv and C57BL/6. Behav Brain Res. 2009;201:59–65.

54. Koblinger K, Füzesi T, Ejdrygiewicz J, Krajacic A, Bains JS, Whelan PJ. Characterization of A11 neurons projecting to the spinal cord of mice. PLoS One. 2014;9:1–12.

3

Reasons for discontinuation of subcutaneous interferon β-1a three times a week among patients with multiple sclerosis: a real-world cohort study

Meritxell Sabidó-Espin[1]* and Rick Munschauer[2]

Abstract

Background: Continuation of interferon (IFN) β-based therapies is important for maximum treatment effectiveness in patients with multiple sclerosis (MS); however, few real-world data are available on discontinuation from IFN β. The aim of this cohort analysis was to estimate real-world discontinuation rates up to 3 years among MS patients in the United States taking subcutaneous (sc) IFN β-1a three times a week (tiw) and to identify whether the factors associated with discontinuation change over time.

Methods: Patient data were pooled from the MarketScan© Commercial and Medicare Supplemental healthcare claims databases. Patients with ≥1 multiple sclerosis diagnosis who were sc IFN β-1a tiw naïve, had ≥1 year of continuous eligibility before treatment, and ≥1 prescription were followed from first prescription (index date) until date of discontinuation, switch, or end of observation. Treatment status was analysed at exactly 1, 2 or 3 years after index. Multivariable models were used to identify drivers of discontinuation.

Results: Data from 5956 patients were included; 2862 patients (48.1%) discontinued therapy. Discontinuation rates were 36.9% (1 year), 49.5% (2 years) and 55.8% (3 years). A greater proportion of discontinuing patients had poor adherence (<80% [94.0%] versus ≥80% [51.7%]) or were taking additional medication at follow-up versus the overall population. Factors independently associated with discontinuation irrespective of time on therapy were increasing number of magnetic resonance imaging scans (1 year adjusted odds ratio 1.45, 95% confidence interval 1.26–1.67; 2 years 1.18, 1.06–1.32; 3 years 1.20, 1.07–1.34) and adherence <80% versus ≥80% (1 year 180.95, 135.84–241.03; 2 years 135.80, 100.10–184.23; 3 years 174.89, 115.27–265.38). Factors associated only with early discontinuation (at 1 year) were ≥3 sets of laboratory investigations versus none (2.54, 1.20–5.38), and anxiolytic use at follow-up (1.40, 1.06–1.82). Factors associated only with later discontinuation (at 2 years and/or at 3 years) were antidepressant use at follow-up (2 years 1.46, 1.10–1.94) and greater number of relapses (2 years 1.60, 1.11–2.30; 3 years 2.31, 1.27–4.22).

Conclusions: Potential drivers of discontinuation change over time. Improved awareness of the drivers of discontinuation could lead to targeted interventions to improve adherence.

Keywords: Interferon β-1a, Multiple sclerosis, Adherence, Discontinuation

* Correspondence: meritxell.sabido-espin@merckgroup.com
[1]Frankfurter Str. 250, HPC: F135/201, Darmstadt 64293, Germany
Full list of author information is available at the end of the article

Background

The chronic nature of multiple sclerosis (MS) necessitates long-term treatment with a disease-modifying drug (DMD) to delay the progression of MS-related disability, reduce the frequency of relapses and prevent the formation of new brain lesions in patients with the relapsing-remitting form of the disease [1]. Adherence is defined as the ability and willingness to follow a prescribed treatment regimen correctly [2]. Good adherence to DMDs is essential, as it is associated with better clinical outcomes, such as reduced use of health care resources, lower costs, and improvements in patient quality of life [3–6].

Of the DMDs available for the treatment of MS, interferon (IFN) β-based therapies are some of the most widely prescribed [7]. Continued treatment with IFN-β therapy is important to achieve maximum treatment efficacy, [8] but data from clinical trials and registries show that IFN-β therapies have a treatment discontinuation rate of between 14 and 44%, which may lead to disease reactivation [9]. The causes of IFN-β discontinuation may also change as a function of time. A retrospective hospital-chart-based study recently showed a clear difference in stopping patterns of IFN-β therapy according to the length of time on treatment, with patients stopping IFN-β therapy due to side effects after a median of 13 months, while those discontinuing due to failure of therapy stopped after a median of 36 months [10].

The aim of this cohort analysis was to estimate IFN-β discontinuation rates among MS patients in the United States (US) receiving subcutaneous (sc) IFN β-1a three times a week (tiw), and to identify factors associated with stopping patterns according to time on treatment in a real-world setting, by using data from claims databases. This analysis has the potential to provide insights on potential strategies to improve medication-taking behaviour and help health care providers anticipate how the challenges associated with long-term therapy change over time.

Methods

Data sources

Data were pooled from two sources. The first was the longitudinal Truven MarketScan© Commercial Claims and Encounters database, which contains claims for more than 138 million health plan members from the year 2000 onwards and is considered to be representative of the US commercially insured population. The second source was the Medicare Supplemental and Coordination of Benefits (Medicare) databases, which contain the pooled claims data of approximately 2.5 million claimers in the US annually who have Medicare Supplemental Insurance paid for by employers.

Patients

Patient data were included in the retrospective analysis if patients were ≥18 years old on the year of the index date, had a diagnosis of MS (presence of ≥1 medical claim with a primary or secondary International Classification of Diseases, 9th revision, Clinical Modification [ICD-9-CM] diagnosis code for MS [340]) and had initiated treatment with sc IFN β-1a tiw during the study period (January 1, 2007 to December 31, 2013), had no record of previous sc IFN β-1a tiw treatment recorded in the database for at least 1 year before the index date, had ≥1 pharmacy claim for sc IFN β-1a tiw after the index date (captured through National Drug Codes), and had ≥1 year of continuous eligibility of treatment initiation with sc IFN β-1a tiw. Patients with a prescription for sc IFN β-1a tiw without a recorded diagnosis code for MS were excluded, as were pregnant women. Patients were followed from first prescription for sc IFN β-1a tiw until therapy switch or discontinuation, end of insurance eligibility, or end of observation period, whichever occurred first.

Data were fully compliant with the Health Insurance Portability and Accountability Act of 1996 (HIPPA). Given that the study only involved de-identified data, Institutional Review Board review or approval was not required.

Study measures

Patient demographics were captured at the time of the index prescription claim, with baseline characteristics based on the year preceding sc IFN β-1a tiw initiation (baseline period). Health care utilisation, adherence, persistence, sc IFN β-1a tiw treatment duration, and use of corticosteroids and other symptomatic therapies were measured during follow-up (≥1 prescription fill), including the index date.

Annualised relapse rates were calculated using a validated algorithm [11, 12] that defined an MS-related relapse as a claim in the primary position at any time during an in-patient hospitalisation, or a claim with an MS diagnosis code in the primary or secondary outpatient setting (including emergency room visits) in addition to a pharmacy or medical claim for a qualifying corticosteroid on the day of, or within 7 days after, the visit. Comorbidity burden was evaluated using the Charlson Comorbidity Index score [13].

Treatment adherence was operationalised as the number of days of medication supplied within a refill interval in relation to the number of days in the refill interval, also referred to as the medication possession ratio [14]. Treatment persistence was defined as the proportion of patients who continued on sc IFN β-1a tiw for a period of 1 year without a gap in therapy of ≥90 days, [15] and treatment duration was calculated as the time (in months) elapsed from index date to switch or complete discontinuation.

Statistical analysis

All statistical analyses were performed using SAS 9.4 (SAS institute Inc., Cary, NC, USA). Frequency distributions for categorical variables and mean (standard deviation) or median (interquartile range [IQR]) for continuous variables were calculated.

Overall discontinuation (%) was measured using the total sample of patients and with variable follow-up time. Discontinuation at 1 year, 2 years, and 3 years was calculated using patients who were followed-up for at least 1, 2, and 3 years, respectively. The proportion of patients who discontinued, including those who switched to another drug after discontinuation, at 1 year, 2 years and 3 years was calculated for patients who were followed-up for at least 1, 2 and 3 years, respectively. Among patients who continued or discontinued, the mean (standard deviation [SD]) number of relapses per year and the proportion of patients with a high number of relapses was calculated for the patients who were followed-up for at least 1, 2 and 3 years respectively.

To identify potential factors associated with discontinuation, bivariate and multivariate logistic regression models were used, and results were expressed as odds ratios (OR) with 95% confidence interval (CI). Variables with an unadjusted OR at the 0.15 level were included in the initial multivariable model and a stepwise fitted procedure was used; a variable was retained in the model if the p value was <0.05. Kaplan-Meier curves were used to estimate time to discontinuation by relapsing activity for those with ≥2 sc IFN β-1a claims. The models were also run without adherence to examine the relationship of other independent variables with adherence.

Results

Patient characteristics

Overall, data from 5956 patients were included in this retrospective cohort analysis (Fig. 1). Baseline demographics and clinical characteristics are shown in Table 1. Most patients received specialist neurological care, rather than general or emergency medical care (Additional file 1: Table S1).

Discontinuation of sc IFN β-1a tiw

In total, 2862 patients (48.1%) discontinued sc IFN β-1a tiw; the median treatment duration was 6 months (Table 1). The clinical characteristics of the patients who discontinued were similar to those reported for the total sample, although a greater proportion of discontinuing patients presented with low adherence (adherence <80%, 94.0% versus 51.7%, respectively). In addition, a greater proportion were taking additional medication at follow-

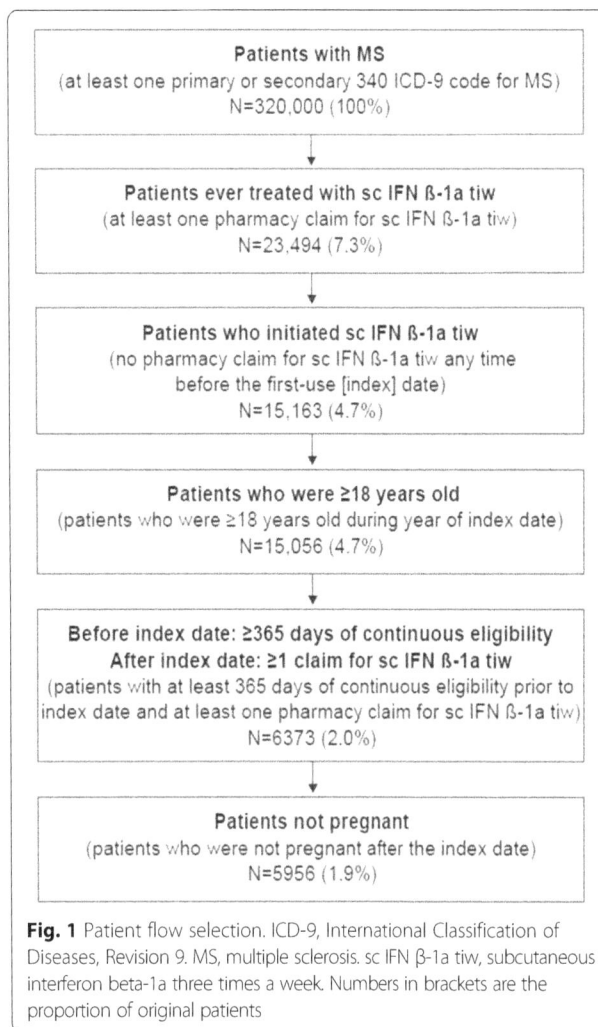

Fig. 1 Patient flow selection. ICD-9, International Classification of Diseases, Revision 9. MS, multiple sclerosis. sc IFN β-1a tiw, subcutaneous interferon beta-1a three times a week. Numbers in brackets are the proportion of original patients

up versus the overall population (non-steroidal anti-inflammatory drugs, 65.1% versus 54.1%; antidepressants, 58.8% versus 50.7%; anxiolytics, 26.3% versus 20.6%; corticosteroids, 47.6% versus 37.3%) (Table 1).

The discontinuation rates at 1, 2 and 3 years were 36.9% (1470 of 3975 patients)), 49.5% (1282 of 2592 patients), and 55.8% (928 of 1664 patients), respectively. Among those who discontinued, 20.6% did not switch to another drug at 1 year, 22.9% at 2 years, and 23.9% at 3 years. The proportion who discontinued and switched to another drug was 16.4% at 1 year, 26.6% at 2 years, and 31.9% at 3 years.

Factors associated with sc IFN β-1a tiw discontinuation

Factors independently associated with sc IFN β-1a tiw discontinuation at 1 year, 2 years, and 3 years are summarised in Table 2 and Additional file 1: Table S2. Two factors were identified that were independently associated with discontinuation irrespective of time on therapy. The first was increasing number of magnetic

Table 1 Demographic and clinical characteristics of patients with multiple sclerosis initiating subcutaneous interferon β-1a, three times weekly, by discontinuation status

Characteristics	sc IFN β-1a tiw			
	Total sample (N = 5956)		Discontinued (N = 2862)	
	n	%	n	%
Female sex	4447	74.7	2177	76.1
Age, mean (SD) years	44 (10.7)		44 (10.8)	
Region				
Northeast	999	16.8	481	16.8
North Central	1764	29.6	766	26.8
South	2156	36.2	1066	37.2
West	968	16.3	517	18.1
Unknown	69	1.2	32	1.1
Charlson comorbidity index				
Index = 0	3974	66.7	1887	65.9
Index = 1	1102	18.5	552	19.3
Index = 2	501	8.4	242	8.5
Index ≥ 3	379	6.4	181	6.3
Relapse per year, mean (SD)	0.21 (0.57)		0.25 (0.55)	
High relapse (≥2 relapses)[a]	271	4.6	154	5.4
DMD use history	2162	36.3	1143	39.9
Treatment duration, median (IQR) months	9 (3–22)		6 (2–15)	
Persistence	5634	94.6	2645	92.4
Adherence to treatment <80% (vs. ≥80%)	3078	51.7	2691	94.0
Baseline corticosteroid use	2384	40.0	1194	41.7
Follow-up				
NSAID use	3221	54.1	1862	65.1
Antidepressant use	3020	50.7	1682	58.8
Anxiolytic use	1229	20.6	753	26.3
Corticosteroid use	2222	37.3	1362	47.6

DMD disease-modifying drug, *NSAID* non-steroidal anti-inflammatory drugs, *IFN* interferon, *IQR*, interquartile range, *SC* subcutaneous, *SD* standard deviation, Tiw three times a week

[a]High relapse activity defined as having ≥2 relapses in the first year prior to start of subcutaneous interferon β-1a, three times weekly

resonance imaging (MRI) scans (per one additional scan), with adjusted OR (AORs) at 1, 2 and 3 years of 1.45 (95% confidence interval [CI] 1.26–1.67), 1.18 (95% CI 1.06–1.32) and 1.20 (95% CI 1.07–1.34), respectively; the second was adherence <80% versus adherence ≥80%, with AORs at 1, 2 and 3 years of 180.95 (95% CI 135.84–241.03), 135.80 (95% CI 100.10–184.23), and 174.89 (95% CI 115.27–265.38), respectively.

Factors associated only with early discontinuation (at 1 year) were three or more sets of laboratory investigations versus no laboratory investigations (AOR 2.54,

95% CI 1.20–5.38) and anxiolytic use at follow-up (AOR 1.40, 95% CI 1.06–1.82). Factors associated only with later discontinuation (at 2 years and/or at 3 years) were antidepressant use at follow up versus no antidepressant use (AOR at 2 years 1.46, 95% CI 1.10–1.94) and a greater number of relapses (AOR at 2 years 1.60, 95% CI 1.11–2.30; AOR at 3 years 2.31, 95% CI 1.27–4.22). Results from multivariable regression when adherence was removed from the model are shown in Additional file 1: Table S3.

At 1, 2, and 3 years, patients who had ≥1 relapse were more likely to discontinue sc IFN β-1a tiw than those who had no relapses (Fig. 2a–c); at each time point, those who discontinued had a high mean number of relapses per year (≥2 relapses) in the year prior to starting treatment with sc IFN β-1a tiw than those patients who continued (Table 3).

Discussion

In this retrospective cohort study, discontinuation rates among US patients with MS receiving sc IFN β-1a tiw increased over time, from 36.9% at the first year to 55.8% at 3 years after treatment initiation. Poor adherence was the main factor associated with discontinuation of this therapy, irrespective of the length of time on treatment. The discontinuation rates seen in the current study are in agreement with those reported previously,[16] although other studies report a wide variation in discontinuation in patients with MS. In a respective cohort study of pharmacy claims in Germany, at 2 years post-initiation, overall persistence to one of the four first-line injected therapies was 32.3%, [17] while in a similar study approximately half of patients with MS had discontinued DMDs at the same time point [18].

Treatment adherence describes the successful self-administration of medicine by a patient, taking into account correct treatment usage with regard to administration schedule and treatment regimen (compliance) over time (persistence) [6]. Poor adherence is a common problem among patients with many types of chronic disease, including MS, and improvements in treatment adherence may have a larger effect on society and health than most therapeutic advances [2, 19]. Many factors that contribute to poor adherence to long-term therapy in patients with MS are recognised; [6] indeed, recent retrospective [7, 20] and prospective [19] observational studies indicate that the most common reasons to discontinue IFN-β therapy in real-world settings are adverse events (such as influenza-like symptoms, depression and injection-site reactions) and increased disease activity (including radiographic progression, relapses, and disability progression). Although in this study indices of disability progression were not reported, an association between relapses and discontinuation was

Table 2 Adjusted odds ratios of factors associated with discontinuation of subcutaneous interferon β-1a, three times weekly, at 1, 2, and 3 years, respectively

Adjusted odds ratio (95% confidence interval)	sc IFN β-1a tiw		
	Discontinuation at 1 year ($n = 3975$)	Discontinuation at 2 years ($n = 2592$)	Discontinuation at 3 years ($n = 1664$)
Female sex (vs. male)	NS	NS	1.48 (0.98–2.22)
Region (vs. unknown)	NS	NS	NS
Age in years (continuous)	NS	NS	NS
Charlson comorbidity index (≥1 vs. 0)	NS	NS	NS
Relapses per year (continuous)	NS	1.60 (1.11–2.30)	2.31 (1.27–4.22)
High relapses (≥2 relapses) (vs. no)[a]	NS	NS	NS
DMD use history (vs. no)	NS	NS	NS
Months of treatment duration (continuous)	NS	NS	NS
No persistence (vs. yes)	NS	NS	NS
Adherence <80% (vs. ≥80%)	180.95 (135.84–241.03)	135.80 (100.10–184.23)	174.90 (115.27–265.38)
Health resource usage			
Hospital visits (1 vs. 0, 2 vs. 0, and ≥3vs. 0)	NS	NS	NS
Emergency room visits 1 vs. 0, 2 vs. 0, and ≥3vs. 0)	NS	NS	NS
Nurse visits (1 vs. 0, 2 vs. 0, and ≥3vs. 0)	NS	NS	NS
Neurologist visits (vs. 10+)			
1	0.84 (0.57–1.25)	NS	NS
2	0.67 (0.47–0.97)	NS	NS
3+	1.11 (0.84–1.48)	NS	NS
Psychologist visits (1 vs. 0, 2 vs. 0, and ≥3vs. 0)	NS	NS	NS
Psychiatrist visits (1 vs. 0, 2 vs. 0, and ≥3vs. 0)	NS	NS	NS
Speech Therapy visits (1 vs. 0, 2 vs. 0, and ≥3vs. 0)	NS	NS	NS
Outpatients (1 vs. 0, 2 vs. 0, and ≥3vs. 0)	NS	NS	NS
Increasing number of MRI scans (one additional scan versus no increase in number of MRI scans)	1.45 (1.26–1.67)	1.18 (1.06–1.32)	1.20 (1.07–1.34)
Laboratory investigations (vs. 0)			
1	0.61 (0.30–1.25)	NS	NS
2	0.93 (0.38–2.26)	NS	NS
3+	2.54 (1.20–5.38)	NS	NS
Baseline corticosteroid use (No = 0, Yes = 1)	NS	NS	NS
Follow-up			
NSAID use (vs. no)	NS	NS	NS
Antidepressants use (vs. no)	NS	1.46 (1.10–1.94)	NS
Anxiolitics use (vs. no)	1.40 (1.06–1.82)	NS	NS
Corticosteroid use (vs. no)	NS	NS	NS

DMD disease-modifying drug, *IFN* interferon, *MRI* magnetic resonance imaging, *NS* no significant association with discontinuation, *NSAID* non-steroidal anti-inflammatory drug, *sc* subcutaneous, *tiw* three times a week

[a]High relapse activity defined as having ≥2 relapses in the first year prior to start of subcutaneous interferon β-1a, three times weekly

observed at years 2 and 3, and the association with an increasing number of MRI scans may be an indicator of radiographic progression. Despite the development of strategies to help mitigate these factors, [10, 21] sustained adherence to DMDs in patients with MS remains low [16, 18].

When we compared factors associated with discontinuation in models including and excluding adherence, the only variable associated in both models was the number of laboratory investigations at 1 year (one laboratory investigation versus no laboratory investigations was inversely associated with discontinuation in the model

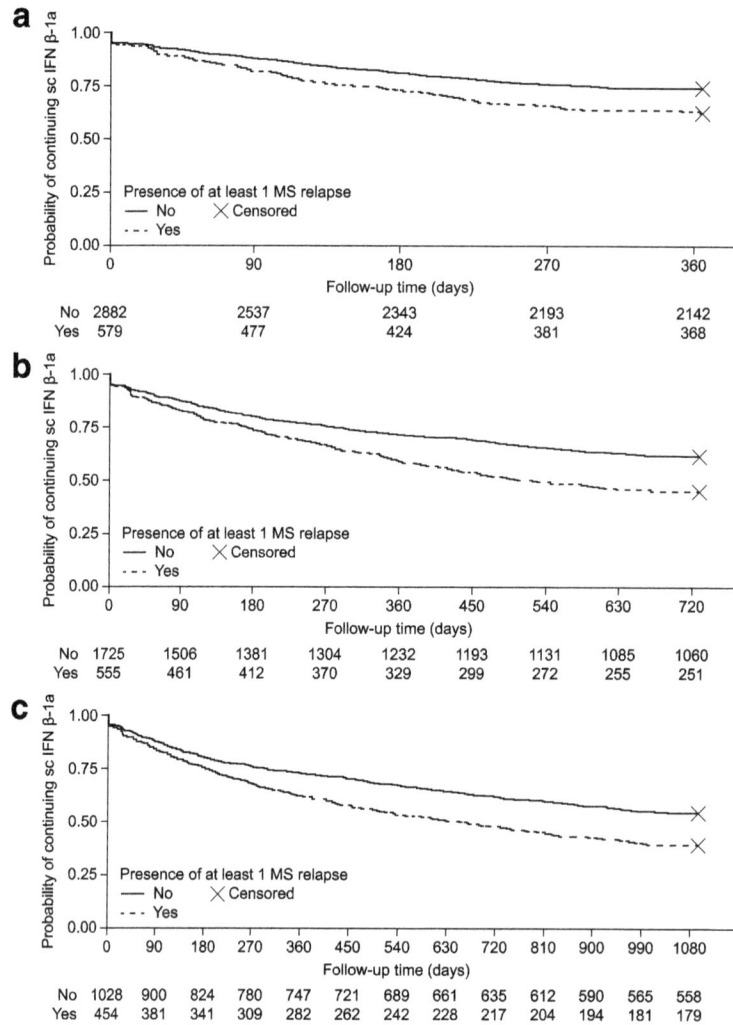

Fig. 2 Kaplan-Meier curves of probability of sc IFN β-1a tiw continuation by follow-up time in days. **a** Data are truncated at 1 year from the index date. Kaplan-Meier curves are stratified by the presence of one or more relapses (red line) or no relapses (blue line). 3975 patients were included in the analysis; 3461 patients had two or more sc IFN β-1a tiw claims during this period. **b** Data are truncated at 2 years from the index date. Kaplan-Meier curves are stratified by the presence of one or more relapses (red line) or no relapses (blue line). 2592 patients were included in the analysis; 2280 patients had two or more sc IFN β-1a tiw claims during this period. **c** Data are truncated at 3 years from the index date. Kaplan-Meier curves are stratified by the presence of one or more relapses (red line) or no relapses (blue line). 1664 patients were included in the analysis; 1482 patients had two or more sc IFN β-1a tiw claims during this period

Table 3 Relapse characteristics according to discontinuation status at 1, 2 and 3 years

	sc IFN β-1a tiw					
	Follow-up at 1 year		Follow-up at 2 years		Follow-up at 3 years	
	Continued	Discontinued	Continued	Discontinued	Continued	Discontinued
Total patients, n (%)	2505 (63.0)	1470 (37.0)	1310 (50.5)	1282 (49.5)	736 (44.2)	928 (55.8)
Relapses per year, mean (SD)	0.18 (0.52)	0.32 (0.67)	0.14 (0.34)	0.26 (0.49)	0.12 (0.26)	0.23 (0.42)
Patients with high relapses, n (%)[a]	97 (3.9)	84 (5.7)	46 (3.5)	73 (5.7)	21 (2.9)	52 (5.6)

IFN, interferon, *sc* subcutaneous, *SD* standard deviation, *tiw* three times a week
[a]High relapse activity defined as having ≥2 relapses in the first year prior to start of subcutaneous interferon β-1a, three times weekly

without adherence [AOR 0.16]; three or more laboratory investigations versus no laboratory investigations was associated with discontinuation in the model that includes adherence [AOR 2.54]). For the other factors, which were significantly associated with discontinuation in only one of the models, we cannot exclude a relationship with adherence. Furthermore, the high AORs for adherence were driven by the very low proportion of patients who had adherence ≥80% but still discontinued sc IFN β-1a tiw (1 year, $n = 68$; 2 years, $n = 66$; 3 years, $n = 41$).

In this retrospective analysis, there was no significant association between age, sex, and initial DMD, respectively, and discontinuation of sc IFN β-1a tiw, which is in line with previous studies [22]. Furthermore, although overall time on treatment was not associated with discontinuation, a change was observed in the drivers of discontinuation as time on therapy increases. In the short-term (up to and including 1 year), the main drivers (an increase in laboratory investigations and an increase in the use of anxiolytics) could be associated with the common emergent adverse effects of treatment with sc IFN β-1a tiw [7]. Even though the adverse-event profile of sc IFN β-1a tiw is well-documented, consistent and stable during both clinical trials and in real-world experience, [7] adverse events can still lead to considerable discomfort and patient anxiety. Pharmacological and non-pharmacological approaches to prevent discontinuation due to adverse events have not been widely implemented in patients who discontinue sc IFN β-1a tiw therapy, resulting in missed opportunities to improve retention [16]. In the long-term (at 2 years and/or at 3 years), factors associated only with later discontinuation were antidepressant use at follow-up versus no antidepressant use and a greater number of relapses. Depression and anxiety are both comorbid conditions in patients with MS, [23] and the presence of both can contribute to poor adherence to DMDs [24]. Indeed, the 12-month prevalence of depression in patients with MS has been reported as 25.7%, and estimates of lifetime prevalence of depression are as high as 50% [25]. MS patients with comorbid depression are about half as likely to be adherent to a DMD than MS patients without depression [26]. In addition, in a real-world US health insurance-claims-based study of more than 8000 patients, depression was also a recognised adverse effect of treatment with IFN therapy (incidence rate 7.75 [95% CI 7.32–8.20]) [7]. As the current analysis shows, further investigation is required to corroborate the validity of new prescriptions of antidepressants as a driver of discontinuation at and beyond 2 years, or whether this is associated with a decrease in quality of life as a consequence of increased disease activity.

The relation between discontinuation and relapse is not straightforward. The association between the increase in the number of relapses and later discontinuation (Table 3) could be the result of the absence of perceived benefit of long-term treatment, leading to poor adherence; however, any theories on the precise nature of this association require further investigation. Although the exact causes of increased disease activity are not investigated in this retrospective real-world cohort study, there are several other possible reasons that could be investigated further, including the development of neutralising antibodies, which were shown in a European prospective multicentre centre study to develop in almost a quarter of patients on any IFN β-based regimen at a median of 23.8 months on treatment. The development of neutralising antibodies may abrogate treatment effectiveness, leading to clinical and radiological disease progression [27].

The number of patients who discontinued and switched to a different therapy increased over each of the time periods studied. Although data on the drugs to which patients switched was not analysed, the period of analysis overlaps with the date from which the oral MS drug dimethyl fumarate first became available in the USA (March 28, 2013) [28]. This also corresponds to an increase in market-based reports of dimethyl fumarate use in the final quarter of 2013 [29]. It is possible that, in response to the momentum of pre-marketing demand for an oral therapy, data collected during this study period may have included patients who switched from injected to oral therapies. Additionally, the current study showed that patients who had a history of using other DMDs may be more likely to switch to another medication after discontinuing sc IFN β-10 tiw. However, this period of overlap (9 months) is too short to assess the impact on discontinuation of sc IFN β-1a tiw.

One limitation of this retrospective study is that, as an analysis of administrative health care claims data, it does not take into account all clinical information (such as MS subtype and disease severity), socioeconomic status, enrolment in patient-support programmes, and other factors that might influence discontinuation. However, claims database analyses may have an advantage over retrospective chart review for identifying the causes for discontinuation over time, as they provide a precise record of the duration of treatment in the broader patient population and do not have the biases associated with reporting in clinical trials or post-marketing observational studies [7].

Conclusion

In conclusion, increased awareness among physicians of the clinical significance of the length of time on treatment could foster a culture where patients are actively asked by physicians whether they are experiencing any time-specific adverse events, rather than reliance on emergent or retrospective reporting by patients. Such improved awareness could lead to earlier access to disease-management strategies and patient-support services and could inform proactive preventive treatment strategies to improve long-term treatment adherence in patients with MS.

Acknowledgements
Data analysis was provided by Genesis Group, Woodcliff Lake, NJ, USA. The study was sponsored by Merck KGaA, Darmstadt, Germany. The authors would like to thank the US patients whose data contributed to this study. Medical writing assistance was provided by Steven Goodrick of inScience Communications, UK, and funded by Merck KGaA, Darmstadt, Germany.

Authors' contributions
MS designed the study and performed the research. MS and RM wrote the manuscript and agreed on the submitted version. Both authors read and approved the final manuscript.

Competing of interests
M Sabidó Espin is an employee of Merck KGaA, Darmstadt, Germany. At the time of the analysis, R Munschauer was an employee of EMD Serono, a business of Merck KGaA, Darmstadt, Germany.

Author details
[1]Frankfurter Str. 250, HPC: F135/201, Darmstadt 64293, Germany. [2]EMD Serono, Rockland, MA, USA.

References
1. Wingerchuk DM, Carter JL. Multiple sclerosis: current and emerging disease-modifying therapies and treatment strategies. Mayo Clin Proc. 2014;89:225–40.
2. WHO. Adherence to long-term therapies: evidence for action. Geneva: WHO; 2003.
3. Kappos L, Kuhle J, Multanen J, Kremenchutzky M, Verdun di Cantogno E, Cornelisse P, Lehr L, Casset-Semanaz F, Issard D, Uitdehaag BM. Factors influencing long-term outcomes in relapsing-remitting multiple sclerosis: PRISMS-15. J Neurol Neurosurg Psychiatry. 2015;86(11):1202–7.
4. Steinberg SC, Faris RJ, Chang CF, Chan A, Tankersley MA. Impact of adherence to interferons in the treatment of multiple sclerosis: a non-experimental, retrospective, cohort study. Clin Drug Investig. 2010;30(2):89–100.
5. Tan H, Yu J, Tabby D, Devries A, Singer J. Clinical and economic impact of a specialty care management program among patients with multiple sclerosis: a cohort study. Mult Scler. 2010;16(8):956–63.
6. Treadaway K, Cutter G, Salter A, Lynch S, Simsarian J, Corboy J, Jeffery D, Cohen B, Mankowski K, Guarnaccia J, et al. Factors that influence adherence with disease-modifying therapy in MS. J Neurol. 2009;256(4):568–76.
7. Smith MY, Sabido-Espin M, Trochanov A, Samuelson M, Guedes S, Corvino FA, Richy FF. Postmarketing safety profile of subcutaneous interferon beta-1a given 3 times weekly: a retrospective administrative claims analysis. J Manag Care Spec Pharm. 2015;21(8):650–60.
8. Zhornitsky S, Greenfield J, Koch MW, Patten SB, Harris C, Wall W, Alikhani K, Burton J, Busche K, Costello F, et al. Long-term persistence with injectable therapy in relapsing-remitting multiple sclerosis: an 18-year observational cohort study. PLoS One. 2015;10(4):e0123824.
9. Portaccio E, Amato MP. Improving compliance with interferon-beta therapy in patients with multiple sclerosis. CNS Drugs. 2009;23(6):453–62.
10. Patti F. Optimizing the benefit of multiple sclerosis therapy: the importance of treatment adherence. Patient Prefer Adherence. 2010;4:1–9.
11. Ollendorf DA, Jilinskaia E, Oleen-Burkey M. Clinical and economic impact of glatiramer acetate versus beta interferon therapy among patients with multiple sclerosis in a managed care population. J Manag Care Pharm. 2002;8(6):469–76.
12. Chastek BJ, Oleen-Burkey M, Lopez-Bresnahan MV. Medical chart validation of an algorithm for identifying multiple sclerosis relapse in healthcare claims. J Med Econ. 2010;13(4):618–25.
13. Charlson M, Szatrowski TP, Peterson J, Gold J. Validation of a combined comorbidity index. J Clin Epidemiol. 1994;47(11):1245–51.
14. Steiner JF, Prochazka AV. The assessment of refill compliance using pharmacy records: methods, validity, and applications. J Clin Epidemiol. 1997;50(1):105–16.
15. Cramer JA, Roy A, Burrell A, Fairchild CJ, Fuldeore MJ, Ollendorf DA, Wong PK. Medication compliance and persistence: terminology and definitions. Value Health. 2008;11(1):44–7.
16. Bruce JM, Lynch SG. Multiple sclerosis: MS treatment adherence–how to keep patients on medication? Nat Rev Neurol. 2011;7(8):421–2.
17. Hansen K, Schussel K, Kieble M, Werning J, Schulz M, Friis R, Pohlau D, Schmitz N, Kugler J. Adherence to disease modifying drugs among patients with multiple sclerosis in Germany: a retrospective cohort study. PLoS One. 2015;10(7):e0133279.
18. Wong J, Gomes T, Mamdani M, Manno M, O'Connor PW. Adherence to multiple sclerosis disease-modifying therapies in Ontario is low. Can J Neurol Sci. 2011;38(3):429–33.
19. Hupperts R, Ghazi-Visser L, Martins Silva A, Arvanitis M, Kuusisto H, Marhardt K, Vlaikidis N. The STAR Study: a real-world, international, observational study of the safety and tolerability of, and adherence to, serum-free subcutaneous interferon beta-1a in patients with relapsing multiple sclerosis. Clin Ther. 2014;36(12):1946–57.
20. Gobbi C, Zecca C, Linnebank M, Muller S, You X, Meier R, Borter E, Traber M. Swiss analysis of multiple sclerosis: a multicenter, non-interventional, retrospective cohort study of disease-modifying therapies. Eur Neurol. 2013;70(1–2):35–41.
21. Remington G, Rodriguez Y, Logan D, Williamson C, Treadaway K. Facilitating medication adherence in patients with multiple sclerosis. Int J MS Care. 2013;15(1):36–45.
22. Evans C, Tam J, Kingwell E, Oger J, University of British Columbia MSCN, Tremlett H. Long-term persistence with the immunomodulatory drugs for multiple sclerosis: a retrospective database study. Clin Ther. 2012;34(2):341–50.
23. Wallin MT, Wilken JA, Turner AP, Williams RM, Kane R. Depression and multiple sclerosis: review of a lethal combination. J Rehabil Res Dev. 2006;43(1):45.
24. Marrie RA, Reingold S, Cohen J, Stuve O, Trojano M, Sorensen PS, Cutter G, Reider N. The incidence and prevalence of psychiatric disorders in multiple sclerosis: a systematic review. Mult Scler. 2015;21(3):305–17.
25. Siegert RJ, Abernethy DA. Depression in multiple sclerosis: a review. J Neurol Neurosurg Psychiatry. 2005;76(4):469–75.
26. Tarrants M, Oleen-Burkey M, Castelli-Haley J, Lage MJ. The impact of comorbid depression on adherence to therapy for multiple sclerosis. Mult Scler Int. 2011;2011:271321.
27. Govindappa K, Sathish J, Park K, Kirkham J, Pirmohamed M. Development of interferon beta-neutralising antibodies in multiple sclerosis–a systematic review and meta-analysis. Eur J Clin Pharmacol. 2015;71(11):1287–98.
28. Yao S. FDA approves new multiple sclerosis treatment: Tecfidera [Press release]. Retrieved from: http://www.fda.gov/newsevents/newsroom/pressannouncements/ucm345528.htm. Accessed 18 Jan 2016.
29. Biogen Idec. Biogen Idec total revenues increased 32% to $1.8 billion in the third quarter; company raise 2013 financial guidance [Press release]. Retrieved from http://media.biogen.com/press-release/investor-relations/biogen-idec-total-revenues-increased-32-18-billion-third-quarter-co. Accessed 18 Jan 2016. [http://media.biogen.com/press-release/investor-relations/biogen-idec-total-revenues-increased-32-18-billion-third-quarter-co].

4

High dose vitamin D supplementation does not affect biochemical bone markers in multiple sclerosis

Trygve Holmøy[1,2][*] (iD), Jonas Christoffer Lindstrøm[2,3], Erik Fink Eriksen[2,4], Linn Hofsøy Steffensen[5,6]
and Margitta T. Kampman[5]

Abstract

Background: People with multiple sclerosis have high risk of osteoporosis and fractures. A poor vitamin D status is a risk factor for MS, and vitamin D supplementation has been recommended both to prevent MS progression and to maintain bone health.

Methods: We assessed the effect of 20,000 IU vitamin D_3 weekly compared to placebo on biochemical markers of bone metabolism in 68 persons with relapsing remitting multiple sclerosis.

Results: Serum levels of 25-hydroxyvitamin D more than doubled in the vitamin D group, and parathyroid hormone decreased in the vitamin D group compared to the placebo group at week 48 and week 96. There was however no effect on bone formation as measured by procollagen type I N propeptide (PINP), or on bone resorption as measured by C-terminal cross-linking telopeptide of type I collagen (CTX1). Neither PINP nor CTX1 predicted bone loss from baseline to week 96.

Conclusions: These findings corroborate the previously reported lack of effect of weekly high dose vitamin D supplementation on bone mass density in the same patients, and suggest that such vitamin D supplementation does not prevent bone loss in persons with MS who are not vitamin D deficient.

Keywords: Multiple sclerosis, vitamin D, osteoporosis, randomized controlled trial

Background

Low levels of vitamin D are associated with increased future risk of developing multiple sclerosis and with increased disease activity [1–3]. Vitamin D is also essential for bone health. Several studies have shown that people with multiple sclerosis (MS) are at increased risk of developing osteoporosis [4, 5]. Physical disability is likely the main driver of accelerated bone loss in MS, but also disease duration and lifetime steroid dose are associated with low bone mineral density (BMD) [4, 6]. Low BMD is however prevalent also in ambulatory persons with

MS even shortly after clinical onset [6, 7], suggesting that shared etiological factors such as low vitamin D may operate in both MS and osteoporosis.

The combination of osteoporosis and high risk of falling may add to the burden of disease through increased risk of fractures. In line with this, large population based studies have shown that persons with MS have a marked increase of fractures compared to the general population [8–12]. Data from the Danish MS Registry and The National Hospital Discharge Registry showed that the risk of fractures of tibia, hip and femur in persons with MS was three to six times higher than in the general population [10].

Although the role of vitamin D supplementation on disease activity in MS is unclear [13], several authors have suggested that vitamin D should be monitored to

* Correspondence: Trygve.holmoy@medisin.uio.no
[1]Department of Neurology, Akershus University Hospital, Lørenskog, Norway
[2]Institute of Clinical Medicine, University of Oslo, Oslo, Norway
Full list of author information is available at the end of the article

prevent osteoporosis and fractures [5, 14–16]. The optimal intake of vitamin D and serum level of 25-hydroxyvitamin D is however controversial. Whereas the National Institute of Medicine considers a serum level of 25-hydroxyvitamin (25(OH)D) at 50 nmol/L and a daily intake of 600 IU vitamin D adequate for the general population [17], others argue that the serum level needed for both optimal bone health and for the potentially beneficial non-calcemic effects is at least 75 nmol/L [18–20]. There is, however limited evidence on the effect of vitamin D supplementation on bone heath in MS.

We have previously reported a randomized controlled trial (RCT) of weekly supplementation with 20,000 IU vitamin D_3 compared to placebo in fully ambulatory (expanded disability status scale ≤4.5) persons with relapsing remitting MS living above the Arctic Circle [21]. This dose has proven safe in several RTCs in the same area [22]. Even though people with MS may need more vitamin D than others to reach the same 25-hydroxyvitamin D (25(OH)D) serum concentration, [23], we expected that this dose would bring the vast majority of patients to 25(OH)D levels considered optimal for bone health and also within the range associated with decreased disease activity. Although bone mineral density (BMD) decreased significantly in the placebo group and not in the vitamin D treated group, the primary outcome (difference in percentage change in BMD between groups) was negative [21].

The markers of bone formation procollagen type I N propeptide (PINP) and bone resorption C-terminal cross-linking telopeptide of type I collagen (CTX1) have been shown to predict fracture risk and to reflect the response to osteoporosis treatment [24]. These markers are recommended as reference markers in observational and treatment studies in osteoporosis by the International Osteoporosis Foundation and the International Federation of Clinical Chemistry and Laboratory Medicine [25], and could be more sensitive for treatment effects than BMD. The aim of the current study was to examine if CTX and PINP predict bone loss, and if vitamin D_3 supplementation affect these markers of bone formation and turnover in persons with MS.

Methods
The design of the RCT have been reported previously [21, 26]. Briefly, 71 RRMS patients from Troms and Finnmark (the northernmost counties in Norway), aged 18–50 years and with Kurtzke's Expanded Disability Status Scale (EDSS) score ≤4.5 were included in the original study [21]. The exclusion criteria comprised a history of conditions or diseases affecting bone, pregnancy or lactation the past 6 months, use of bone-active medications other than intravenous methylprednisolone for treatment

of MS relapses, a history of nephrolithiasis during the previous 5 years, or menopause.

The participants were randomized to receive either once-weekly oral 20,000 IU vitamin D_3 (Dekristol™; SWISS CAPS AG, Kirchberg, Switzerland) or placebo. All participants also received 500 mg calcium daily (calcium carbonate, Weifa AS, Oslo, Norway). Participants who had gastrointestinal side effects attributed to Weifa calcium switched to Calcium Sandoz™ effervescent tablets (calcium lactate-gluconate and calcium carbonate, Sandoz A/S, Odense, Denmark), or discontinued the calcium supplement if their estimated dietary calcium intake as measured by a validated food frequency questionnaire exceeded 800 mg/day [27]. By capsule count, all subjects were ≥80% (mean 98%, range 80–100%) adherent to the study medication [21].

Measurement of BMD at the hip (mean of left and right), the spine (anterior–posterior spine L1–L4), and the non-dominant ultra-distal radius by DXA (dual X-ray absorptiometry) was performed by trained technicians at the University Hospital of North-Norway, using a Lunar Prodigy advanced densitometer (Lunar Radiation Corp., Madison, WI, USA.). The long-term precision was 0.26–0.28%, obtained by daily calibration of the densitometer. One fourth of the patients had low BMD (z-scores blow −2) at baseline [6].

Serum samples were collected at baseline (January or February for all participants) and at week 48 and 96 (randomly to intake of vitamin D supplementation), and frozen at −70 °C until batch analyses. 25(OH)D was measured by spectroscopy detecting total concentrations of both 25(OH)D$_2$ and 25(OH)D$_3$ at the Hormone laboratory at Haukeland University Hospital. The coefficient of variat4ion (CV) was 5.3% at 20 nmol/L and 4.0% at 239 nmol/L 25(OH)D. PINP and CTX1 were measured by electrochemiluminiscence at the Hormone laboratory at Oslo University Hospital. The CVs were 11% for PINP and 12% for CTX1, and the detection limits were 5–1200 µg/l and 0,07–6,00 µg/l respectively.

The associations between bone markers and BMD at baseline, and whether the concentrations of PINP and CTX1 at baseline predicted BMD change from baseline to week 96, were analyzed with linear regression. The longitudinal changes in CTX1, PINP and PTH were modelled with two separate linear mixed models. The models included time of measurement, treatment arm, time-treatment interaction, and a random intercept for each participant. The markers were log-transformed, making the estimated differences interpretable as percentages. The models formed the basis for all inferences on the relationship between vitamin D and the markers. To investigate whether disease modifying drugs could influence the results, we also used a model which included the drug treatment status at each sample time.

Table 1 Baseline characteristics

		Vitamin D group (N = 35)	Placebo group (N = 33)
Females	N (%)	24 (69)	24 (73)
Age (years)	Mean (range)	40 (21–50)	41 (26–50)
Body mass index	Mean (range)	25.9 (21.0–40.7)	26.4 (18.4–39.9)
Ongoing smoking	N (%)	15 (43)	14 (42)
EDSS	Median (range)	2.5 (0–4.5)	2.0 (0–4.5)
Annualised relapse rate	Mean (range)	0.11 (0–0.54)	0.15 (0–1.10)
Immunomodulatory treatment	N (%)	17 (49)[a]	17 (52)[b]
Serum 25(OH)D (nmol/L)	Mean (SD)	55.6 (29.0)	57.3 (21.8)
Hip BMD (mg/cm^2)	Mean (SD)	1018.8 (98.8)	968.9 (119.9)
Spine BMD (mg/cm^2)	Mean (SD)	1205.2 (117.7)	1165.7 (135.6)
Distal radius BMD (mg/cm^2)	Mean (SD)	484.8 (67.1)	472.8 (80.6)

[a]16 patients on IFN-β and one on glatiramer acetate
[b]15 patients on IFN-β, one on glatiramer acetate and one on natalizumab

Results

Serum samples for measurement of bone markers were available from 68 participants who completed the study. Baseline characteristics of the study population are shown in Table 1. As reported previously [28] there were no group differences in age, body mass index (BMI), smoking, use of disease modifying drugs, disability as measured by EDSS, calcium intake or relapse rate the previous year. The serum concentration of 25(OH)D increased to 123.2 ± 34.2 nmol/L at week 96 in the vitamin D group, and to 61.8 ± 25.2 nmol/L in the placebo group. Ionized calcium was similar and unchanged at baseline and week 96 in both groups (1.2 ± 0.0 nmol/L).

The concentrations of CTX1, PINP and PTH did not differ significantly between the groups at baseline (Table 2). The concentrations of CTX1 and PINP remained similar between treatment groups throughout the study group, whereas PTH was lower in the vitamin D group at both week 48 and at week 96.

The associations between the bone markers and BMD are presented in Table 3. There was a weak negative association between CTX1 and PINP and hip BMD at baseline, and between CTX1 and spine BMD at baseline ($p < 0.05$). The baseline marker concentrations did not predict change in BMD from baseline to week 48 or week 96.

The effect of vitamin D supplementation was finally analyzed using a linear mixed model for each bone marker with random patient-wise intercepts. There was no significant difference between treatment groups in the change of CTX1, PINP or PTH from baseline to week 48 or from baseline to week 96 (Table 4). These results did not change substantially when immune modulatory treatment was included in the model (results not shown). In total 14 patients received methylprednisolone for MS attack. Of these two in the placebo and two in the vitamin D groups were treated during the last 6 months prior to the first blood sampling, and three in the vitamin D group and one in the placebo group during the last 6 months prior to the last blood sampling. Excluding the 14 patients treated with methylprednisolone did not alter the results (data nor shown).

Discussion

To our knowledge the effect on vitamin D supplementation on markers of bone formation and resorption in persons with MS has not been reported previously. We found that increasing mean 25(OH)D levels from 56 to 123 nmol/L with weekly high dose vitamin D supplementation did not influence biochemical markers of bone formation or turnover in persons with MS receiving calcium supplementation. This concurs with the previously negative

Table 2 Bone markers and PTH throughot the study period

	CTX1 (µg/l)			PINP (µg/l)			PTH pmol/L		
	Placebo	Vitamin D	p-value*	Placebo	Vitamin D	p-value*	Placebo	Vitamin D	p-value*
Baseline. mean (SD)	0.20 (0.10)	0.22 (0.11)	0.59	43.10 (15.1)	40.32 (10.0)	0.57	4.75 (1.08)	4.68 (1.29)	0.66
Week 48. mean (SD)	0.22 (0.16)	0.21 (0.11)	0.79	43.36 (17.2)	38.56 (10.6)	0.43	3.68 (1.04)	3.13 (0.96)	0.017
Week 96. mean (SD)	0.23 (0.17)	0.23 (0.12)	0.98	42.54 (15.0)	43.52 (10.6)	0.22	3.96 (1.27)	3.39 (1.00)	0.046

*Obtained from linear mixed model

Table 3 Association between bone markers at baseline and BMD (regression coefficients)

BMD	CTX1	PINP
Baseline hip	−279.4*	−2.42*
Baseline spine	−385.0*	−2.12
Baseline distal radius	91.3	1.05
DELTA hip	−7.6	0.10
DELTA spine	61.5	0.40
DELTA distal radius	−30.9	0.30

*$p < 0.05$; DELTA indicated the difference in BMD from baseline to week 96

results on BMD in the same cohort [21], and also with data obtained in healthy persons [29]. Moreover, we here showed that neither CTX1 nor PINP at baseline predicted BMD loss the subsequent 96 weeks. This is in contrast with a previous study comprising 29 MS patients followed for 3.1 ± 1.9 years, reporting a decline in BMD in the hip but not in the lumbar spine correlated inversely with bone turnover markers [30]. Whereas the patients included in these studies were fairly comparable regarding disease duration, BMI and disability levels, all known to be important for bone health in MS, only 50% of our patients received immunomodulatory treatment compared to 100% in the previous study [30]. Immunomodulatory drugs, including interferon beta which was most commonly used by our patients, could affect bone loss [31]. The use of immunomodulatory treatment did however not influence the effect of vitamin D on bone markers, and was not associated with BMD at baseline in our patients [32]. Other possible explanations for this discrepancy include differences in sample sizes and duration of follow up.

The vitamin D measurements in this study were performed in January and February and should therefore represent the seasonal nadir fairly well [33]. At this time point 18 of 35 patients in the treatment group had 25(OH)D levels above 50 nmol/L, which are considered adequate for maintenance of good bone health by the Institute of Medicine. Clear evidence of vitamin D deficiency (25(OH)D below 25 nmol) were only recorded in nine patients in each treatment group. It is conceivable that people with vitamin deficiency have a better effect of vitamin D supplementation on bone health than people with adequate vitamin D status, and that the low

proportion of patients with vitamin D deficiency contributed to the negative results.

RCTs of vitamin D supplementation have not shown a consistent effect on BMD or fracture risk in the general population [17]. This does not exclude that particular subgroups with increased risk of osteoporosis due to immobilization, inadequate nutrition, medication or disease may need vitamin D supplementation to maintain bone health [8]. Our study population had rather low disease activity and their ambulation was only moderately impaired. MS patients with more advanced disability are more prone to both accelerated bone loss and vitamin D deficiency D [34], and could benefit more from vitamin D supplementation than those included in this study.

There are several strengths and limitations of this study. The randomized design minimized the risk of selection bias, and rigorous follow-up throughout the study period ensured adherence to the study medication. The optimal 25(OH)D level for bone health is not known, but the dose used in this trial was well above 800 IU per day which has been suggested to prevent fracture in meta-analysis [35], and brought 25(OH)D in most patients above 75–100 nmol/L which has been suggested by several experts to be adequate [19, 36]. The main weakness of the study is the limited size, which was not sufficient to perform subgroup analyses or to detect minor yet relevant effects of vitamin D supplementation. Moreover, patients were allowed to continue use of vitamin D supplements, and more than 50% of the patients in the placebo group reported a vitamin D intake exceeding 7.5 μg/day. This concurs with the generally favorable vitamin D status of our patients. It is conceivable that depriving the patients from their vitamin D supplements could have increased the chance for a positive result, but it would expose patients in the placebo group to the risks of vitamin D deficiency, and would be particularly problematic in a population living north of the Arctic Circle. Another potential weakness is the use of weekly dosing of vitamin D3. Although weekly dosing leads to a stable serum concentration of 25(OH)D, which has a long half-life, the effect on other vitamin D metabolites is different. Notably, the serum concentration of native vitamin D, which likely plays an important role as substrate for synthesis of active 1,25-dihydroxyvitamin D in several tissues, peaks after six to 8 h and thereafter falls rapidly [37]. It is therefore

Table 4 Effect of high dose vitamin D supplementation compared to placebo on bone markers

	Week 48		Week 96	
	Change from baseline, percent difference (95% CI)	p-value*	Change from baseline, percent difference (95%CI)	p-value*
PINP	-5.10% (−17.77, 7.56)	0.43	10.26% (−2.48 22.99)	0.12
CTX1	-6.68% (−33.62, 20.25)	0.63	−3.60% (−30.67, 23.48)	0.80
PTH	-13.69% (−29.55, 2.12)	0.09	−10.9% (−26.81, 5.03)	0.17

*Obtained from linear mixed model

possible that daily supplementation is better than weekly supplementation of vitamin D.

Conclusions

Our results do not support that high dose weekly vitamin D supplementation is beneficial for bone health in ambulatory persons with MS, and suggest that weekly vitamin D supplementation alone is not sufficient to prevent bone loss in persons with MS who are not vitamin D deficient.

Abbreviations

25(OH)D: 25-hydroxyvitamion D; BMD: Bone mineral density; CTX1: C-terminal cross-linking telopeptide of type I collagen; CV: Coefficient of variation; MS: Multiple sclerosis; PINP: Procollagen type 1 N-terminal propeptide; PTH: Parathyroid hormone

Acknowledgements

Not applicable.

Funding

The study was funded by The University of Oslo.

Authors' contributions

TH planned the study, collected data, and wrote the manuscript. JCV analyzed the data and revised the manuscript. EFE planned the study and revised the manuscript. LSH and MTK planned the study, collected data and revised the manuscript. All authors read and approved the final manuscript.

Competing interests

On behalf of all authors, the corresponding author states that there is no competing interest.

Author details

[1]Department of Neurology, Akershus University Hospital, Lørenskog, Norway. [2]Institute of Clinical Medicine, University of Oslo, Oslo, Norway. [3]Helse Øst Health Services and Research Centre, Akershus University Hospital, Lørenskog, Norway. [4]Department of Endocrinology, Oslo University Hospital, Oslo, Norway. [5]Department of Neurology, University Hospital of North Norway, Tromsø, Norway. [6]Department of Clinical Medicine, University of Tromsø, Tromsø, Norway.

References

1. Munger KL, Levin LI, Hollis BW, Howard NS, Ascherio A. Serum 25-hydroxyvitamin D levels and risk of multiple sclerosis. JAMA. 2006;296:2832–8.
2. Løken-Amsrud KI, Holmøy T, Bakke SJ, Beiske AG, Bjerve KS, Bjørnarå BT, et al. Vitamin D and disease activity in multiple sclerosis before and during interferon beta treatment. Neurology. 2012;79:267–73.
3. Simpson Jr S, Taylor B, Blizzard L, Ponsonby AL, Pittas F, Tremlett H, et al. Higher 25-hydroxyvitamin D is associated with lower relapse risk in multiple sclerosis. Ann Neurol. 2010;68:193–203.
4. Huang Z, Qi Y, Du S, Chen G, Yan W. Bone mineral density levels in adults with multiple sclerosis: A meta-analysis. Int J Neurosci. 2015;125:904–12.
5. Gupta S, Ahsan I, Mahfooz N, Abdelhamid N, Ramanathan M, Weinstock-Guttman B. Osteoporosis and multiple sclerosis: risk factors, pathophysiology, and therapeutic interventions. CNS Drugs. 2014;28:731–42.
6. Steffensen LH, Mellgren SI, Kampman MT. Predictors and prevalence of low bone mineral density in fully ambulatory persons with multiple sclerosis. J Neurol. 2010;257:410–8.
7. Moen SM, Celius EG, Sandvik L, Nordsletten L, Eriksen EF, Holmoy T. Low bone mass in newly diagnosed multiple sclerosis and clinically isolated syndrome. Neurology. 2011;77:151–7.
8. Silk LN, Greene DA, Baker MK, Jander CB. The effect of calcium and vitamin D supplementation on bone health of male Jockeys. J Sci Med Sport. 2016; doi:10.1016/j.jsams.2016.08.004.
9. Bazelier MT, van Staa TP, Uitdehaag BM, Cooper C, Leufkens HG, Vestergaard P, et al. The risk of fracture in patients with multiple sclerosis: the UK general practice research database. J Bone Miner Res. 2011;26:2271–9.
10. Bazelier MT, de Vries F, Bentzen J, Vestergaard P, Leufkens HG, van Staa TP, et al. Incidence of fractures in patients with multiple sclerosis: the Danish National Health Registers. Mult Scler. 2012;18:622–7.
11. Bazelier MT, van Staa TP, Uitdehaag BM, Cooper C, Leufkens HG, Vestergaard P, et al. Risk of fractures in patients with multiple sclerosis: a population-based cohort study. Neurology. 2012;78:1967–73.
12. Ramagopalan SV, Seminog O, Goldacre R, Goldacre MJ. Risk of fractures in patients with multiple sclerosis: record-linkage study. BMC Neurol. 2012;12:135. doi:10.1186/1471-2377-12-135.
13. James E, Dobson R, Kuhle J, Baker D, Giovannoni G, Ramagopalan SV. The effect of vitamin D-related interventions on multiple sclerosis relapses: a meta-analysis. Mult Scler. 2013;19:1571–9.
14. Hearn AP, Silber E. Osteoporosis in multiple sclerosis. Mult Scler. 2010;16:1031–43.
15. Dobson R, Ramagopalan S, Giovannoni G. Bone health and multiple sclerosis. Mult Scler. 2012;18:1522–8.
16. Kampman MT, Eriksen EF, Holmoy T. Multiple sclerosis, a cause of secondary osteoporosis? What is the evidence and what are the clinical implications? Acta Neurol Scand Suppl. 2011:44–9.
17. RossCA TCL, Yaktine AL, Del Valle HB. Institute of Medicine. Daily reference values for calcium and vitamin D. Washington DC: The National Academic Press; 2011.
18. Priemel M, von DC, Klatte TO, Kessler S, Schlie J, Meier S, et al. Bone mineralization defects and vitamin D deficiency: histomorphometric analysis of iliac crest bone biopsies and circulating 25-hydroxyvitamin D in 675 patients. J Bone Miner Res. 2010;25:305–12.
19. Vieth R. Why the minimum desirable serum 25-hydroxyvitamin D level should be 75 nmol/L (30 ng/ml). Best Pract Res Clin Endocrinol Metab. 2011;25:681–91.
20. Pludowski P, Holick MF, Grant WB, Konstantynowicz J, Mascarenhas MR, Haq A, et al. Vitamin D supplementation guidelines. J Steroid Biochem Mol Biol. 2017; doi:10.1016/j.jsbmb.2017.01.021.
21. Steffensen LH, Jorgensen L, Straume B, Mellgren SI, Kampman MT. Can vitamin D(3) supplementation prevent bone loss in persons with MS? A placebo-controlled trial. J Neurol. 2011;258:1624–31.
22. Jorde R, Grimnes G, Hutchinson MS, Kjaergaard M, Kamycheva E, Svartberg J. Supplementation with vitamin D does not increase serum testosterone levels in healthy males. Horm Metab Res. 2013;45:675–81.
23. Bhargava P, Steele SU, Waubant E, Revirajan NR, Marcus J, Dembele M, et al. Multiple sclerosis patients have a diminished serologic response to vitamin D supplementation compared to healthy controls. Mult Scler. 2016;22:753–60.
24. Johansson H, Oden A, Kanis JA, McCloskey EV, Morris HA, Cooper C, et al. A meta-analysis of reference markers of bone turnover for prediction of fracture. Calcif Tissue Int. 2014;94:560–7.
25. Vasikaran S, Eastell R, Bruyere O, Foldes AJ, Garnero P, Griesmacher A, et al. Markers of bone turnover for the prediction of fracture risk and monitoring of osteoporosis treatment: a need for international reference standards. Osteoporos Int. 2011;22:391–420.
26. Kampman MT, Steffensen LH, Mellgren SI, Jorgensen L. Effect of vitamin D3 supplementation on relapses, disease progression and measures of function in persons with multiple sclerosis: exploratory outcomes from a double-blind randomised controlled trial. Mult Scler. 2012;18:1144–51.
27. Hjartaker A, Andersen LF, Lund E. Comparison of diet measures from a food-frequency questionnaire with measures from repeated 24-hour dietary recalls. The Norwegian Women and Cancer Study. Public Health Nutr. 2007;10:1094–103.
28. Rosjo E, Lossius A, Abdelmagid N, Lindstrom JC, Kampman MT, Jorgensen L, et al. Effect of high-dose vitamin D3 supplementation on antibody responses against Epstein-Barr virus in relapsing-remitting multiple sclerosis. Mult Scler Mult Scler. 2017;23:395–402.
29. Aloia J, Bojadzievski T, Yusupov E, Shahzad G, Pollack S, Mikhail M, et al. The relative influence of calcium intake and vitamin D status on serum parathyroid hormone and bone turnover biomarkers in a double-blind, placebo-controlled parallel group, longitudinal factorial design. J Clin Endocrinol Metab. 2010;95:3216–24.
30. McKenna MJ, Murray B, Lonergan R, Redmond JM. Immunomodulators for multiple sclerosis may ameliorate spinal bone loss. Ir J Med Sci. 2013;182:29–32.

31. Abraham AK, Ramanathan M, Weinstock-Guttman B, Mager DE. Mechanisms of interferon-beta effects on bone homeostasis. Biochem Pharmacol. 2009;77:175762.

32. Kampman MT, Steffensen LH. Comment on Shuhaibar et al: Favourable effect of immunomodulator therapy on bone mineral density in multiple sclerosis. Ir J Med Sci. 2009;178:235–6.

33. Saltyte Benth J, Myhr KM, Loken-Amsrud KI, Beiske AG, Bjerve KS, Hovdal H, et al. Modelling and prediction of 25-hydroxyvitamin D levels in Norwegian relapsing-remitting multiple sclerosis patients. Neuroepidemiology. 2012;39:84–93.

34. Huang Z, Qi Y, Du S, Chen G, Yan W. BMI levels with MS Bone mineral density levels in adults with multiple sclerosis: a meta-analysis. Int J Neurosci. 2015;125:904–12.

35. Bischoff-Ferrari HA, Willett WC, Orav EJ, Lips P, Meunier PJ, Lyons RA, et al. A pooled analysis of vitamin D dose requirements for fracture prevention. N Engl J Med. 2012;367:40–9.

36. Souberbielle JC, Body JJ, Lappe JM, Plebani M, Shoenfeld Y, Wang TJ, et al. Vitamin D and musculoskeletal health, cardiovascular disease, autoimmunity and cancer: Recommendations for clinical practice. Autoimmun Rev. 2010;9:709–15.

37. Hollis BW, Wagner CL. Clinical review: The role of the parent compound vitamin D with respect to metabolism and function: Why clinical dose intervals can affect clinical outcomes. J Clin Endocrinol Metab. 2013;98:4619–28.

5

Peripheral blood lymphocytes immunophenotyping predicts disease activity in clinically isolated syndrome patients

Helena Posová[1]* ⓘ, Dana Horáková[2], Václav Čapek[1], Tomáš Uher[2], Zdenka Hrušková[1] and Eva Havrdová[2]

Abstract

Background: Clinically isolated syndrome (CIS) represents first neurological symptoms suggestive of demyelinating lesion in the central nervous system (CNS). Currently, there are no sufficient immunological or genetic markers predicting relapse and disability progression, nor there is evidence of the efficacy of registered disease modifying treatments (DMTs), such as intramuscular interferon beta1a. The aim of the study is to evaluate immunological predictors of a relapse or disability progression.

Methods: One hundred and eighty one patients with CIS were treated with interferon beta1a and followed over the period of 4 years. Lymphocyte subsets were analyzed by flow cytometry. A Kaplan-Meier estimator of survival probability was used to analyze prognosis. For statistical assessment only individual differences between baseline values and values at the time of relapse or confirmed disability progression were analysed.

Results: Higher levels of B lymphocytes predicted relapse-free status. On the other hand, a decrease of the naïve subset of cells (CD45RA+ in CD4+) after 12, 24, and 36 months of follow-up were associated with an increased risk of confirmed disability progression. Conclusion: Our data suggest that the quantification of lymphocyte subsets in patients after the first demyelinating event suggestive of MS may be an important biomarker.

Keywords: Clinically isolated syndrome, Multiple sclerosis, Lymphocyte subpopulations, Flow cytometry

Background

Clinically isolated syndrome (CIS) is the first manifestation of multiple sclerosis (MS), a chronic inflammatory autoimmune disease of the central nervous system (CNS) affecting over 2.5 million people worldwide. [1] After CIS, the delay in manifestation of a new relapse, which corresponds to the clinically definite MS (CDMS) according to McDonald's criteria 2005 [2], varies from several months to more than 10 years and should be associated with the brain and spinal cord pathology at the time of a relapse [3]. In about a third of the cases, CIS patients will not experience a new relapse activity over long-term follow-up [4].

Different clinical and brain imaging predictors have been evaluated for their sensitivity and specificity to predict occurrence of a relapse during follow-up. In this context, a number of studies have shown that abnormal MRI findings are the most informative predictors of future disease activity [5, 6].

On the other hand, the role of cerebrospinal fluid (CSF) biomarkers for the prediction of a relapse remains to be explored. It is also unclear if MRI predictors together with CSF biomarkers may improve prediction of CDMS when applied in a single model. Apart from oligoclonal bands (OCBs), several markers in the CSF appear to be more specific for neuro-inflammatory and neuro-degenerative pathophysiological processes in MS, such as inflammation and immune dysfunction, or cell type, such as B cells [7]. Some of these markers have been shown to predict conversion to MS in patients with

---

* Correspondence: hmare@lf1.cuni.cz
[1]Institute of Immunology and Microbiology, First Faculty of Medicine, Charles University and General University Hospital in Prague, Prague, Czech Republic
Full list of author information is available at the end of the article

CIS, e.g. polyspecific intrathecal B-cell response of IgG antibodies against neurotropic viruses such as measles, rubella, and varicella zoster [8]. CSF IgG heavy-chain bias was detected in patients with CIS who converted to MS within 6 months of the CIS presentation [9], and increased CSF concentrations of B cell recruiting chemokine CXCL13 were shown to be a good predictor of conversion to MS in patients with CIS over 2 years of follow-up [10]. It has been suggested that Tau and neurofilaments, CSF markers of axonal damage, might be even more specific than MRI for predicting conversion of CIS to MS. [11] Shorter time to CDMS conversion was also associated with high concentrations of CSF chitinase 3-like 1, which is up-regulated during inflammation [12].

Nevertheless, up to date none of these CSF markers can be recommended for routine implementation in clinical practice, mainly because of methodological limitations, invasiveness of the spinal tap, absence of conclusive data from small studies or other technical problems. Therefore large multicentre studies are needed to confirm the importance of CSF biomarkers as a tool in the clinical practice [13]. CSF is the compartment in the closest proximity to CNS parenchyma and might reflect immunopathology in CNS. However, studies usually fail to provide longitudinal CSF data because repeated lumbar punctures are difficult to justify. Therefore, single CSF samples are only snapshots of immune response at the time of collection.

In this context, peripheral blood as a mirror of immune reaction in CNS is much easier to measure longitudinally. CD4+ T cells and later CD4 + Th1 cells are the most studied cell populations in MS [14] because of their potential role in the pathogenesis of the disease, as well as they are used to assess the effect of different therapies used in MS. More recently, regulatory subpopulations such as Th2 cells, regulatory CD4+ T cells and NK cells were studied for their relationship in disease prognosis [15] and radiologically confirmed MS activity. Changes in their effector populations were described [16]. The association of CD4 + CD45RO+ IL-17A+ cells to clinical and radiological disease activity was reported. [17, 18] Differences in naive CD4 T-cell biology, notably in TCR and TLR signalling pathways, identified patients with MS with more rapid conversion to secondary progression [19].

In CIS patients, the most intriguing finding was published by Vilar et al. [20], who showed the possibility of using an analysis of peripheral blood CD5 + CD19+ subsets as a predictive factor for CDMS conversion.

In our study, we followed-up patients with CIS who were treated with interferon beta, irrespective of the further disease course (patients with both subsequent relapse and no relapse were included) for at least 48 months. Peripheral blood immunophenotyping was used to find early changes in lymphocyte subsets, which could predict the development of relapse.

Methods
Study population
The study enrolled patients after first clinical event suggestive of MS within 4 months from the first clinical event. The inclusion criteria were:18–55 years of age, enrolled within 4 months from the clinical event, Expanded Disability Status Scale (EDSS) ≤3.5, presence of ≥2 T2-hyperintense lesions on diagnostic MRI, and presence of ≥2 oligoclonal bands in CSF obtained at the screening visit prior to steroid treatment. The exclusion criteria were: occurrence of a second relapse before the baseline visit, pregnancy and symptoms that could possibly be attributed to neurological diseases different from MS (e.g. neuromyelitis optica).

All patients included with CIS were treated with intravenous steroids (3–5 g of methylprednisolone) following screening and preceding baseline, and subsequently at baseline started the treatment with 30 mg of intramuscular IFNb-1a once a week. Two hundred and twenty CIS patients were enrolled in the study; analyses in this laboratory part of study were limited to 191 subjects with immunophenotyping flow cytometry data available. Clinical assessments (EDSS) and peripheral blood assessments were obtained at baseline, 6, 12, 24, 36 and 48 months. In the case of relapses, patients were evaluated within 4 days from the onset of new symptoms.

The study protocol was approved by the Medical Ethics Committee of the General University Hospital in Prague and First Faculty of Medicine, Charles University in Prague for grant MZ ČR NT 13108–4.

Study outcomes
We used two clinical outcomes in this analysis – 1) development of a new clinical relapse, and 2) confirmed disability progression. A new clinical relapse was defined as patient-reported symptoms or objectively observed signs typical for an acute inflammatory demyelinating event in the central nervous system with duration of at least 24 h, in the absence of fever or infection. [21] Confirmed disability progression (CDP) was defined as an increase in EDSS by 1.0 point (if baseline EDSS >0) or 1.5 points (if baseline EDSS = 0) confirmed after 6 months [22].

Immunophenotyping
Whole peripheral blood (PB) samples (2 ml/subject) were collected in ethylenediamine tetra-acetic acid (EDTA) test tubes. The following monoclonal antibodies from BD Biosciences (San Jose, CA, USA) were used: CD3 FITC, CD4 PE-Cy7, CD5 FITC, CD8 APC Cy7,

CD19 PE, CD45RA FITC, HLA-DR PE Cy7, CD16 + 56 PE and CD45 PerCP. Whole PB samples were labelled with appropriate volumes of conjugated MoAb for 20 min at room temperature, and then lysed with 2 ml of lysis solution (FACS Lysis Solution, BD). Cells were washed twice and analyzed on a standard FACSCanto instrument (BD) with DIVA software (BD). All results were expressed as percentages of each subset out of total lymphocytes.

Statistical methods

Percentages of lymphocyte populations do not have normal distribution and therefore, the parametric tests cannot be applied. Moreover, the results at the end of the study were influenced by different treatment modalities in study patients. For statistical assessment, only individual differences between baseline values and values at the time of relapse were used and compared with various indicators.

Predictive values of measured variables were investigated through receiver operating characteristic (ROC) curves. Based on these curves, thresholds which maximised the sum of sensitivity and specificity for each measured parameter were defined. A Kaplan-Meier estimator of survival probability and an asymptotic log-rank test were used to test differences between subsets of patients. For each lymphocyte population and the clinical outcome (relapse or CDP) three different indicators were considered: a) the population relative value, b) the population relative value change compared to baseline and c) the population relative value change compared to a measurement one year before.

For all indicators the following analyses were performed:

1. An ROC curve to predict the clinical outcome at one year was constructed and an optimal threshold was chosen.
2. At every time-point a cohort of patients was divided into two groups according to the chosen threshold and survival curves (Kaplan-Meier estimators) were constructed for each of these groups. Further, an asymptotic log-rank test was performed to test difference between these survivals probability curves (see Figures and Tables). P-values less than 0.05 were considered as statistically significant.

The ROC curves were constructed from all the time points at once. As a predicted outcome we considered a relapse or disease progression, respectively that appeared in (and only in) a year after the corresponding measurement. The events were analysed from the year end. The same threshold applied to measurements before baseline, at baseline, at 6 M, etc. Every time it divided patients into two groups. For those groups the survival probability curves were constructed and compared.

Analyses were conducted using R statistical package, version 3.1.2, R Core Team (2014).

Results
Clinical data
Of the 220 patients enrolled in the study, 191 had available clinical and laboratory follow-up data (181 till the end of study, not only till relapse or disability progression) and were included in the analysis. During the first year of follow-up, second disease relapse was observed in 55 patients, during the second year additional 25 patients relapsed, and 21 and 13 patients, respectively, relapsed during the third and the fourth year of the follow-up. At 48 months, 114 (59.6%) patients experienced the second clinical attack, 69 (36.1%) experienced the third clinical attack and 37 (19.3%) had confirmed disability progression (CDP).

Laboratory data
Representation of different lymphocyte subpopulations in patients who did not experience a relapse was compared to patients who relapsed within the respective time period (6, 12, 24, 36 and 48 months). The same comparison was done for patients who showed CDP. Patients who underwent both events (relapse and CDP) were included in both subgroups. Table 1a, b shows the number of patients in each subgroup and median ± standard deviation of measured lymphocyte subpopulations. Absolute counts of lymphocyte subpopulations are shown in Table 2a, b.

The results are shown for a better orientation and to complement the statistical analysis, but a few trends were observed in the results, the most noticeable ones were the increase in B lymphocytes and the decrease in NK cells. These trends were present in all subgroups, regardless of the clinical status (conversion to CDMS or no conversion). However, a profound decrease in B lymphocytes and an increase in NK cells was observed between the study entry and the baseline results and of at least 30 days prior to initiation of interferon therapy (of at least 30 days after steroid administration).

Statistical analysis
We aimed to test the possibility of finding a threshold value that would distinguish patients with a higher or lower probability of relapse or CDP (the "value" in Figs. 1-4). More importantly, we aimed to measure changes in lymphocyte subpopulations longitudinally in each patient separately so that the disease course could be predicted. Therefore, we tested the ratio of current values versus values obtained a year before compared to baseline (Ratio vs. LY and Ratio vs. BL Figs. 1-4).

For the assessment of lymphocyte subpopulations, relative percentage is usually used, but absolute counts

Table 1 a, b Median ± standard deviation of lymphocyte subpopulations (in % of all lymphocytes) in different subgroups

a

	n	T ly	CD4+	CD8+	B ly	NK cells	CD5+
all patients at first relapse	191	71.8 ± 7	44.6 ± 7	23 ± 6	11.1 ± 4	14 ± 7	72 ± 7
all patients at baseline (BL)[a]	191	71.5 ± 7	43 ± 8	24 ± 7	9.3 ± 4	16.1 ± 7	71 ± 9
all patients at 48 months (48)[b]	181	72.5 ± 7	45 ± 7	21.7 ± 6	15.3 ± 6	9.6 ± 5	73.9 ± 6
patients without relapse at BL	77	71.2 ± 7	42.3 ± 8	23.4 ± 7	9.3 ± 4	16.5 ± 8	71.2 ± 8
patients without relapse at 48[b]	77	73 ± 6	46.2 ± 6	22.1 ± 6	14.8 ± 5	9.45 ± 4	74.5 ± 5
patients with relapse at BL	114	71.7 ± 8	43.5 ± 7	24.5 ± 6	9.3 ± 4	15.4 ± 7	70.7 ± 10
patients with relapse at 48[b]	104	72.1 ± 8	45.9 ± 8	21.4 ± 6	15.8 ± 7	9.8 ± 5	73.6 ± 7.
patients without CDP at BL	154	71.3 ± 8	42.2 ± 8	24.5 ± 7	9.1 ± 4	17 ± 7	70.8 ± 9
patients without CDP at 48[b]	148	72.5 ± 7	45.7 ± 8	22.2 ± 6	15.3 ± 6	9.9 ± 5	73.6 ± 6
patients with CDP at BL	37	73.4 ± 6	47 ± 7	23.1 ± 6	10 ± 4	13 ± 6	72.8 ± 6
patients with CDP at 48[b]	33	74.6 ± 7	47.8 ± 7	20.5 ± 5	16.3 ± 6	8.4 ± 3	75.3 ± 6

b

	n	DR+ in T ly	CD45RA+	CD45RA+ in CD4+	CD5+ in B ly	CD5+ B ly
all patients at first relapse	191	10.8 ± 9	65.4 ± 11	58.8 ± 19	20 ± 16	2.1 ± 2
all patients at baseline (BL)[a]	191	12.1 ± 11	65.2 ± 10	56.4 ± 20	18.1 ± 19	1.7 ± 2
all patients at 48 months (48)[b]	181	12.2 ± 6	65.1 ± 8	44.8 ± 12	11.1 ± 7	1.7 ± 1
patients without relapse at BL	77	12.9 ± 11	64.9 ± 9	57.5 ± 20	23.3 ± 18	1.9 ± 3
patients without relapse at 48[b]	77	12.1 ± 6	64.3 ± 8	45.2 ± 12	11.4 ± 8	1.9 ± 2
patients with relapse at BL	114	11.8 ± 10	63.4 ± 11	55.6 ± 21	18 ± 14	1.7 ± 2
patients with relapse at 48[b]	104	12.8 ± 5	66.2 ± 8	44.8 ± 13	10 ± 6	1.7 ± 2
patients without CDP at BL	154	12.5 ± 10	64.8 ± 10	54.9 ± 20	18.1 ± 20	1.7 ± 2
patients without CDP at 48[b]	148	12.4 ± 6	66.1 ± 8	45.8 ± 13	11.6 ± 8	1.9 ± 1
patients with CDP at BL	37	9.8 ± 9	62.4 ± 12	60.5 ± 23	16.7 ± 14	1.9 ± 2
patients with CDP at 48[b]	33	11.1 ± 5	62.7 ± 9	40.7 ± 11	9.7 ± 5	1.4 ± 1

Double positive populations (HLA-DR + CD3+, CD45RA + CD4+, CD5 + CD19+) are expressed as the percentage of the first mentioned subpopulation in the basic population. CD5+ B lymphocytes are expressed as the originally measured value (percentage of total lymphocytes) to enable comparison with previously published results. [20]
[a]The laboratory test were done before intravenous steroids treatment, interval between this examination and baseline was 2–3 months
[b]The results at 48 months of following should be influenced by treatment (natalizumab n = 18, fingolimod n = 3, copaxone n = 6)
T ly – T lymphocytes (CD3+), B ly – B lymphocytes (CD19+), NK cells (CD3-CD16 + 56+)

can be also calculated. As interferon beta decreases the overall lymphocyte count, including absolute values of respective subpopulations, we selected relative values for the statistical analysis. Since only results obtained before a relapse or CDP were statistically assessed, no other treatment than interferon beta could have influenced the parameters, and treatment was the same in all patients. The results obtained from patients after therapy escalation (18 natalizumab, 3 fingolimod) and also after changing for copaxone (6 patients) were excluded from this part of our study. Also methylprednisolone pulses were the same in all patients and the treatment was given at least 30 days before baseline.

No significant changes were observed in cytotoxic (CD8+) T lymphocytes, CD5+ cells and CD5+ B lymphocytes (CD19+) subpopulations as well as in activated T lymphocytes (DR+).

Only a few statistically significant changes in CD3+ T lymphocytes and CD4+ T lymphocytes were found in Kaplan-Meier estimators, while ROC curves did not show any clinically relevant predictive values of a new relapse or CDP.

The results assessing CD19+ cells, NK cells and naïve CD4+ T lymphocytes showed a much higher significance of these populations as a prediction of a clinical event.

B lymphocytes (CD19+)

In B lymphocytes, higher levels (the population relative value in our study was 9.5% of the total count of lymphocytes) were a positive predictive factor. (Figure1) The decrease of B lymphocytes below this level increased the probability of a relapse from month 6 until the end of the follow-up.

Table 2 a, b Median ± standard deviation of lymphocyte subpopulations (absolute count in 10^3/ml) in different subgroups

a

	n	T ly	CD4+	CD8+	B ly	NK cells	CD5+
all patients at first relapse	191	1.3 ± 0.4	0.8 ± 0.3	0.4 ± 0.2	0.2 ± 0.1	0.2 ± 0.1	1.3 ± 0.4
all patients at baseline (BL)[a]	191	1.3 ± 0.4	0.8 ± 0.3	0.5 ± 0.2	0.2 ± 0.1	0.3 ± 0.2	1.3 ± 0.4
all patients at 48 months (48)[b]	181	1.3 ± 0.5	0.8 ± 0.3	0.4 ± 0.2	0.3 ± 0.2	0.2 ± 0.1	1.3 ± 0.5
patients without relapse at BL	77	1.3 ± 0.3	0.8 ± 0.2	0.4 ± 0.2	0.2 ± 0.1	0.3 ± 0.2	1.3 ± 0.3
patients without relapse at 48[b]	77	1.3 ± 0.4	0.8 ± 0.2	0.4 ± 0.2	0.3 ± 0.1	0.2 ± 0.1	1.4 ± 0.4
patients with relapse at BL	114	1.3 ± 0.5	0.8 ± 0.3	0.5 ± 0.2	0.2 ± 0.1	0.3 ± 0.1	1.3 ± 0.5
patients with relapse at 48[b]	104	1.3 ± 0.5	0.8 ± 0.3	0.4 ± 0.2	0.2 ± 0.2	0.2 ± 0.1	1.3 ± 0.6
patients without CPD at BL	154	1.3 ± 0.4	0.8 ± 0.3	0.4 ± 0.2	0.2 ± 0.1	0.2 ± 0.1	1.3 ± 0.4
patients without CPD at 48[b]	148	1.3 ± 0.5	0.8 ± 0.3	0.4 ± 0.2	0.3 ± 0.2	0.2 ± 0.1	1.4 ± 0.5
patients with CPD at BL	37	1.2 ± 0.4	0.8 ± 0.2	0.3 ± 0.2	0.2 ± 0.1	0.2 ± 0.1	1.2 ± 0.4
patients with CPD at 48[b]	33	1.1 ± 0.5	0.8 ± 0.3	0.3 ± 0.2	0.3 ± 0.2	0.1 ± 0.1	1.2 ± 0.6

b

	n	DR+ CD3+	CD45RA+	CD45RA+ CD4+	CD5+ B ly
all patients at first relapse	191	0.1 ± 0.1	1.1 ± 0.4	0.5 ± 0.2	0.04 ± 0.05
all patients at baseline (BL)[a]	191	0.2 ± 0.1	1.2 ± 0.4	0.5 ± 0.3	0.03 ± 0.05
all patients at 48 months (48)[b]	181	0.2 ± 0.1	1.1 ± 0.5	0.4 ± 0.2	0.03 ± 0.03
patients without relapse at BL	77	0.2 ± 0.1	1.2 ± 0.3	0.5 ± 0.2	0.03 ± 0.05
patients without relapse at 48[b]	77	0.2 ± 0.1	1.1 ± 0.4	0.4 ± 0.2	0.03 ± 0.04
patients with relapse at BL	114	0.2 ± 0.1	1.2 ± 0.5	0.5 ± 0.3	0.03 ± 0.04
patients with relapse at 48[b]	104	0.1 ± 0.1	1.1 ± 0.6	0.4 ± 0.2	0.03 ± 0.03
patients without CDP at BL	154	0.2 ± 0.1	1.2 ± 0.4	0.5 ± 0.3	0.04 ± 0.05
patients without CPD at 48[b]	148	0.1 ± 0.1	1.1 ± 0.5	0.4 ± 0.2	0.03 ± 0.03
patients with CPD at BL	37	0.1 ± 0.2	1 ± 0.4	0.4 ± 0.2	0.04 ± 0.04
patients with CPD at 48[b]	33	0.1 ± 0.1	1 ± 0.6	0.3 ± 0.2	0.02 ± 0.03

[a]The laboratory test were done before intravenous steroids treatment, interval between this examination and baseline was 2–3 months
[b]The results at 48 months of following should be influenced by treatment (natalizumab $n = 18$, fingolimod $n = 3$, copaxone $n = 6$)
T ly – T lymphocytes (CD3+), B ly – B lymphocytes (CD19+), NK cells (CD3-CD16 + 56+)

NK cells (CD3-CD16 + 56+)
Analysis of NK cells (Fig. 2) stressed the importance of long-term follow-up of representation of this population. The decrease of NK cells below 10.8% of the total count of lymphocytes increased the probability of CDP. Overall, a decreasing trend in the percentage of this population in peripheral blood was present, but transient more significant increase (of more than 28.7%) increased the probability of EDSS worsening in the first and third year of follow-up.

Naive cells (CD45RA+)
Percentages of naïve (CD45RA+) lymphocytes did not vary much (Table 1), but the statistical analysis revealed a significant relationship between this particular population and EDSS worsening. (Fig. 3) The probability of CDP was lower if the percentage of naïve lymphocytes was higher than 64.65% of total count of lymphocytes, and this was valid from the first year of follow-up. A more prominent decrease (to less than 95.9% of the baseline value) was a negative factor. However, the results were not significant when assessed with regard to the second relapse.

Naive helper cells (C45RA+ in CD4+)
Due to the fact that different subpopulations were included within CD45RA+ lymphocytes that may vary and influence the total results, we focused on one of the subpopulations – CD4+ naïve cells. (Fig. 4) In this subpopulation, the results were also statistically more significant when related to EDSS worsening. The percentage above 52.3% of total count of lymphocytes seemed to be important for protection against the clinical deterioration and the decrease of more than 30.5% as compared to the baseline value was a negative prognostic factor. No significant results were found in the context of the relapse.

The explanation for the fact that we found more significant changes in case of the CDP assessment than in

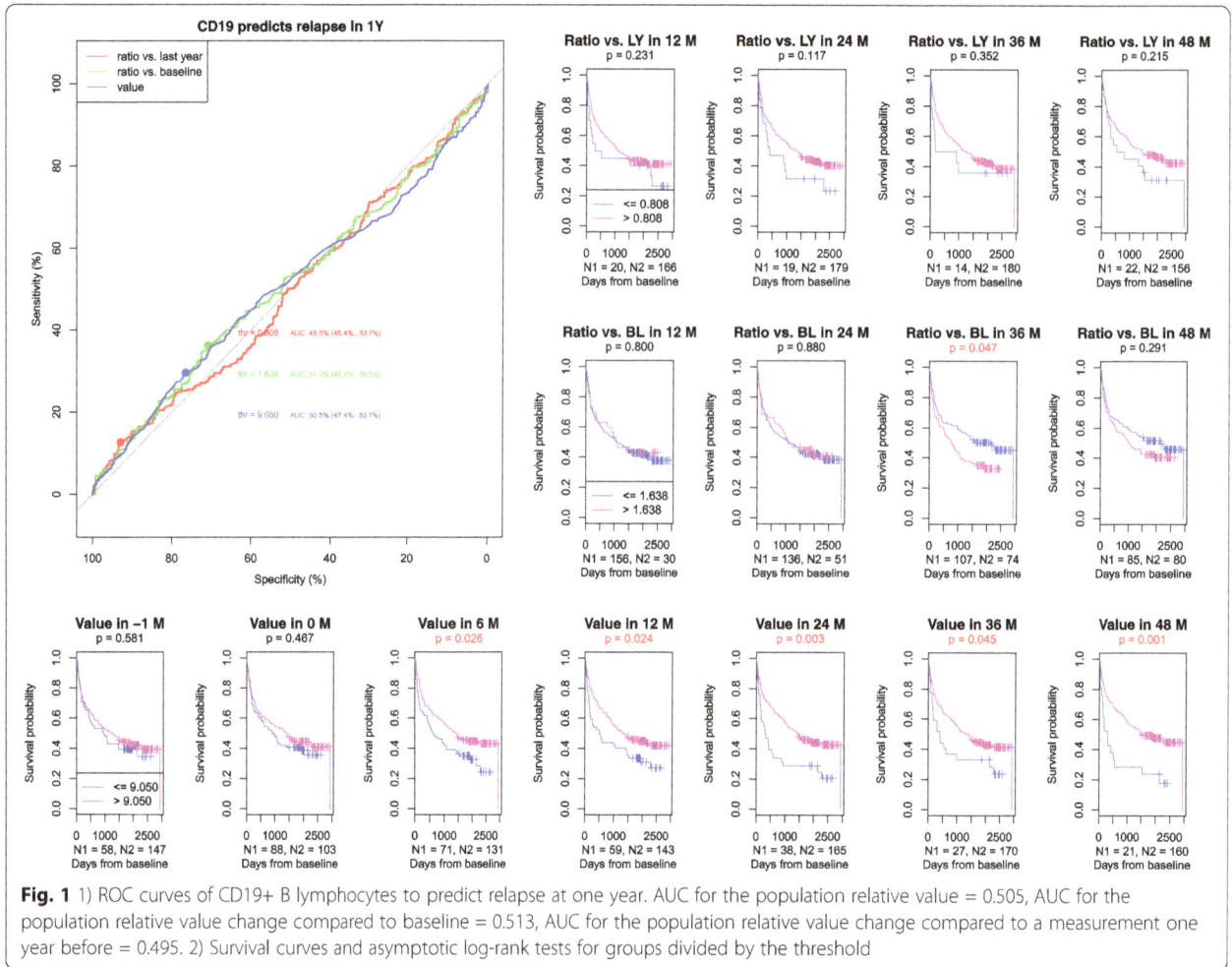

Fig. 1 1) ROC curves of CD19+ B lymphocytes to predict relapse at one year. AUC for the population relative value = 0.505, AUC for the population relative value change compared to baseline = 0.513, AUC for the population relative value change compared to a measurement one year before = 0.495. 2) Survival curves and asymptotic log-rank tests for groups divided by the threshold

the relapse one could be our incapability to guarantee examination at the same interval from relapse, as the examination was performed in predefined (yearly) intervals, irrespective of the presence and/or timing of relapse. We discovered CDP parameter to be more consistent for such an evaluation.

Discussion

Various immunological markers with a potential of predicting conversion to CDMS or a relapse were not the only parameters analysed during a long-term follow-up of the CIS patients, which complemented results of radiological investigation of the same cohort. [6].

The results of our study corresponded with our long-time observation of immunophenotyping patterns in MS patients, i.e. higher level of CD4+ lymphocytes with a decreased expression of CD45RA molecules and lower proportion of B lymphocytes and NK cells. Almost all these results fit within normal values because of wide variability of these parameters. The same problem makes parametric statistical tests impossible for use in our and all such studies and this is the reason why we cannot

use the value of these subsets as a MS diagnostic marker. We therefore decided to look at our data at an individual patient level and compared individual differences in observed subsets during 48 months of follow up in patients with newly diagnosed CIS treated with methylprednisolone at the beginning of the study and treated with interferon β either for the whole study (48 months) or until the time of a relapse or disability progression (before treatment escalation).

The key role in MS pathogenesis had been assigned to CD4+ cells for a long time and so this population was the most studied one, but low numbers of patients and different methods caused rather conflicting results [23]. In general, the levels of CD4+ cell population in MS patients (unless influenced by treatment (e.g. fingolimod)), are at the upper limit of normal range. Values of CD4+ T lymphocytes in our CIS patients at baseline were lower than we commonly found in MS patients in our laboratory and so we assumed significant augmentation in this subset during the disease progression to CDMS, but only a tendency to increase during the whole time of follow-up was found in all groups. This supports our

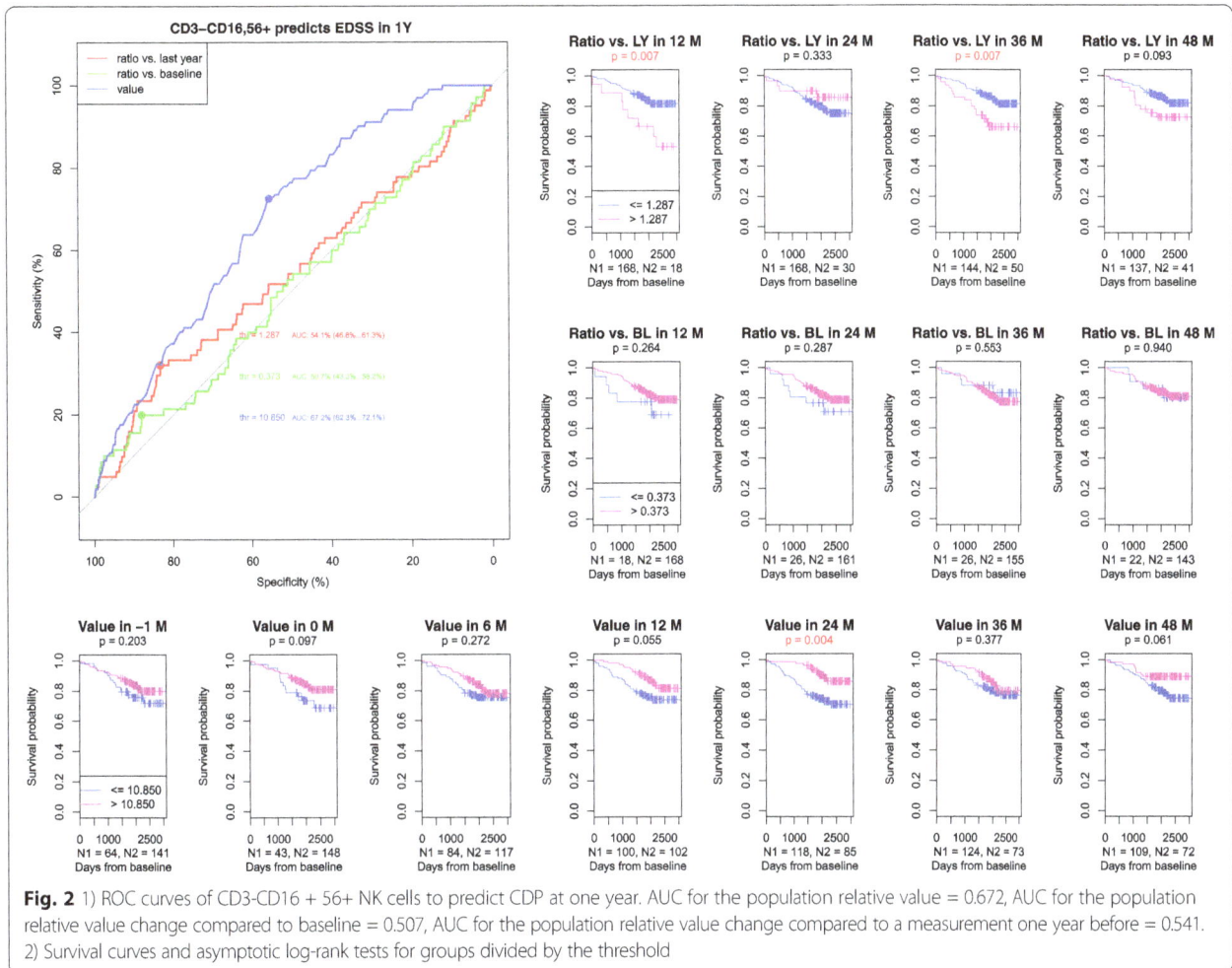

Fig. 2 1) ROC curves of CD3-CD16 + 56+ NK cells to predict CDP at one year. AUC for the population relative value = 0.672, AUC for the population relative value change compared to baseline = 0.507, AUC for the population relative value change compared to a measurement one year before = 0.541. 2) Survival curves and asymptotic log-rank tests for groups divided by the threshold

anticipation, but we cannot designate whole CD4 + CD3+ lymphocyte subpopulation as a predictive factor for conversion to MS.

In 1986, *Mossman and Coffman* [24] presented the concept of distinct T helper cell subsets and MS was later considered a CD4+ Th1-mediated autoimmune disease [15] but not surprisingly the T-cell biology in vivo is more complex than a simple dichotomy. In addition to Th1/Th2, the Th17 subset and different classes of regulatory T cells (Treg) are involved in MS. Recent studies have shown that the T cells mediating MS can be heterogeneous, with Th17 cells predominating in some individuals and Th1 cells in others [25] The plasticity of different T cell subsets and emerging evidence that subset-signature cytokine expression is not as stable as initially believed [26] strongly support our attempt to find a more reliable marker as a predictor of conversion to CDMS.

In 1996 *Bomgioanni* [23] confirmed previous results [27] and showed a significantly decreased percentage of CD4 + CD45RA+ cells in peripheral blood during a relapse in RR-MS. Decrease in CD4+ CD45RA+ subset was also detectable one month before clinical relapse.

[28] Up regulation of naive CD45RA+ T- lymphocytes and parallel down regulation of memory CD45RO+ cells seemed to be one of the main mechanisms by which Linomide inhibited the MS activity. [29] Also in this study, the higher levels of naive CD4+ cells seem to be a positive prognostic marker.

The above-mentioned studies prove the significance of monitoring naive CD4+ cell in the follow-up of our patients and our results are in agreement with them. Higher levels of naive CD4+ cells were shown to be a positive prognostic factor in our study, specifically more than 52.3% of naive cells in CD4+ cells and 64.6% of all naive lymphocytes. A reduction of naive helper cells by one third (exactly 30.5% in relationship to baseline) and only a slight reduction of total CD45RA+ lymphocytes (4.1% in relationship to baseline, statistically significant in the first, third and fourth year of follow-up) was associated with clinical worsening (CDP). According to these results, we could use monitoring of naïve CD4 + changes as an important predictive factor, but further studies will be required to examine the optimal frequency of (monitoring) measurement.

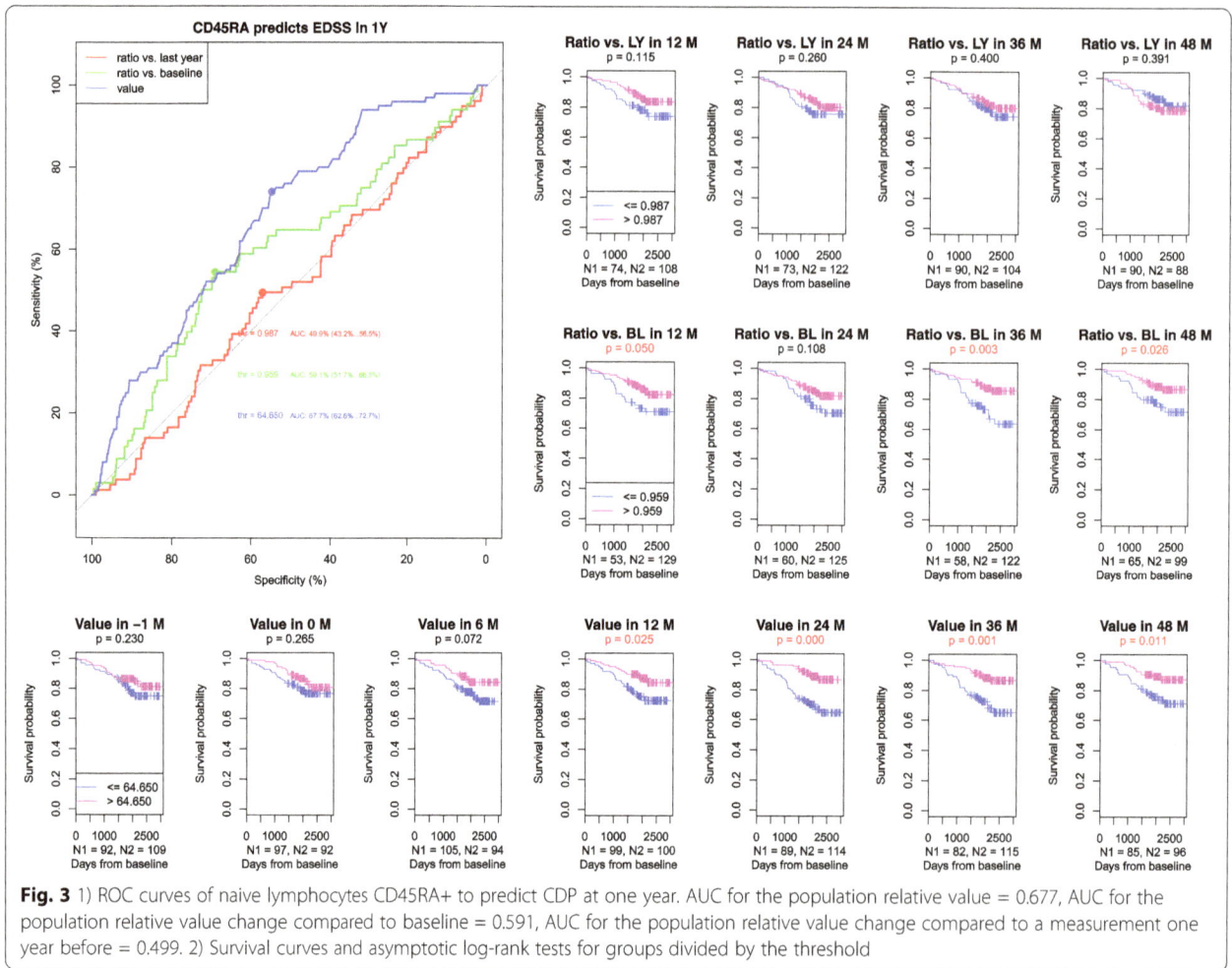

Fig. 3 1) ROC curves of naive lymphocytes CD45RA+ to predict CDP at one year. AUC for the population relative value = 0.677, AUC for the population relative value change compared to baseline = 0.591, AUC for the population relative value change compared to a measurement one year before = 0.499. 2) Survival curves and asymptotic log-rank tests for groups divided by the threshold

The contribution of B cells to the mechanisms of conversion to MS is shown not only by CSF B-cell associated biomarkers, but also by peripheral B cells. *Kreutzfelder* in 1992 [30] showed a reduction of CD19+ peripheral blood in MS patients. This observation combined with the reduced percentage of CD19+ circulating cells in patients with a stable RR form of MS *Bomgioanni* [23] suggested that such a decrease is due to the sequestration of cells within the CNS. *Lee-Chang* [31] supported this theory by finding an up-regulation of α4 integrin on peripheral B cells that may enhance B-cell accumulation within the CSF at the time of CIS.

Our results confirm reduction of B cells in PB as a negative predictive factor. The cut off level of 9.5% CD19+ cells of lymphocytes was calculated and a decrease below it increased the relapse probability. Overall augmentation of B cells during our study corresponded with the finding that circulating B cells became distinctly reallocated by long-term treatment with IFN-beta, which is compatible with the protective effects attributed to this drug [32]. Studies of the RR MS patients treated with IFN-1b confirmed that its in vivo therapeutic effects include: the inhibition of B

cell stimulatory capacity and the B cells cytokine secretion changes, which may selectively inhibit Th17-mediated autoimmune response in RR MS. [33, 34] Given this, we could also conclude that lower levels of B cells in patients converting to CDMS were associated with lower responsiveness to interferon beta treatment and B cells analysis could predict need of treatment escalation so that relapse would be prevented.

Completely different results were found in one CD5+ B lymphocyte subpopulations. Earlier, this subpopulation was thought to be a potential source of autoantibodies, but its role in autoimmunity is still being investigated. Elevated CD5+ expression on peripheral B lymphocytes correlated with MS disease activity expressed by a number of gadolinium-enhancing lesions on MRI and inversely correlated with disease duration [35] and a recent study performed in blood of MS patients found an increase of CD5+ memory B cells in remitting stage of the disease [36]. *Villar* [20] concluded that increased percentages of blood CD5+ B cells were associated with further elevated risk of conversion to MS and relapse rate in these patients independently of cerebrospinal

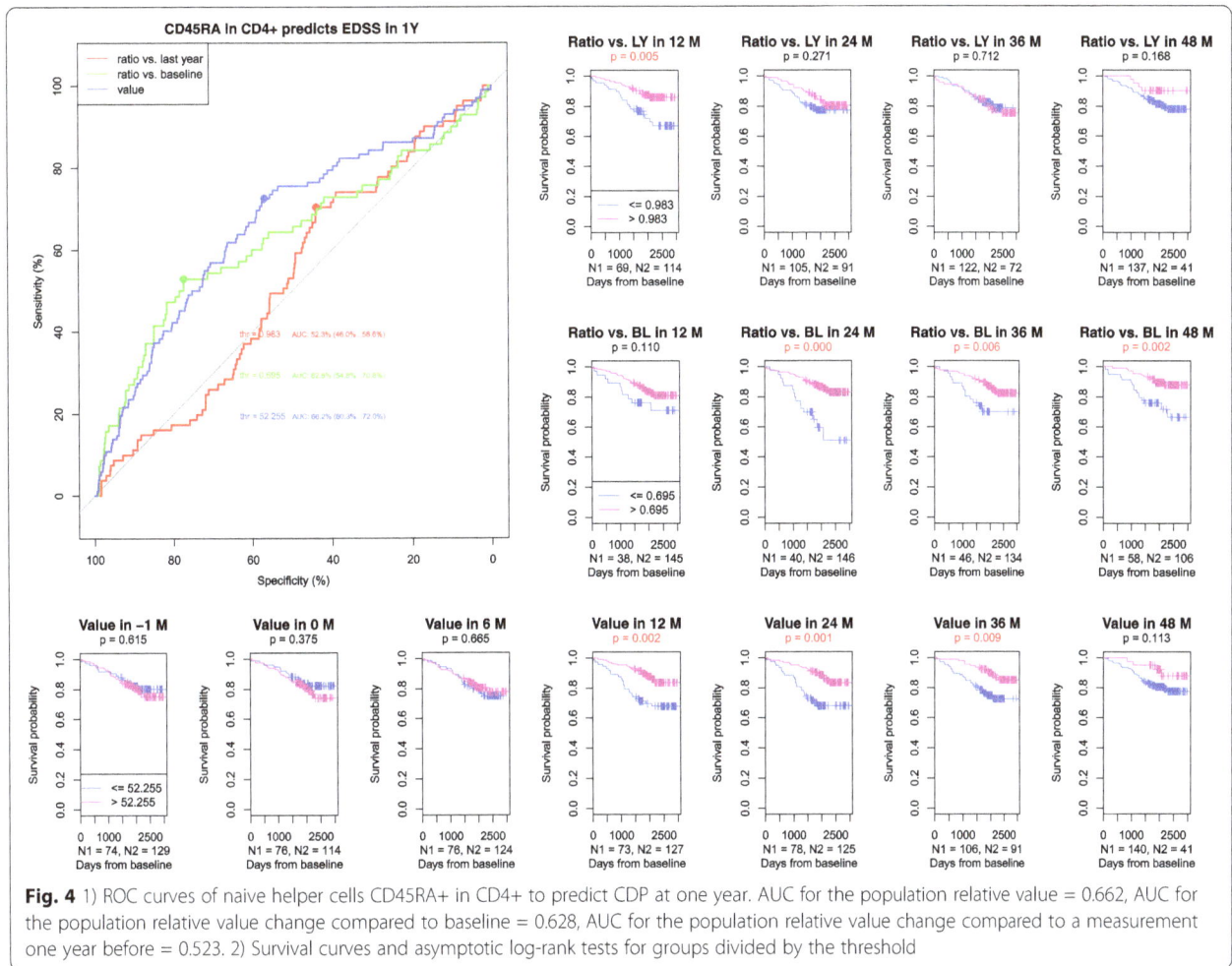

Fig. 4 1) ROC curves of naive helper cells CD45RA+ in CD4+ to predict CDP at one year. AUC for the population relative value = 0.662, AUC for the population relative value change compared to baseline = 0.628, AUC for the population relative value change compared to a measurement one year before = 0.523. 2) Survival curves and asymptotic log-rank tests for groups divided by the threshold

fluid oligoclonal bands presence and MRI. She calculated a cut off value of 3.5% of this subset for relapse risk. This value was based on mean +/− 2 SD of the percentage of blood CD5+ B cells of the control group. The association of blood CD5+ B cells with the conversion to MS suggests that this lymphocyte subset plays an important role in early phases of the disorder. We planned to use the same method for a cut off calculation, but, as we were looking for an individual predicted outcome, we used a different one.

Number of CD5 + CD19+ lymphocytes was generally lower in our study (Table 1b) and we were not able to confirm Vilar's results neither by presented statistical calculation nor by former one [20]. We did not find significant changes in this population in relationship to the second relapse or CDP.

A recent phenotyping study that performed cytometric staining for multiple cell surface markers revealed lower frequencies of circulating CD8lowCD56 + CD3-CD4- cells in untreated patients with relapsing–remitting multiple sclerosis or clinically isolated demyelinating syndrome than in healthy controls [37]. The MS relapses

and new brain lesions detected by magnetic resonance imaging are often preceded by a reduction in PB NK cell functional activity [38], but similar percentages of PB NK cells were detected in treated MS patients when compared to non-MS patients despite decreased frequency of CSF NK cells [39].

There was a slight gradual decrease of the NK cells in our study during the whole 4 year follow-up and the value of 10.8% could be considered as a critical point. Contrary to this, an increase at year one (and three) should predict CDP. This inconsistent result could be related to the changes in NK subpopulation: CD56bright NK cells. [40] During a follow-up we observed a decrease in the NK cells minor subpopulation, which lead to a lower control of T lymphocytes. Inter-annual increase of the NK cells preceding CDP could be caused by a transient increase of major CD56low population, which is found in chronic inflammatory process.

Nevertheless, in our study, we only assessed the total population of CD3-CD16 + 56+ NK cells as the representation of CD56bright NK cells was low in our patients, and we therefore did not consider this population suitable for a long-term assessment and statistical analysis. However, in recent years, some publications described the necessity of examination of this subpopulation.

Daclizumab-induced increased frequencies of circulating CD56bright NK cells were related to the therapeutic benefit of the drug [40]. Likewise, during therapy with IFNb, the total number of circulating natural killer cell declined slightly [41] or did not change [42] but there was a marked increase in the proportion of CD56high NK cells in both 12 month follow up studies. One of the possible mechanisms of action of IFN-β in MS is the enhancement of NK activity, especially CD56bright NK cells [38]. Given this finding, the analysis of NK cells seems to be a good predictive factor, in particular in combination with CD56bright subset analysis.

Conclusions

In conclusion, our results confirm the potential role of monitoring early changes in immunophenotyping of peripheral blood lymphocytes for the prediction of a relapse and disability progression in patients after a first demyelinating event suggestive of MS. According to our results we can conclude that some changes in selected subpopulations should be considered as a signal for more frequent clinical and laboratory monitoring of our patients. More specifically, a decrease in B cells and NK cells populations (or a significant increase) and a marked reduction of naive CD4+ helper cells were the best predictors of a relapse or disability progression. Their predictive role has to be investigated and confirmed in further prospective studies. This study also shows difficulties of statistical assessment, and points to the fact that examination of inter-individual comparison of the measured parameters may be necessary instead of the comparison of whole groups of patients.

Abbreviations

CDMS: Clinically definite MS; CIS: Clinically isolated syndrome; CNS: Central nervous system; CSF: Cerebrospinal fluid; DMTs: Disease modifying treatments; EDSS: Expanded Disability Status Scale; EDTA: Ethylenediamine tetra-acetic acid; IFNb: Interferon beta; IL: Interleukin; MoAb: Monoclonal antibody; MRI: Magnetic resonance imaging; MS: Multiple sclerosis; NK: Natural killer; OCBs: Oligoclonal bands; PB: Peripheral blood; TCR: T cell receptor; TLR: Toll like receptor; Treg: Regulatory T cells

Acknowledgements
Not applicable.

Funding
This study was financial supported by grant MZ ČR NT 13108–4 and Progres Q25/LF1.

Disclosures
Dr. Horakova received compensation for travel, speaker honoraria and consultant fees from Biogen Idec, Novartis, Merck Serono, Bayer Shering, Genzyme, and Teva, as well as support for research activities from Biogen Idec. Dr. Havrdova received speaker honoraria and consultant fees from Biogen Idec, Merck Serono, Novartis, Genzyme and Teva, as well as support for research activities from Biogen Idec and Merck Serono. Dr. Uher received financial support for conference travel and honoraria from Biogen Idec, Novartis, Merck Serono and Genzyme.

Authors´ contributions
HP - study design, laboratory data acquisition and analysis. DH - clinical data acquisition and analysis. VČ - statistical analysis. TU - clinical data acquisition and analysis. ZH - laboratory data acquisition and analysis. EH - final approval of data interpretation. All authors have read and approved the final manuscript.

Competing interests
Dr. Horakova received compensation for travel, speaker honoraria and consultant fees from Biogen Idec, Novartis, Merck Serono, Bayer Shering, Genzyme, and Teva, as well as support for research activities from Biogen Idec. Dr. Havrdova received speaker honoraria and consultant fees from Biogen Idec, Merck Serono, Novartis, Genzyme and Teva, as well as support for research activities from Biogen Idec and Merck Serono. Dr. Uher received financial support for conference travel and honoraria from Biogen Idec, Novartis, Merck Serono and Genzyme.

Author details
[1]Institute of Immunology and Microbiology, First Faculty of Medicine, Charles University and General University Hospital in Prague, Prague, Czech Republic. [2]Department of Neurology and Centre of Clinical Neuroscience First Faculty of Medicine, Charles University and General University Hospital in Prague, Prague, Czech Republic.

References
1. Comi G, Martinelli V, Rodegher M, Moiola L, Bajenaru O, Carra A, Elovaara I, Fazekas F, Hartung H, Hillert J. Effect of glatiramer acetate on conversion to clinically definite multiple sclerosis in patients with clinically isolated syndrome (PreCISe study): a randomised, double-blind, placebo-controlled trial. Lancet. 2009;374(9700):1503–11.
2. Polman CH, Reingold SC, Edan G, Filippi M, Hartung HP, Kappos L, Lublin FD, Metz LM, McFarland HF, O'Connor PW. Diagnostic criteria for multiple sclerosis: 2005 revisions to the "McDonald criteria". Ann Neurol. 2005;58(6):840–6.
3. Thouvenot É. Update on clinically isolated syndrome. Presse Med. 2015; 44(4):e121–36.
4. Fisniku L, Brex P, Altmann D, Miszkiel K, Benton C, Lanyon R, Thompson A, Miller D. Disability and T2 MRI lesions: a 20-year follow-up of patients with relapse onset of multiple sclerosis. Brain. 2008;131(3):808–17.
5. Dobson R, Rudick RA, Turner B, Schmierer K, Giovannoni G. Assessing treatment response to interferon-β is there a role for MRI. Neurology. 2014;82(3):248–54.
6. Uher T, Horakova D, Bergsland N, Tyblova M, Ramasamy DP, Seidl Z, Vaneckova M, Krasensky J, Havrdova E, Zivadinov R. MRI correlates of disability progression in patients with CIS over 48 months. NeuroImage: Clinical. 2014;6:312–9.
7. Tumani H, Hartung H-P, Hemmer B, Teunissen C, Deisenhammer F, Giovannoni G, Zettl UK, Group BS. Cerebrospinal fluid biomarkers in multiple sclerosis. Neurobiol Dis. 2009;35(2):117–27.
8. Brettschneider J, Tumani H, Kiechle U, Muche R, Richards G, Lehmensiek V, Ludolph AC, Otto M. IgG antibodies against measles, rubella, and varicella zoster virus predict conversion to multiple sclerosis in clinically isolated syndrome. PLoS One. 2009;4(11):e7638.
9. Bennett JL, Haubold K, Ritchie AM, Edwards SJ, Burgoon M, Shearer AJ, Gilden DH, Owens GP. CSF IgG heavy-chain bias in patients at the time of a clinically isolated syndrome. J Neuroimmunol. 2008;199(1):126–32.
10. Brettschneider J, Czerwoniak A, Senel M, Fang L, Kassubek J, Pinkhardt E, Lauda F, Kapfer T, Jesse S, Lehmensiek V. The chemokine CXCL13 is a prognostic marker in clinically isolated syndrome (CIS). PLoS One. 2010;5(8):e11986.
11. Brettschneider J, Petzold A, Süssmuth S, Ludolph A, Tumani H. Axonal damage markers in cerebrospinal fluid are increased in ALS. Neurology. 2006;66(6):852–6.

12. Comabella M, Fernández M, Martin R, Rivera-Vallvé S, Borrás E, Chiva C, Julià E, Rovira A, Cantó E, Alvarez-Cermeño JC. Cerebrospinal fluid chitinase 3-like 1 levels are associated with conversion to multiple sclerosis. Brain. 2010; 133(4):1082–93.

13. Tintore M, Rovira À, Río J, Otero-Romero S, Arrambide G, Tur C, Comabella M, Nos C, Arévalo MJ, Negrotto L: Defining high, medium and low impact prognostic factors for developing multiple sclerosis. Brain 2015:awv105.

14. Lassmann H, Ransohoff RM. The CD4–Th1 model for multiple sclerosis: a crucial re-appraisal. Trends Immunol. 2004;25(3):132–7.

15. Sospedra M, Martin R. Immunology of multiple sclerosis. Annu Rev Immunol. 2005;23:683–747.

16. Rinaldi L, Gallo P, Calabrese M, Ranzato F, Luise D, Colavito D, Motta M, Guglielmo A, Del Giudice E, Romualdi C. Longitudinal analysis of immune cell phenotypes in early stage multiple sclerosis: distinctive patterns characterize MRI-active patients. Brain. 2006;129(8):1993–2007.

17. Kebir H, Ifergan I, Alvarez JI, Bernard M, Poirier J, Arbour N, Duquette P, Prat A. Preferential recruitment of interferon-γ–expressing TH17 cells in multiple sclerosis. Ann Neurol. 2009;66(3):390–402.

18. Durelli L, Conti L, Clerico M, Boselli D, Contessa G, Ripellino P, Ferrero B, Eid P, Novelli F. T-helper 17 cells expand in multiple sclerosis and are inhibited by interferon-β. Ann Neurol. 2009;65(5):499–509.

19. Zastepa E, Fitz-Gerald L, Hallett M, Antel J, Bar-Or A, Baranzini S, Lapierre Y, Haegert DG. Naive CD4 T-cell activation identifies MS patients having rapid transition to progressive MS. Neurology. 2014;82(8):681–90.

20. Villar LM, Espiño M, Roldán E, Marín N, Costa-Frossard L, Muriel A, Álvarez-Cermeño JC. Increased peripheral blood CD5+ B cells predict earlier conversion to MS in high-risk clinically isolated syndromes. Mult Scler J. 2011;17(6):690–4.

21. Polman CH, Reingold SC, Banwell B, Clanet M, Cohen JA, Filippi M, Fujihara K, Havrdova E, Hutchinson M, Kappos L. Diagnostic criteria for multiple sclerosis: 2010 revisions to the McDonald criteria. Ann Neurol. 2011;69(2):292–302.

22. Kappos L, De Stefano N, Freedman MS, Cree BA, Radue E-W, Sprenger T, Sormani MP, Smith T, Häring DA, Meier DP. Inclusion of brain volume loss in a revised measure of 'no evidence of disease activity'(NEDA-4) in relapsing–remitting multiple sclerosis. Mult Scler J. 2015;1352458515616701

23. Bongioanni P, Fioretti C, Vanacore R, Bianchi F, Lombardo F, Ambrogi F, Meucci G. Lymphocyte subsets in multiple sclerosis a study with two-colour fluorescence analysis. J Neurol Sci. 1996;139(1):71–7.

24. Mosmann TR, Cherwinski H, Bond MW, Giedlin MA, Coffman RL. Two types of murine helper T cell clone. I. Definition according to profiles of lymphokine activities and secreted proteins. J Immunol. 1986;136(7):2348–57.

25. Constantinescu CS, Gran B. The essential role of T cells in multiple sclerosis: a reappraisal. Biom J. 2014;37(2):34.

26. Raphael I, Nalawade S, Eagar TN, Forsthuber TG. T cell subsets and their signature cytokines in autoimmune and inflammatory diseases. Cytokine. 2015;74(1):5–17.

27. Eoli M, Ferrarini M, Dufour A, Heltaj S, Bevilacqua L, Comi G, Cosi V, Filippini G, Martinelli V, Milanese C. Presence of T-cell subset abnormalities in newly diagnosed cases of multiple sclerosis and relationship with short-term clinical activity. J Neurol. 1993;240(2):79–82.

28. Calopa M, Bas J, Mestre M, Arbizu T, Peres J, Buendia E. T cell subsets in multiple sclerosis: a serial study. Acta Neurol Scand. 1995;92(5):361–8.

29. Lehmann D, Karussis D, Mizrachi-Koll R, Linde AS, Abramsky O. Inhibition of the progression of multiple sclerosis by linomide is associated with upregulation of CD4+/CD45RA+ cells and downregulation of CD4 +/CD45RO+ cells. Clin Immunol Immunopathol. 1997;85(2):202–9.

30. Kreuzfelder E, Shen G, Bittorf M, Scheiermann N, Thraenhart O, Seidel D, Grosse-Wilde H. Enumeration of T, B and natural killer peripheral blood cells of patients with multiple sclerosis and controls. Eur Neurol. 1992;32(4):190–4.

31. Lee-Chang C, Zéphir H, Top I, Dubucquoi S, Trauet J, Prin L, Vermersch P. B-cell subsets up-regulate α4 integrin and accumulate in the cerebrospinal fluid in clinically isolated syndrome suggestive of multiple sclerosis onset. Neurosci Lett. 2011;487(3):273–7.

32. Haas J, Bekeredjian-Ding I, Milkova M, Balint B, Schwarz A, Korporal M, Jarius S, Fritz B, Lorenz H-M, Wildemann B. B cells undergo unique compartmentalized redistribution in multiple sclerosis. J Autoimmun. 2011;37(4):289–99.

33. Disanto G, Morahan J, Barnett M, Giovannoni G, Ramagopalan S. The evidence for a role of B cells in multiple sclerosis. Neurology. 2012;78(11):823–32.

34. Ramgolam VS, Sha Y, Marcus KL, Choudhary N, Troiani L, Chopra M, Markovic-Plese S. B cells as a therapeutic target for IFN-β in relapsing–remitting multiple sclerosis. J Immunol. 2011;186(7):4518–26.

35. Seidi O, Semra Y, Sharief M. Expression of CD5 on B lymphocytes correlates with disease activity in patients with multiple sclerosis. J Neuroimmunol. 2002;133(1):205–10.

36. Niino M, Hirotani M, Miyazaki Y, Sasaki H. Memory and naive B-cell subsets in patients with multiple sclerosis. Neurosci Lett. 2009;464(1):74–8.

37. De Jager PL, Rossin E, Pyne S, Tamayo P, Ottoboni L, Viglietta V, Weiner M, Soler D, Izmailova E, Faron-Yowe L. Cytometric profiling in multiple sclerosis uncovers patient population structure and a reduction of CD8low cells. Brain. 2008;131(7):1701–11.

38. Martinez-Rodriguez J, Lopez-Botet M, Munteis E, Rio J, Roquer J, Montalban X, Comabella M. Natural killer cell phenotype and clinical response to interferon-beta therapy in multiple sclerosis. Clin Immunol. 2011;141(3):348–56.

39. Hamann I, Dörr J, Glumm R, Chanvillard C, Janssen A, Millward JM, Paul F, Ransohoff RM, Infante-Duarte C. Characterization of natural killer cells in paired CSF and blood samples during neuroinflammation. J Neuroimmunol. 2013;254(1):165–9.

40. Bielekova B, Catalfamo M, Reichert-Scrivner S, Packer A, Cerna M, Waldmann TA, McFarland H, Henkart PA, Martin R. Regulatory CD56bright natural killer cells mediate immunomodulatory effects of IL-2Rα-targeted therapy (daclizumab) in multiple sclerosis. Proc Natl Acad Sci. 2006;103(15):5941–6.

41. Saraste M, Irjala H, Airas L. Expansion of CD56Bright natural killer cells in the peripheral blood of multiple sclerosis patients treated with interferon-beta. Neurol Sci. 2007;28(3):121–6.

42. Vandenbark AA, Huan J, Agotsch M, La Tocha D, Goelz S, Offner H, Lanker S, Bourdette D. Interferon-beta-1a treatment increases CD56 bright natural killer cells and CD4+ CD25+ Foxp3 expression in subjects with multiple sclerosis. J Neuroimmunol. 2009;215(1):125–8.

6

Long-term efficacy and safety of fingolimod in Japanese patients with relapsing multiple sclerosis: 3-year results of the phase 2 extension study

Takahiko Saida[1,2,3]*, Yasuto Itoyama[4], Seiji Kikuchi[5], Qi Hao[1], Takayoshi Kurosawa[6], Kengo Ueda[6], Lixin Zhang Auberson[7], Isao Tsumiyama[6], Kazuo Nagato[8] and Jun-ichi Kira[9]

Abstract

Background: The low level of disease activity and manageable safety profile seen with fingolimod versus placebo in a 6-month, phase 2, randomized controlled trial in Japanese patients with relapsing multiple sclerosis were maintained in the initial 6-month observational study extension. Here, we report long-term safety and efficacy results of the 3-year follow-up to the phase 2 study extension.

Methods: The 6-month core study was completed by 147 patients, of whom 143 entered the extension and took at least one dose of fingolimod. Those originally randomized to placebo were re-randomized to fingolimod 1.25 mg ($n = 23$) or 0.5 mg ($n = 27$). During the extension, the patients taking fingolimod 1.25 mg ($n = 46$) were switched to open-label fingolimod 0.5 mg, and those originally randomized to fingolimod 0.5 mg ($n = 47$) continued with open-label fingolimod 0.5 mg.

Results: Continuous fingolimod treatment was associated with a sustained low level of MRI and relapse activity for the duration of the extension phase; 75–100% (range across all assessment time points up to end of study) of patients remained free of Gd-enhanced T1 lesions, 88–100% remained free of new/newly enlarged T2 lesions, and 45–62% remained relapse-free. In patients who switched to the active treatment, a 79.5% decrease in annualized relapse rate (ARR; from 1.131 before switch to 0.232 6-months after switch) was observed in the first 6 months of the extension phase and thereafter remained low until the end of study (0.16–0.31 across all assessment time points after switch up to end of study). The mean number of Gd-enhanced T1 and new/newly enlarged T2 lesions decreased up to month 9 and thereafter remained low until the end of study (0.0–0.1 and 0.0–0.3, respectively, across all assessment time points after switch up to end of study). Fingolimod was generally well-tolerated and the safety profile was consistent with the core and 6-month extension. Serious adverse events were reported in 13.3% of patients during the extension study, with the range in the continuous fingolimod and placebo-fingolimod switch groups (3.7–21.7%) being similar to that reported in the core study for the placebo and fingolimod groups (5.3–20.4%).

Conclusion: Continuous fingolimod treatment over 36 months was associated with maintained efficacy and a manageable safety profile with no new safety signals. These results indicate that fingolimod provides long-term treatment benefit for Japanese patients with relapsing MS.

Keywords: Fingolimod, Multiple sclerosis, Phase 2 study extension, Relapse, Aquaporin 4

* Correspondence: saida_takahiko@maia.eonet.ne.jp
[1]Institute of Multiple Sclerosis Therapeutics, Nishinokyo-Kasugacho 16-44-409, Nakakyo-ku, Kyoto 604-8453, Japan
[2]Kyoto Min-Iren-Central Hospital, Kyoto, Japan
Full list of author information is available at the end of the article

Background

Fingolimod is a once-daily, orally administered therapy for relapsing forms of multiple sclerosis (MS). Currently, it is estimated that fingolimod has been used to treat approximately 155,000 patients in both clinical trials and post-marketing settings, with a total exposure of approximately 343,000 patient-years [1]. In the phase 2 and 3 trials, conducted in predominantly Caucasian populations, fingolimod treatment led to a significant reduction in clinical and magnetic resonance imaging (MRI) measures of disease activity compared with placebo [2–4] or interferon (IFN) beta-1a [5]. Similarly, a 6-month, phase 2, randomized controlled trial in Japanese patients with relapsing MS (ClinicalTrials.gov Identifier NCT00537082) demonstrated that fingolimod 0.5 and 1.25 mg significantly reduced relapse rates and MRI disease activity compared with placebo [6]. In the 6-month observational extension of this study, continuous fingolimod treatment for up to 12 months was associated with maintained or improved efficacy and a manageable safety profile [7]. The extension was continued until fingolimod received marketing authorization in Japan (28 November 2011). Here, we report long-term safety and efficacy results of the 3-year follow-up to the phase 2 extension study of fingolimod in Japanese patients with relapsing MS.

Methods

Study design and patient population

This was an extension of a 6-month, randomized, double-blind study comparing fingolimod 0.5 or 1.25 mg with placebo [6], conducted at 43 centers in Japan between 2008 and 2012. The study design, inclusion criteria and patient population have previously been described [6, 7]. Patients diagnosed with relapsing MS according to the McDonald criteria [8] were eligible to enter the study, and were randomized to fingolimod 0.5 or 1.25 mg, or placebo in a 1:1:1 ratio. Patients with longitudinally extensive spinal cord lesions of at least three vertebral segments (a marker of neuromyelitis optica [NMO]) detected by MRI at screening were excluded. Those who completed the 6-month core study had an option to enter the extension study. In the extension phase, patients originally randomized to placebo were re-randomized to dose-blind fingolimod 0.5 or 1.25 mg, and patients already treated with fingolimod continued on the same dose. Subsequent review of safety and efficacy data from the phase 3 clinical trials [4] revealed a more favorable benefit-risk profile using fingolimod 0.5 than 1.25 mg. Consequently, all patients treated with fingolimod 1.25 mg were switched to this lower dose by 22 February 2010, and the study adopted an open-label design until the end of the study.

Efficacy and safety endpoints

Although no primary efficacy analysis was undertaken owing to the nature of the extension study, several efficacy and safety outcomes were assessed. MRI measures, including the number of lesions (both Gd-enhanced T1 and new or newly enlarged T2) by visit and treatment, and the proportion of patients free from these lesions were assessed at screening and months 3, 6, 9, 12, 18, 24 and 36. ARR and Expanded Disability Status Scale (EDSS) measurements were conducted every 3 months from month 6 onwards. Relapse activity (proportions of patients without relapses, time to the first confirmed relapse and ARR) was determined up to the end of the study. ARR was calculated using the total number of relapses experienced during a specific period of time adjusted to a 1-year period. Confirmed relapse was defined as new, worsening, or recurrent neurological symptoms that occurred at least 30 days after the onset of a preceding relapse, lasted at least 24 h without fever or infection and were accompanied by an increase of at least half a point on the EDSS or an increase of at least one point in two functional systems scores or of at least two points in one functional system score (excluding changes in bowel or bladder function and cognition). Confirmed disability was measured using the EDSS score; 3-month and 6-month confirmed disability progression was defined as a 3-month and 6-month sustained increase from core baseline in the EDSS score, respectively, with progression defined as a 1-point increase from baseline in patients with a baseline EDSS score of 0–5.0, or a 0.5-point increase in patients with a baseline EDSS score of 5.5 or above. All adverse events (AEs) and serious adverse events (SAEs) were summarized by patient group, and pregnancy outcomes were tracked. Regular monitoring of laboratory values and assessments of vital signs, electrocardiograms, physical condition and body weight were undertaken during patient visits. Additional safety assessments as specified per protocol included dermatological examinations, ophthalmic examinations, chest radiography and pulmonary function tests. Anti-aquaporin-4 (AQP4) antibody test results were collected retrospectively from medical records of patients who consented to provide the data during the extension study.

Statistical analyses

All patients who were randomized in the 6-month core study and received at least one dose of study drug were analyzed as the core full analysis set (FAS) in the extension study. Efficacy analyses were performed on the core FAS; all analyses were based on descriptive statistics and no inferential analysis was performed. ARR was calculated by treatment group in the core FAS. A Kaplan-Meier analysis of time to first confirmed relapse from core baseline to end of study estimated the proportion of relapse-free patients at each time point. Data for patients with no confirmed relapse during this time and for those who dropped out or otherwise stopped treatment before a confirmed relapse occurred were all censored (i.e. the time to first onset of the confirmed relapse for these patients was set as the time in study from month 0 to the end of the study). No data imputation for drop-outs or missing values was used in this analysis.

Safety analyses were performed on the extension safety set, which included all patients who received at least one dose of the study drug in the extension period.

Results

Patient characteristics and fingolimod exposure

Of 147 patients who completed the core study, 143 entered the extension study (Fig. 1). Baseline characteristics were similar across treatment groups (placebo-fingolimod 0.5 mg; placebo-fingolimod 1.25 mg; fingolimod 0.5 mg, fingolimod 1.25 mg) (Table 1); approximately two-thirds (67.8%) of patients were female and the mean age was 35.1 years. The extension study was completed by 107 (74.8%) patients and 36 (25.2%) discontinued treatment (Fig. 1). AEs were the most common reason for treatment discontinuation ($n = 21$, [14.7%]), followed by protocol deviations ($n = 4$, [2.8%]), withdrawal of consent ($n = 3$, [2.1%]), administrative problems ($n = 3$, [2.1%]), unsatisfactory therapeutic effect ($n = 3$, [2.1%]) and abnormal laboratory values ($n = 2$, [1.4%]). In patients who received fingolimod 0.5 or 1.25 mg during the core study, and continued with treatment during the extension, the median duration of fingolimod exposure was 1180 and 1070 days, respectively. Patients who received placebo during the core study and then switched to fingolimod 0.5 or 1.25 mg at month 6 had a median duration of fingolimod exposure of 857 and 820 days, respectively (Additional file 1: Table S1).

Efficacy evaluation

The high proportion of patients reported free from Gd-enhanced T1 or new or newly enlarged T2 lesions from 6 months in those receiving continuous treatment [6], and from 12 months in those switching to fingolimod [7], was maintained during the 3-year extension and ranged from 85.7–92.0 to 90.5–92.0%, respectively, at month 36 (ranges provided are across all treatment groups and assessment time points during the extension; Fig. 2). Similarly, the reductions in mean numbers of Gd-enhanced or new or newly enlarged T2 lesions achieved at 12 months in both continuous and switch groups [7] ranged from 0.0–0.1 to 0.0–0.3, respectively, during the 3-year extension (Fig. 2).

Continuous fingolimod 0.5 or 1.25 mg treatment during the extension phase resulted in reductions in ARR compared with the core phase (Fig. 3a). A reduction in ARR was observed at months 6–12 (fingolimod 0.5 mg, from 0.539 to 0.227 [57.9% reduction]; fingolimod 1.25 mg, from 0.404 to 0.284 [29.7% reduction]; Fig. 3a); the reduction in both groups was sustained to the end of study (month 0–end of study [EoS]: fingolimod 0.5 mg, 0.247; fingolimod 1.25 mg, 0.208; Fig. 3a). After switching to active treatment, a 79.5% decrease in ARR was observed in the placebo-fingolimod group in the first 6 months of the extension (from 1.131 to 0.232). Overall, 45–62% of patients in the continuous fingolimod groups and 48% of patients in the placebo-fingolimod group were relapse-free at the end of study based on Kaplan-Meier estimates (Fig. 3b).

Among patients treated continuously with fingolimod, disability levels remained stable in the extension study

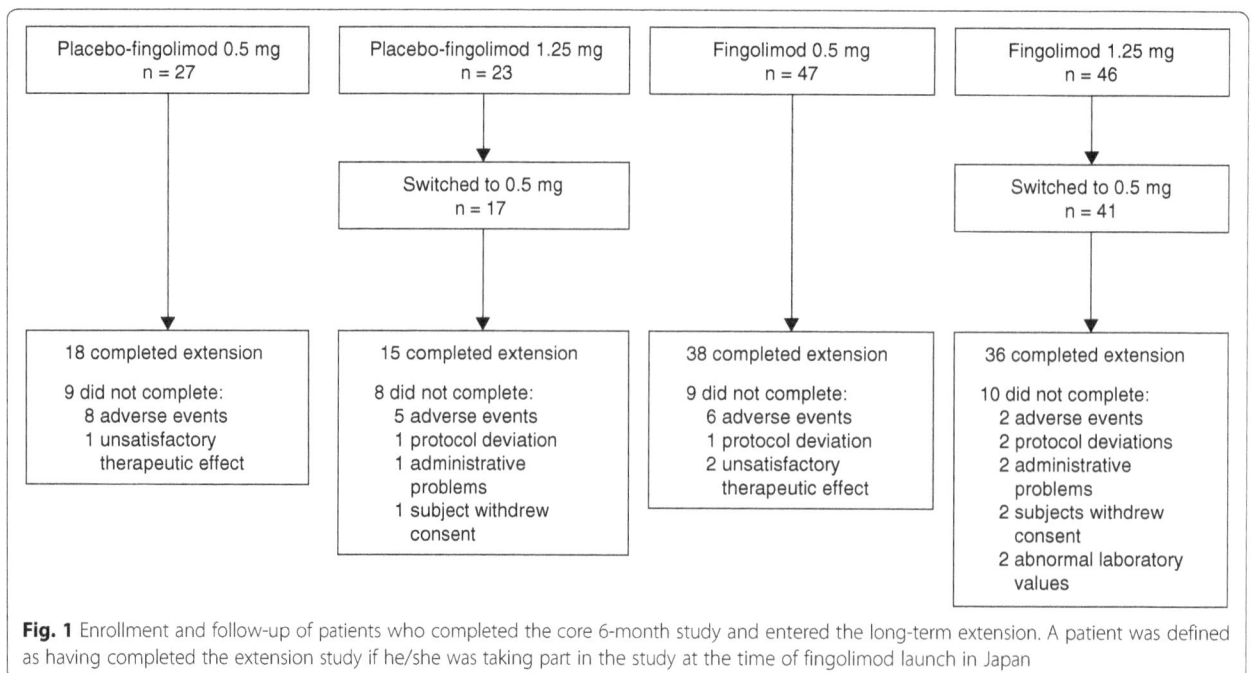

Fig. 1 Enrollment and follow-up of patients who completed the core 6-month study and entered the long-term extension. A patient was defined as having completed the extension study if he/she was taking part in the study at the time of fingolimod launch in Japan

Table 1 Baseline demographics and clinical characteristics of patients at entry to the core study (extension randomized population)

Characteristic	Placebo-fingolimod 0.5 mg (n = 27)	Placebo-fingolimod 1.25 mg (n = 23)	Fingolimod 0.5 mg (n = 47)	Fingolimod 1.25 mg (n = 46)
Age, years				
Mean (SD)	34.2 (9.1)	35.5 (8.4)	34.9 (9.0)	35.7 (8.8)
Median (range)	34.0 (18–52)	34.0 (21–51)	34.0 (19–52)	36.0 (18–55)
Female, n (%)	19 (70.4)	14 (60.9)	33 (70.2)	31 (67.4)
BMI, kg/m²				
Mean (SD)	21.0 (2.6)	20.7 (3.1)	21.8 (3.2)	22.0 (3.9)
Median (range)	20.8 (15.0–26.2)	20.2 (13.8–28.8)	21.5 (15.1–32.6)	21.1 (18.1–36.2)
Duration of MS since first symptom, years				
Mean (SD)	8.4 (8.1)	8.4 (7.2)	8.2 (6.6)	7.6 (5.5)
Median (range)	5.4 (1–27)	5.9 (1–24)	6.4 (1–26)	6.2 (0–21)
Number of relapses within previous year				
Mean (SD)	2.1 (2.1)	1.4 (0.7)	1.4 (0.9)	1.5 (1.0)
Median (range)	2.0 (1–12)	1.0 (0–3)	1.0 (0–3)	1.0 (0–4)
EDSS score				
Mean (SD)	1.9 (1.6)	2.4 (1.6)	2.4 (1.9)	1.9 (1.7)
Median (range)	1.5 (0.0–5.0)	2.0 (0.0–5.5)	2.0 (0.0–6.0)	2.0 (0.0–6.0)
Patients free of Gd-enhancing lesions				
n (%)	13 (48.1)	17 (73.9)	28 (59.6)	22 (47.8)
Number of Gd-enhancing lesions				
Mean (SD)	1.7 (2.5)	0.7 (1.5)	1.0 (1.6)	1.7 (2.42)
Median (range)	1.0 (0–9)	0.0 (0–5)	0.0 (0–5)	1.0 (0–9)
Number of T2 lesions				
Mean (SD)	28.9 (23.2)	33.3 (23.1)	30.3 (22.8)	34.6 (24.2)
Median (range)	23.0 (3–98)	35.0 (1–91)	24.0 (4–100)	29.5 (5–119)

Abbreviations: *BMI* body mass index, *EDSS* Expanded Disability Status Scale, *Gd* gadoliunium, *MS* multiple sclerosis, *SD* standard deviation

(month 6 vs EoS: fingolimod 0.5 mg, mean EDSS score = 2.30 vs 2.24; fingolimod 1.25 mg, mean EDSS score = 1.70 vs 1.54). Among patients who switched from placebo to fingolimod, disability levels were lower in the extension study compared with the core phase (month 6 vs EoS: mean EDSS score = 2.20 vs 1.80). In addition, 74.3% (fingolimod 0.5 mg) and 90.6% (placebo-fingolimod) of patients were free from 3 month confirmed disability progression and 87.1% (fingolimod 0.5 mg) and 92.3% (placebo-fingolimod) of patients were free from 6 month confirmed disability progression at last EDSS assessment.

Safety and tolerability

The majority of AEs were mild or moderate in severity. SAEs were reported in 19 (13.3%) patients during the extension study, with the range in the continuous fingolimod and placebo-fingolimod switch groups (3.7–21.7%) being similar to that reported in the core study for the placebo and fingolimod groups (5.3–20.4%) [6]. During the extension, bradycardia was the only SAE reported in more than one patient (placebo-fingolimod 1.25 mg,

n = 2 [8.7%]). One case of macular edema was reported as an SAE in a patient treated continuously with fingolimod 0.5 mg for 27 months, although medical intervention was not required to resolve the event and the case was subsequently unconfirmed on central review by a retina specialist from the data and safety monitoring board. Infections and infestations classified as SAEs were reported in two patients treated in the continuous fingolimod 1.25 mg group (appendicitis, n = 1; urinary tract infection, n = 1). During the extension study, SAEs leading to study drug discontinuation were reported for five patients (3.5%): three in the continuous fingolimod 0.5 mg group (6.4%; breast cancer, central nervous system lymphoma, MS relapse), one in the placebo-fingolimod 1.25 mg group (NMO relapse as leukoencephalopathy) and one in the placebo-fingolimod 0.5 mg group (NMO relapse). NMO relapse SAEs occurred in two patients who were seropositive for anti-AQP4 antibodies; these were both previously described in [7].

The proportion of patients with AEs during the extension study was similar across groups (Table 2) and

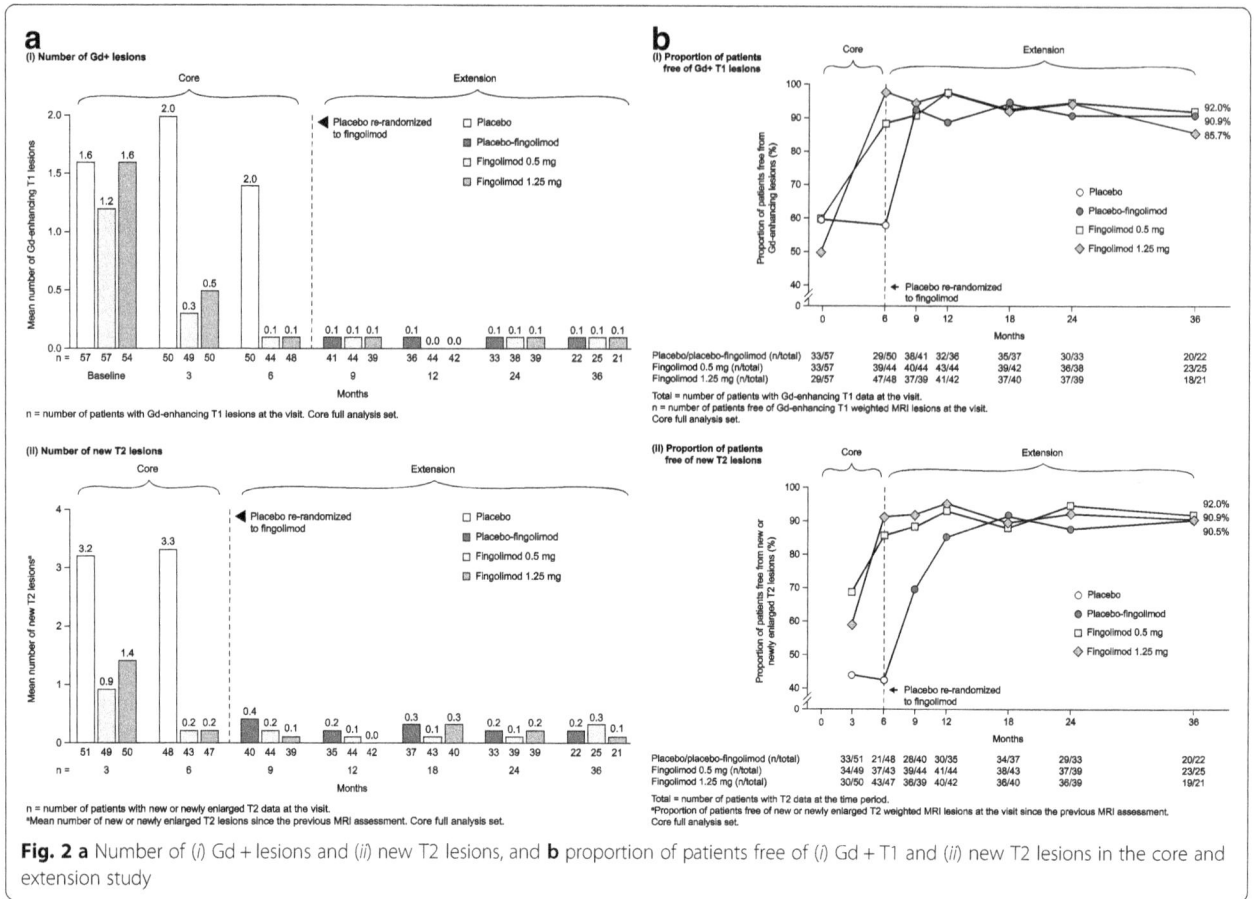

Fig. 2 a Number of (*i*) Gd + lesions and (*ii*) new T2 lesions, and **b** proportion of patients free of (*i*) Gd + T1 and (*ii*) new T2 lesions in the core and extension study

similar to the 6-month core study [6]. Nasopharyngitis was the most common AE (58.7%), followed by abnormal liver function test (21.0%), lymphopenia (13.3%), stomatitis (10.5%) and headache (10.5%; Table 2). Over the course of the extension study, infections and infestations were reported in 114 patients (79.7%); the majority were categorized as mild or moderate. Herpes zoster infections were reported in five patients; two in the

placebo-fingolimod 1.25 mg group, one in the placebo-fingolimod 0.5 mg group, one in the fingolimod 1.25 mg group and one in the fingolimod 0.5 mg group. Influenza occurred in 14 patients, and was more frequent in the continuous and placebo-fingolimod 1.25 mg switch groups (Table 2). There were no reports of infections and infestations AEs leading to study drug discontinuation during the extension study. Cardiac AEs were reported in

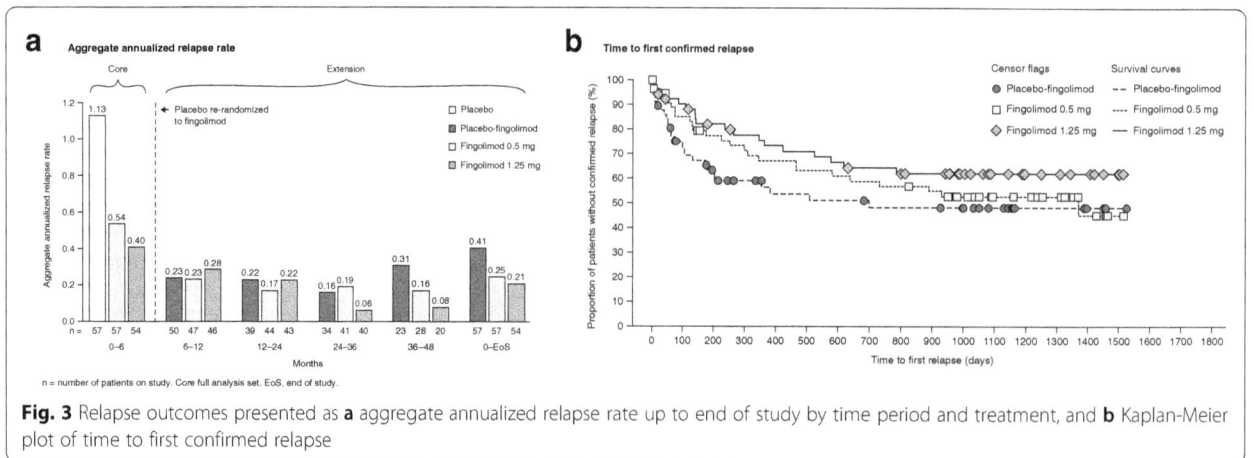

Fig. 3 Relapse outcomes presented as **a** aggregate annualized relapse rate up to end of study by time period and treatment, and **b** Kaplan-Meier plot of time to first confirmed relapse

Table 2 Adverse events and first-dose monitoring events during the extension study

	Placebo-fingolimod 0.5 mg (*n* = 27)	Placebo-fingolimod 1.25 mg (*n* = 23)	Fingolimod 0.5 mg (*n* = 47)	Fingolimod 1.25 mg (*n* = 46)	Total (*n* = 143)
Any AE	27 (100)	23 (100)	45 (95.7)	44 (95.7)	139 (97.2)
AEs leading to study drug discontinuation[a]	8 (29.6)	5 (21.7)	7 (14.9)	2 (4.3)	22 (15.4)
SAEs	1 (3.7)	5 (21.7)	8 (17.0)	5 (10.9)	19 (13.3)
SAEs leading to study drug discontinuation[b]	1 (3.7)	1 (4.3)	3 (6.4)	0 (0.0)	5 (3.5)
Frequent or special-interest adverse events					
Infections and infestations	22 (81.5)	17 (73.9)	37 (78.7)	38 (82.6)	114 (79.7)
Total upper respiratory tract infections	17 (63.0)	12 (52.2)	31 (66.0)	29 (63.0)	89 (62.2)
Nasopharyngitis	15 (55.6)	12 (52.2)	29 (61.7)	28 (60.9)	84 (58.7)
Pharyngitis	1 (3.7)	2 (8.7)	5 (10.6)	4 (8.7)	12 (8.4)
Upper respiratory tract infection	1 (3.7)	0 (0.0)	2 (4.3)	1 (2.2)	4 (2.8)
Influenza viral infections	2 (7.4)	3 (13.0)	3 (6.4)	6 (13.0)	14 (9.8)
Lower respiratory tract and lung infections	1 (3.7)	0 (0.0)	1 (2.1)	2 (4.3)	4 (2.8)
Bronchitis	1 (3.7)	0 (0.0)	1 (2.1)	2 (4.3)	4 (2.8)
Herpes viral infections	2 (7.4)	4 (17.4)	1 (2.1)	3 (6.5)	10 (7.0)
Herpes zoster	1 (3.7)	2 (8.7)	1 (2.1)	1 (2.2)	5 (3.5)
Oral herpes	0 (0.0)	2 (8.7)	0 (0.0)	0 (0.0)	2 (1.4)
Urinary tract infections	2 (7.4)	1 (4.3)	4 (8.5)	9 (19.6)	16 (11.2)
Cystitis	2 (7.4)	1 (4.3)	3 (6.4)	7 (15.2)	13 (9.1)
Vascular disorders	1 (3.7)	1 (4.3)	4 (8.5)	2 (4.3)	8 (5.6)
Hypertension	0 (0.0)	1 (4.3)	3 (6.4)	1 (2.2)	5 (3.5)
Eye disorders	5 (18.5)	3 (13.0)	14 (29.8)	9 (19.6)	31 (21.7)
Macular edema	0 (0.0)	0 (0.0)	1 (2.1)[c]	0 (0.0)	1 (0.7)
Nervous system disorders	4 (14.8)	6 (26.1)	14 (29.8)	9 (19.6)	33 (23.1)
Headache	1 (3.7)	3 (13.0)	8 (17.0)	3 (6.5)	15 (10.5)
Investigations	13 (48.1)	14 (60.9)	15 (31.9)	17 (37.0)	59 (41.3)
Abnormal liver function test	7 (25.9)	9 (39.1)	6 (12.8)	8 (17.4)	30 (21.0)
Alanine aminotransferase increased	2 (7.4)	0 (0.0)	0 (0.0)	1 (2.2)	3 (2.1)
Gamma-glutamyl transferase increased	1 (3.7)	2 (8.7)	1 (2.1)	0 (0.0)	4 (2.8)
Aspartate amino-transferase increased	1 (3.7)	0 (0.0)	0 (0.0)	1 (2.2)	2 (1.4)
Hepatic enzyme increased	1 (3.7)	1 (4.3)	1 (2.1)	0 (0.0)	3 (2.1)
Lymphocyte count decreased	3 (11.1)	2 (8.7)	3 (6.4)	2 (4.3)	10 (7.0)
Gastrointestinal disorders	11 (40.7)	6 (26.1)	22 (46.8)	23 (50.0)	62 (43.4)
Stomatitis	4 (14.8)	1 (4.3)	4 (8.5)	6 (13.0)	15 (10.5)
Diarrhea	1 (3.7)	2 (8.7)	3 (6.4)	6 (13.0)	12 (8.4)
Constipation	1 (3.7)	0 (0.0)	5 (10.6)	2 (4.3)	8 (5.6)
Skin and subcutaneous tissue disorders	8 (29.6)	9 (39.1)	14 (29.8)	16 (34.8)	47 (32.9)
Rash	3 (11.1)	4 (17.4)	1 (2.1)	0 (0.0)	8 (5.6)
Blood and lymphatic system disorders	7 (25.9)	5 (21.7)	10 (21.3)	13 (28.3)	35 (24.5)
Lymphopenia	2 (7.4)	3 (13.0)	6 (12.8)	8 (17.4)	19 (13.3)
Leukopenia	4 (14.8)	1 (4.3)	2 (4.3)	5 (10.9)	12 (8.4)
Respiratory, thoracic and mediastinal disorders	1 (3.7)	4 (17.4)	6 (12.8)	9 (19.6)	20 (14.0)

Table 2 Adverse events and first-dose monitoring events during the extension study *(Continued)*

Metabolism and nutrition disorders	4 (14.8)	1 (4.3)	4 (8.5)	7 (15.2)	16 (11.2)
Hyperlipidemia	2 (7.4)	0 (0.0)	2 (4.3)	5 (10.9)	9 (6.3)
Psychiatric disorders	2 (7.4)	2 (8.7)	8 (17.0)	4 (8.7)	16 (11.2)
Neoplasms benign, malignant and unspecified (including cysts and polyps)	0 (0.0)	1 (4.3)	9 (19.1)	1 (2.2)	11 (7.7)
Skin papilloma	0 (0.0)	0 (0.0)	6 (12.8)	0 (0.0)	6 (4.2)
First-dose monitoring events[d]					
Cardiac disorders	4 (14.8)	7 (30.4)	0 (0.0)	0 (0.0)	11 (7.7)
Atrioventricular block second degree	0 (0.0)	3 (13.0)	0 (0.0)	0 (0.0)	3 (2.1)
Bradycardia	0 (0.0)	3 (13.0)	0 (0.0)	0 (0.0)	3 (2.1)
Serious adverse events[e]					
Infections and infestations	0 (0.0)	0 (0.0)	0 (0.0)	2 (4.3)	2 (1.4)
Appendicitis	0 (0.0)	0 (0.0)	0 (0.0)	1 (2.2)	1 (0.7)
Urinary tract infection	0 (0.0)	0 (0.0)	0 (0.0)	1 (2.2)	1 (0.7)
Cardiac disorders	0 (0.0)	2 (8.7)	0 (0.0)	0 (0.0)	2 (1.4)
Bradycardia	0 (0.0)	2 (8.7)	0 (0.0)	0 (0.0)	2 (1.4)
Neoplasms benign, malignant and unspecified (including cysts and polyps)	0 (0.0)	0 (0.0)	2 (4.3)	0 (0.0)	2 (1.4)
Breast cancer	0 (0.0)	0 (0.0)	1 (2.1)	0 (0.0)	1 (0.7)
CNS lymphoma	0 (0.0)	0 (0.0)	1 (2.1)	0 (0.0)	1 (0.7)
Nervous system disorders	1 (3.7)	2 (8.7)	3 (6.4)	1 (2.2)	7 (4.9)
Status epilepticus	0 (0.0)	0 (0.0)	0 (0.0)	1 (2.2)	1 (0.7)
Convulsion	0 (0.0)	0 (0.0)	1 (2.1)	0 (0.0)	1 (0.7)
Leukoencephalopathy	0 (0.0)	1 (4.3)	0 (0.0)	0 (0.0)	1 (0.7)
Multiple sclerosis relapse	0 (0.0)	0 (0.0)	1 (2.1)	0 (0.0)	1 (0.7)
Myoclonus	0 (0.0)	0 (0.0)	1 (2.1)	0 (0.0)	1 (0.7)
Neuromyelitis optica	1 (3.7)	0 (0.0)	0 (0.0)	0 (0.0)	1 (0.7)
Radiculitis	0 (0.0)	1 (4.3)	0 (0.0)	0 (0.0)	1 (0.7)

Data are patients (*n* [%]) in whom events were reported by at least 10% of patients in one or more treatment group, or were events of special interest. Adverse events listed are classified as system organ class (e.g. infections) followed by high-level term (e.g. total upper respiratory tract infections) and/or preferred term (e.g. upper respiratory tract infection, nasopharyngitis, sinusitis) for the event, as applicable
Abbreviations: *AE* Adverse event, *AQP4* Aquaporin-4, *CNS* Central nervous system, FDM, first dose monitoring, *SAE* Serious adverse event
[a]Any AE leading to study drug discontinuation includes any patient whose primary or secondary reason for discontinuing the study drug was an AE
[b]SAEs leading to study drug discontinuation were neoplasms (breast cancer and CNS lymphoma), and nervous system disorders (MS relapse, leukoencephalopathy and neuromyelitis optica). Leukoencephalopathy and neuromyelitis optica were reported in patients who were anti-AQP4 antibody-positive
[c]Not confirmed on central review by a retina specialist from the data and safety monitoring board
[d]FDM events for placebo-fingolimod switch groups on entry to the extension study
[e]SAE data are *n* (%) for events reported by at least two patients in one or more treatment group, unless otherwise stated

11 patients (7.7%), and all of these events occurred following initiation of fingolimod in patients who switched from placebo. Overall, 22 patients out of 143 (15.4%) discontinued study drug due to AEs. AEs leading to permanent study drug discontinuation were reported more frequently in patients who switched from placebo to fingolimod during the extension phase (21.7–29.6%) than in continuous fingolimod groups (4.3–14.9%). The most frequent causes of discontinuation, which were reported in at least two patients, included leukopenia (2.8%), abnormal liver function test (2.1%), hepatic enzyme increase (1.4%) and decreased lymphocyte count (1.4%).

During the extension study, abnormal liver function test AEs were reported more frequently in the groups that switched from placebo to fingolimod (25.9–39.1%) than in the continuous fingolimod groups (12.8–17.4%; Table 2). In the continuous fingolimod groups, the frequency of abnormal liver function test AEs was lower during the extension study (12.8–17.4%) than during the core study (21.1–33.3%) [6]. Greater mean levels of alanine aminotransferase (ALT), aspartate aminotransferase (AST) and gamma-glutamyl transferase (GGT) were observed at month 6 in patients treated continuously with fingolimod than in patients receiving placebo, but these levels remained stable during the extension (Additional file 1: Table S2). After 15 days of fingolimod therapy in the extension (month 6.5), patients who had switched from placebo had increased levels of ALT, AST and GGT, and these were similar to the levels seen among patients treated with fingolimod during the core study. During months 18–36, levels of ALT, AST and GGT were similar across all patient groups (Additional file 1: Table S2). During the core study, the proportions of patients whose ALT and GGT levels were more than three-times the upper limit of normal (3 × ULN) were greater in those receiving fingolimod than in those receiving placebo; in the extension, the proportions of patients with ALT and GGT levels more than 3 × ULN were similar in the continuous and switch groups (Additional file 1: Table S3).

Lymphocyte counts in the continuous fingolimod 1.25 and 0.5 mg groups reduced to 22.1 and 26.9% of the core baseline levels at month 6 (Fig. 4). Subsequently, lymphocyte counts remained stable during the extension (28.3 and 26.3% of core baseline values, respectively). In patients who switched from placebo to fingolimod 1.25 or 0.5 mg, lymphocyte numbers reduced to 22.0 and 30.4% of core baseline levels at month 6.5, and remained stable thereafter (Fig. 4). At the end of study, the majority of patients in each group had lymphocyte counts greater than 0.20×10^9/L, the threshold at which fingolimod treatment was interrupted in clinical studies (fingolimod 0.5 mg, 72.3%; fingolimod 1.25 mg, 71.7%; placebo-fingolimod 0.5 mg, 81.5%; placebo-fingolimod 1.25 mg, 69.6%). Absolute neutrophil and white blood cell (WBC) counts were reduced to a similar extent in

the continuous and switch groups at study end, however no patient group had a neutrophil count $< 1.0 \times 10^9$/L at any stage in the study and all patient groups had WBC counts that were either normal or between 1.5–2.0×10^9/L (Additional file 1: Table S4).

Throughout the core and extension study, no skin malignancy was detected on dermatological examination. Neoplasms were reported in 11 patients (7.7%). Breast cancer and central nervous system lymphoma were each reported in one patient on continuous fingolimod 0.5 mg. All other cases were reported as benign skin neoplasms (skin papilloma, $n = 6$; melanocytic naevus, $n = 2$; anogenital warts, $n = 1$).

No deaths occurred during the extension study for up to 3 months after study drug discontinuation. A 42-year-old man died approximately 1 year after study drug discontinuation (9 months on fingolimod 0.5 mg); cause of death was Epstein-Barr virus (EBV)-positive diffuse large B-cell lymphoma of the brain, skin, lungs, kidneys and thyroid gland; no MS pathology was detected in this case [7]. A second case of diffuse large B-cell lymphoma was reported in a 38-year old woman who received continuous fingolimod 0.5 mg treatment, with a suspected relationship to the study drug medication (onset 1250 days on fingolimod 0.5 mg). First symptoms of malignant lymphoma, identified retrospectively, were reported on 22 September 2011, 1155 days after the start of study medication. Following a computerized tomography scan of the head, which revealed aggravation of hydrocephalus, the patient was withdrawn from the study and the study drug medication was stopped (26 December 2011; 1250 days after the start of study medication). Following draining for

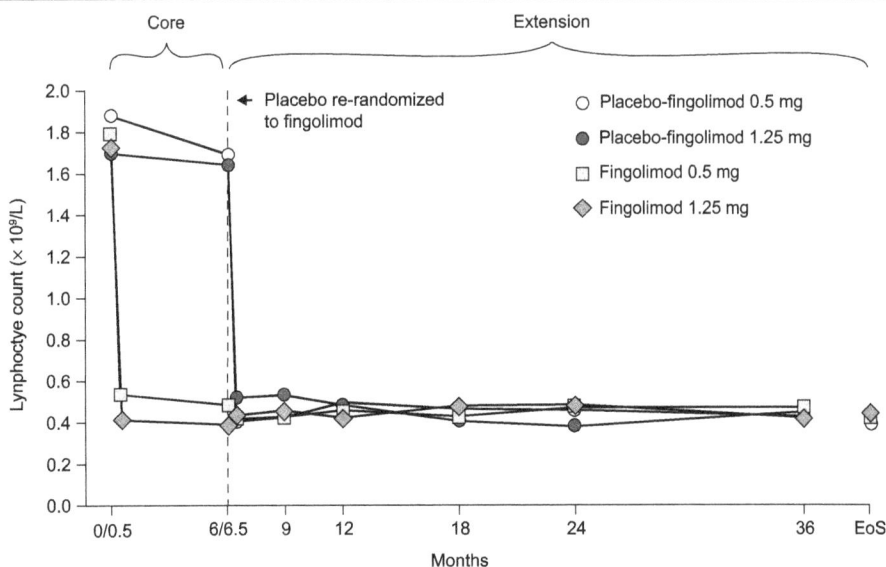

Fig. 4 Change in mean lymphocyte count during the core and extension study (extension safety population). *EoS* (end of study): in this instance is the last non-missing value up to 2 days after the last dose date and is summarized as last assessment on study drug. Data at 0.5 months (day 15) for fingolimod 0.5 mg ($n = 54$) and 1.25 mg ($n = 56$) represent values obtained during the core study (safety population)

hydrocephalus, B-cell lymphoma was confirmed on biopsy analysis (12 January 2012), and chemotherapy was started. Subsequently, multiple lesions previously observed on contrast-enhanced head MRI scan, and sites of aggregation in locations such as the right iliac bone, disappeared and the patient was discharged. During the extension, four patients receiving fingolimod (1.25 mg, $n = 3$; 0.5 mg, $n = 1$) became pregnant and therefore treatment was discontinued immediately. Two of these patients chose to terminate their pregnancies, while the remaining two patients gave birth to infants who were considered healthy. One patient receiving placebo terminated pregnancy during the core study.

Discussion

In this 3-year extension of the original 6-month core study in Japanese patients with MS, fingolimod sustained low levels of disease activity and no new safety signals were observed [6, 7]. These results are important given that genetic, metabolic, lifestyle, incidence and clinical presentation differences exist between Japanese patients with MS and individuals with MS in Western countries [6, 9]. The current study was designed to exclude patients with NMO on the basis of spinal MRI criteria at screening [7], although anti-AQP4-antibody status (a more specific marker for NMO) was not used, hence it is possible that not all cases of NMO were excluded. Notably, results in a small number of patients tested retrospectively for anti-AQP4 antibodies suggested a lack of benefit of fingolimod treatment in patients who tested positive for anti-AQP4 antibodies [7]. However, the overall efficacy and safety findings of fingolimod treatment in this population of Japanese patients with MS were similar to those seen in predominantly Caucasian populations in the original phase 3 pivotal studies and their extensions [2, 4, 5, 9, 10].

A low level of disease activity, based on all efficacy endpoints (ARR, EDSS and MRI outcomes) observed at the end of the core study were sustained until the end of the extension study in patients treated with continuous fingolimod. Reduced MRI and relapse activity were observed within the first 6 months in patients who switched to fingolimod at the start of the extension study, and this was sustained until the end of the study. These findings are similar to those from the 6-month extension study [7], in which continuous fingolimod therapy for 12 months was associated with sustained reductions in relapse rates and MRI lesion activity compared with those in the core study. The current results suggest that continuous treatment with fingolimod provides long-term benefit to the patient.

Fingolimod was generally well tolerated and the safety profile was consistent with results from previous studies [2–5, 10], including those reported in the core and 6-month extension [6, 7]. This was reflected in the high patient retention rate (74.8%) at the end of the 3-year study extension. The incidences of infections and cardiac AEs were low. A case of possible macular edema was unconfirmed and resolved without treatment. A single case of EBV-positive B-cell lymphoma was reported in this extension. One patient died approximately 1 year after study drug discontinuation (0.5 mg fingolimod) due to EBV-positive diffuse large B-cell lymphoma but without any MS pathology, suggesting the existence of brain lymphoma before commencing fingolimod medication. Overall, the incidence of malignancy was low and similar to that in other fingolimod studies [11]. Expected elevations in liver function test enzymes and lymphopenia occurred shortly after initiation of fingolimod therapy, and levels remained stable for the duration of the extension [2, 4, 5]. There was a single case of NMO relapse reported as a SAE during months 7–12 of the extension in one of four AQP4 antibody-positive patients who experienced relapses during the entire study; this case has been discussed previously [7]. NMO exacerbation has been reported in patients treated with MS disease-modifying therapies who were subsequently found to be anti-AQP4 antibody-positive [12], and in whom the initial diagnosis of MS was changed to NMO [13]. As the nature of relapses in all anti-AQP4-positive patients seen after commencing fingolimod appeared to be similar to previous relapses, it is conceivable that fingolimod did not alter but rather enhanced disease activity through an unknown mechanism [7].

In addition to the small sample size, a consequence of the recruitment challenge associated with the low incidence of MS in Japan, a drawback of this extension study that limits conclusions regarding efficacy is the lack of a placebo-control group, and the reduction in comparator groups following the need for all patients receiving fingolimod 1.25 mg to switch to fingolimod 0.5 mg. Nevertheless, continuous fingolimod treatment over 36 months was associated with maintained efficacy and a manageable safety profile.

Conclusion

These results indicate that there is a long-term benefit associated with treating Japanese patients with relapsing MS continuously with fingolimod.

Abbreviations

AE: Adverse event; ALT: Alanine aminotransferase; AQP4: Aquaporin-4; ARR: Annualized relapse rate; AST: Aspartate aminotransferase; BMI: Body mass index; EBV: Epstein-Barr virus; EDSS: Expanded Disability Status Scale; EoS: End of study; FAS: Full analysis set; Gd: Gadolinium; GGT: Gamma-glutamyl transferase; IFN: Interferon; MRI: Magnetic resonance imaging; MS: Multiple sclerosis; NMO: Neuromyelitis optica; RRMS: Relapsing–remitting multiple sclerosis; SAE: Serious adverse event; SD: Standard deviation; SOC: System organ class; ULN: Upper limit of normal; WBC: White blood cell

Acknowledgments
Oxford PharmaGenesis, Oxford, UK provided writing and editorial support for this manuscript.

Funding
This study was funded by Novartis Pharma KK and Mitsubishi Tanabe Pharma Corporation. Funding for medical writing and editorial support from Oxford PharmaGenesis, Oxford, UK was provided by Novartis Pharma KK and Mitsubishi Tanabe Pharma Corporation.

Authors' contributions
The study was designed by Novartis Pharma KK and Mitsubishi Tanabe Pharma Corporation. IT led the statistical analyses. QH conducted the magnetic resonance imaging. TS, YI, SK, QH, TK, KU, LA, IT, KN, JK made substantial contributions to planning of data analyses and data interpretation, and all had final responsibility for the contents and decision to submit for publication. All authors read and approved the final manuscript.

Competing interests
TS has received funding from, held board membership, spoken at scientific meetings, prepared manuscripts and has had consulting agreements in the past years with Novartis Pharma KK, Mitsubishi Tanabe Pharma Corporation, Kaketsuken, Biogen Japan, Astelas Pharma, Bayer, Merck-Serono, Nihon Pharmaceutical, Daiich-Sankyo, Ono Pharmaceutical, TDS Japan, Teijin Farma and Sanofi. YI has received research support from the Ministry of Education, Science and Technology of Japan; the Ministry of Health, Labor and Welfare of Japan, and honoraria from Bayer Schering Pharma and Biogen Idec Japan. SK has received research support from Japan Agency for Medical Research and Development and has received honoraria from Otsuka Pharmaceutical, Mitsubishi Tanabe Pharma Corporation, Abbot Japan, Sumitomo Dainippon Pharma, Nihon Medi-Physics, Fujifilm RI Pharma, GlaxoSmithKline K.K., Eisai, Japan Blood Products Organization, Nihon Pharmaceutical, Kyowa Hakko Kirin and Takeda Pharmaceutical Ltd. QH has no conflicts of interest to disclose. TK KU and IT are employees of Novartis Pharma KK, Japan. LZ-A is an employees of Novartis Pharma AG, Switzerland. KN is an employee of Mitsubishi Tanabe Pharma Corporation Japan. JK is a consultant for Biogen Japan and Novartis Pharma AG and has received honoraria from Bayer Healthcare, Otsuka Pharmaceutical, Novartis Pharma KK and Mitsubishi Tanabe Pharma Corporation, and funding for a trip from Bayer Healthcare. He is funded by grants from the Ministry of Health, Labor and Welfare, Japan, the Japan Science and Technology Agency and the Ministry of Education, Culture, Science, Sports and Technology, Japan, Japan Blood Products Organization, Novartis Pharma KK and Takeda Pharmaceutical Ltd.

Author details
[1]Institute of Multiple Sclerosis Therapeutics, Nishinokyo-Kasugacho 16-44-409, Nakakyo-ku, Kyoto 604-8453, Japan. [2]Kyoto Min-Iren-Central Hospital, Kyoto, Japan. [3]Kyoto University Hospital, Kyoto, Japan. [4]International University of Health and Welfare, 1-7-4 Momochihama, Sawara, Fukuoka City, Fukuoka 814-0001, Japan. [5]Hokkaido Medical Center, National Hospital Organization, 1-1 Yamanote 5-jo 7-chome, Sapporo 063-0005, Japan. [6]Novartis Pharma KK, 1-23-1, Toranomon, Minato-ku, Tokyo 105-6333, Japan. [7]Novartis Pharma AG, Fabrikstrasse 12, 4002 Basel, Switzerland. [8]Mitsubishi Tanabe Pharma Corporation, 17-10, Nihonbashi-Koamicho, Chuo-ku Tokyo 103-8405, Japan. [9]Department of Neurology, Neurological Institute, Graduate School of Medical Sciences, Kyushu University, 3-1-1 Maidashi, Higashi-ku, Fukuoka 812-8582, Japan.

References
1. Novartis: Interim financial report. https://www.novartis.com/sites/www.novartis.com/files/2016-07-interim-financial-report-en.pdf. Accessed 20 Jan 2017.
2. Calabresi PA, Radue EW, Goodin D, Jeffery D, Rammohan KW, Reder AT, Vollmer T, Agius MA, Kappos L, Stites T, et al. Safety and efficacy of fingolimod in patients with relapsing-remitting multiple sclerosis (FREEDOMS II): a double-blind, randomised, placebo-controlled, phase 3 trial. Lancet Neurol. 2014;13(6):545–56.
3. Kappos L, Antel J, Comi G, Montalban X, O'Connor P, Polman CH, Haas T, Korn AA, Karlsson G, Radue EW. Oral fingolimod (FTY720) for relapsing multiple sclerosis. N Engl J Med. 2006;355(11):1124–40.
4. Kappos L, Radue EW, O'Connor P, Polman C, Hohlfeld R, Calabresi P, Selmaj K, Agoropoulou C, Leyk M, Zhang-Auberson L, et al. A placebo-controlled trial of oral fingolimod in relapsing multiple sclerosis. N Engl J Med. 2010;362(5):387–401.
5. Cohen JA, Barkhof F, Comi G, Hartung HP, Khatri BO, Montalban X, Pelletier J, Capra R, Gallo P, Izquierdo G, et al. Oral fingolimod or intramuscular interferon for relapsing multiple sclerosis. N Engl J Med. 2010;362(5):402–15.
6. Saida T, Kikuchi S, Itoyama Y, Hao Q, Kurosawa T, Nagato K, Tang D, Zhang-Auberson L, Kira J. A randomized, controlled trial of fingolimod (FTY720) in Japanese patients with multiple sclerosis. Mult Scler (Houndmills, Basingstoke, England). 2012;18(9):1269–77.
7. Kira J, Itoyama Y, Kikuchi S, Hao Q, Kurosawa T, Nagato K, Tsumiyama I, von Rosenstiel P, Zhang-Auberson L, Saida T. Fingolimod (FTY720) therapy in Japanese patients with relapsing multiple sclerosis over 12 months: results of a phase 2 observational extension. BMC Neurol. 2014;14:21.
8. Polman CH, Reingold SC, Edan G, Filippi M, Hartung HP, Kappos L, Lublin FD, Metz LM, Mcfarland HF, O'Connor PW, et al. Diagnostic criteria for multiple sclerosis: 2005 revisions to the "McDonald criteria". Ann Neurol. 2005;58(6):840–6.
9. Kappos L, O'Connor P, Radue E-W, Polman C, Hohlfeld R, Selmaj K, Ritter S, Schlosshauer R, von Rosenstiel P, Zhang-Auberson L, et al. Long-term effects of fingolimod in multiple sclerosis: the randomized FREEDOMS extension trial. Neurology. 2015;84:1582–91.
10. Cohen JA, Von Rosenstiel P, Gottschalk R, Cappiello L, Zhang Y, Kappos L. Long-term safety of fingolimod: interim evaluation of data from the LONGTERMS trial. Neurology. 2014;82((Meeting Abstracts)):2.
11. Kappos L, Cohen J, Collins W, de Vera A, Zhang-Auberson L, Ritter S, von Rosenstiel P, Francis G. Fingolimod in relapsing multiple sclerosis: an integrated analysis of safety findings. Mult Sclr Rel Dis. 2014;3:495–504.
12. Shimizu J, Hatanaka Y, Hasegawa M, Iwata A, Sugimoto I, Date H, Goto J, Shimizu T, Takatsu M, Sakurai Y, et al. IFNbeta-1b may severely exacerbate Japanese optic-spinal MS in neuromyelitis optica spectrum. Neurology. 2010;75(16):1423–7.
13. Min JH, Kim BJ, Lee KH. Development of extensive brain lesions following fingolimod (FTY720) treatment in a patient with neuromyelitis optica spectrum disorder. Mult Scler (Houndmills, Basingstoke, England). 2012;18(1):113–5.
14. ICH harmonised tripartite guidelines for good clinical practice E6 (R1). International Conference on Harmonization of technical requirements for registration of pharmaceuticals for human use, Geneva (1996) http://www.ich.org/fileadmin/Public_Web_Site/ICH_Products/Guidelines/Efficacy/E6/E6_R1_Guideline.pdf. Accessed 18 July 2016.
15. World Medical Association. Declaration of Helsinki: Ethical principles for medical research involving human subjects. https://www.wma.net/en/30publications/10policies/b3/index.html. Accessed 18 July 2016.

7

Subjective patient-reported versus objective adherence to subcutaneous interferon β-1a in multiple sclerosis using RebiSmart®

Chiara Zecca[1], Giulio Disanto[1], Sarah Mühl[2] and Claudio Gobbi[1,3*]

Abstract

Background: Patient adherence to treatment is key to preventing the worsening of neurological disability in multiple sclerosis (MS). The RebiSmart® autoinjector facilitates self-administration of subcutaneous interferon β-1a (sc IFN β-1a) and records objective adherence data. The CORE study was undertaken to evaluate the relationship between subjectively reported and objective adherence of MS patients using RebiSmart® in Switzerland and explore variables associated with objective adherence.

Methods: Patients with relapsing-remitting MS who were treated with sc IFN β-1a 44 or 22 μg three times weekly using RebiSmart® for at least 9 months participated in this phase IV non-interventional study. Neurologist questionnaires were used at month 0 to collect patient demographics, medical history and estimates of patients' adherence. Patient questionnaires were used to record subjective patient-reported adherence at month 0 and estimates of variables influencing adherence. Objective adherence data were obtained from the RebiSmart® log-files at months 0 and 6.

Results: Of 56 patients who completed the observation period, 53 had evaluable data. Objective adherence differed significantly between self-reported compliant ($n = 33$) and non-compliant groups ($n = 20$) ($p = 0.00001$). Older age, greater disability, patient's perception of the importance of ease of use and storage, being well informed about RebiSmart® features and neurologists' estimations of adherence were all positively associated with treatment adherence.

Conclusions: We showed for the first time that subjective patient-reported adherence in MS was well in line with objective adherence, suggesting that the frequency of administration is reported accurately by patients to their neurologist. This observation may have implications for future treatment monitoring strategies and strategic medical decisions. Patients, particularly those who are younger and with lower levels of disability, may benefit from being better informed of the importance of being adherent to their treatments and receiving information about their medication and the device they are using.

Keywords: Multiple sclerosis, RebiSmart®, Autoinjector, Subcutaneous interferon β-1a, sc IFN β-1a, Adherence, Patient adherence, Self-reported adherence, Subjective adherence, Objective adherence

* Correspondence: Claudio.Gobbi@eoc.ch
[1]Multiple Sclerosis Center, Neurocenter of Southern Switzerland, Ospedale Regionale di Lugano, Lugano, Switzerland
[3]Multiple Sclerosis Center, Neurocenter of Southern Switzerland, Ospedale Regionale di Lugano, Via Tesserete 46, 6903 Lugano, Switzerland
Full list of author information is available at the end of the article

Background

The importance of patient adherence to therapy for the effective management of chronic disease is well documented [1]. Poor adherence to treatment in chronic diseases may be exacerbated due to the need for treatment over the long-term. In some cases, the absence of symptoms over a period of time may be a reason for not adhering to, or even discontinuing, treatment. In other cases, progressive disability during the course of disease may lead to a perception of lack of treatment efficacy or increase difficulty or discomfort when self-administering treatment [2].

In multiple sclerosis (MS), patient adherence is a key factor to ensure improved clinical outcomes and has been associated with a reduced risk of relapse [3, 4], disability progression, hospitalization, MS-related medical costs [4, 5], and an improved quality of life [6]. Obtaining good adherence rates among patients is challenging, with rates as low as 30–40% observed in a retrospective study of patients with MS 2 years after initiating treatment with disease-modifying therapy [7].

Although reliable data are limited, evidence supports the use of tailored intervention strategies to improve patient adherence to therapy [8]. RebiSmart® (Merck Serono S.A., Geneva, Switzerland) is an electronic, multidose, autoinjector for subcutaneous (sc) self-injection of interferon (IFN) β-1a. RebiSmart® was designed to facilitate and increase the comfort level of self-injection for patients by manipulation of various comfort settings. The electronic log-file provides read-outs of objective adherence data, providing patients and physicians with reliable information about levels of compliance [9]. Thus, noncompliance can be easily detected and drive alternative treatment decisions.

The aims of this study were therefore to compare for the first time subjective patient-reported adherence with objectively recorded dosing history using RebiSmart® and to identify factors influencing MS therapy adherence in a Swiss population.

Methods

CORE was a Swiss, practice survey-based study involving 11 centers. Patients with relapsing remitting MS (RRMS) who had received sc IFN β-1a 44 or 22 µg three times weekly (tiw) using RebiSmart® for at least 9 months, and regularly self-injecting the therapy, were included. They were treated according to the physician's evaluation and decision.

All patients provided written informed consent and the responsible ethics committees were notified before study start.

Neurologist questionnaires (Additional file 1: Appendix I) were used to collect patient demographics and medical history at month 0 (M0). Patient questionnaires (Additional file 1: Appendix II) were used to record subjective adherence at M0 and after a 6-month observational period (M6). Patients reporting that they did not miss any injection during the study were defined as "self-reported adherent"; all remaining patients were "self-reported non-adherent". Objective adherence data were collected from RebiSmart® device log-files for the 9-month period preceding M0 (retrospective adherence) and then between M0 and M6 (prospective adherence).

Objective adherence was calculated as the percentage of scheduled injections completed for each patient. Patients were grouped into three categories based on objective adherence data at M0: low (< 90%), medium (90–99.9%) and high (100%).

Objective adherence in self-reported adherent patients was compared to that in non-adherent patients using the Mann-Whitney U test (primary aim). As a secondary aim, retrospective and prospective objective adherence were compared using the Wilcoxon matched paired test. Furthermore, variables potentially associated with a greater objective adherence at M0 were explored using ordinal regression with low versus medium versus high objective adherence groups as the predicted variable.

Adverse drug reactions (ADRs) were reported by the treating physician and MS nurses.

Results

Of 56 patients who completed the observation period, data were available for 53 (non-evaluable patient questionnaires, $n = 2$; treatment for < 9 months, $n = 1$). Patients had a median age of 49 years and most (77.4%) were female. At baseline, the median duration of treatment with sc IFN β-1a prior to study enrolment was 24 months (Table 1).

Median objective adherence was significantly higher in self-reported adherent (100% [interquartile range, IQR: 98.8–100%], $n = 33$) than in self-reported non-adherent patients (93.4% [77.2–97.5%], $n = 20$) ($p = 0.00001$). There was no difference between retrospective (98.8%

Table 1 Patient characteristics at baseline, $N = 53$

Patient characteristic	Median (IQR) or n (%)
Age, years	49.0 (38.0–55.0)
Female, n	41.0 (77.4%)
Last known EDSS score[a]	2.0 (1.5–3.3)
Time since diagnosis, years[b]	6.5 (3.0–12.0)
Duration of therapy, months[c]	47.0 (30.8–96.3)
Duration of therapy with sc IFN β-1a, months	24.0 (20.0–36.0)
Patients with relapse during past 9 months, n	8.0 (15.1%)

EDSS expanded disability status scale, *IFN* interferon, *IQR* interquartile range expressed as Q1–Q3, *sc* subcutaneous
[a]Data missing for 2 patients
[b]Data missing for 1 patient
[c]Data missing for 5 patients

[IQR: 93–100%]) and prospective (98.8% [88.5–100%]) objective adherence (p = 0.75).

Fifteen (28.3%) patients had low objective adherence, 18 (34.0%) had medium adherence and 20 (37.7%) had high adherence at M0. Factors associated with significantly higher objective adherence were older age and greater expanded disability status scale (EDSS) score, neurologist's subjective estimate of adherence, patient's perceived importance of ease of use and ease of storage, and the patient feeling well informed about the features of RebiSmart®; previous MS therapy and perceived importance of treatment in delaying disease progression or importance of administration frequency were not associated (Table 2, Additional file 2). Fifteen cases of ADRs were reported in 11 patients, of which two were serious (depression and sarcoma; Additional file 3: Table S1).

Discussion

In this Swiss MS population, objectively-measured adherence to sc IFN β-1a administered by RebiSmart® was very high, even with a median treatment duration of 2 years. These data were largely consistent with subjective self-reported adherence using questionnaires. Objective adherence was similarly high in the retrospective and prospective study periods, indicating overall good adherence levels before patients were included in the study, and thus suggesting that adherence was not greatly influenced by awareness of being monitored. These real-life adherence data are consistent with findings from other recent trials, in which similarly high levels of objective adherence have been reported for patients using RebiSmart®. In a large study conducted at various sites across Europe (SMART), mean objective adherence among 912 patients with RRMS, over a 12-month study period, was 97.1% [10]; another retrospective study in Italy of 114 RRMS patients using RebiSmart® and followed up during a 1.536 ± 0.961 year period reported a mean objective adherence of 95.0 ± 9.0% [11]; while a more recent long-term retrospective study in Spain of 110 patients with MS, reported median adherence of 96.5% for a median period of 2.7 years [12]; and a smaller study in Finland reported 93.5% objective adherence for 29 patients with RRMS followed up over 24 weeks [13]. The long-term RIVER study showed median overall objective adherence of 85.2% for 57 patients over a mean 20.5 month observational period [14].

Ordinal regression analysis indicated that adherence estimated by the treating neurologist was well in line with objective adherence, suggesting that the frequency of administration is reported accurately by patients to their neurologist and thus that the neurologists were generally aware of their patients' adherence. This observation, together with our finding that objectively measured adherence was consistent with self-reported adherence, has implications in treatment decision making, i.e. supporting the need for switching disease modifying treatment or initiating strategies to improve patient compliance (such as frequent MS nurse monitoring) when poor adherence is suspected.

Ordinal regression analyses additionally showed that older age and greater disability were in this study associated with greater objective adherence to RebiSmart®. In another survey-based study of 708 patients in the U.S., patients who were older at diagnosis of MS were also

Table 2 Factors impacting adherence

Factor	Objective adherence group			Ordinal regression		
	Low n = 15	Medium n = 18	High n = 20	OR	95% CI	p
Patient age, years	41.0 (31.5–48.0)	48.5 (36.5–54.8)	53.5 (42.0–63.0)	1.064	1.016–1.114	**0.008**
Last known EDSS score[a]	1.5 (1.0–2.0)	2.0 (1.5–3.3)	3.0 (2.0–3.8)	1.937	1.197–1.937	**0.008**
Neurologists' estimations of adherence	10.0 (8.0–10.0)	9.0 (9.0–10.0)	10.0 (9.0–10.0)	1.528	1.019–2.291	**0.04**
Previous MS therapy	20.0%	33.0%	0.0%	0.344	0.089–1.340	0.124
Patient's perceived relevance of ease of administration with RebiSmart®	9.0 (7.5–9.5)	10.0 (9.3–10.0)	10.0 (10.0–10.0)	1.578	1.080–2.307	**0.018**
Patient's perceived relevance of storage of RebiSmart®	8.0 (5.5–8.0)	8.0 (5.3–10.0)	10.0 (8.0–10.0)	1.528	1.019–2.291	**0.04**
Being well informed about features of RebiSmart®	10.0 (9.0–10.0)	10.0 (10.0–10.0)	10.0 (10.0–10.0)	3.638	1.201–11.018	**0.022**
Patient's perceived relevance of treatment in delaying progression of disease	10.0 (10.0–10.0)	10.0 (10.0–10.0)	10.0 (10.0–10.0)	1.063	0.644–1.753	0.812
Importance of frequency of administration	8.0 (7.0–9.0)	8.5 (6.3–10.0)	10.0 (5.0–10.0)	1.008	0.808–1.259	0.941

Data were analyzed by ordinal regression and are reported as median (interquartile range, Q1–Q3), with the exception of 'Previous MS therapy' which is reported as percentage of 'yes' responses. P-values that were considered significant (p < 0.05) are in bold type
Low adherence group: < 90%; medium adherence group: 90%–99.9%; high adherence group: > 99.9%
CI confidence interval, *EDSS* expanded disability status scale, *IFN* interferon, *OR* odds ratio, *sc* subcutaneous, *SD* standard deviation
[a]Data missing for 2 patients

found to have better adherence to treatment [15]. Furthermore, in a large prospective MS study in Australia, younger age at treatment initiation was predictive of discontinuation of disease-modifying therapy over a median follow-up period of 2 years [16]. However, patients with a higher EDSS score (greater disability) were also found to be more likely to discontinue treatment in the Australian study [16]. In a previous multicenter 12-month retrospective study of 384 RRMS patients in Italy, younger patients (≤ 25 years old) and those with EDSS score ≥ 4 at baseline again showed poorest adherence to sc IFN β-1a (79 and 71.4% of patients, respectively, with $\geq 80\%$ completed doses), the most adherent patients being those aged 26–40 years at baseline and with EDSS score < 4 (over 90% of patients adherent) [17]. We hypothesize that older patients may have an increased awareness of the importance of treatment adherence for the prevention of further neurological disturbances. This may also be true for patients with greater disability in our study, despite the potential difficulties in performing self-injections in individuals with reduced physical capacity. The different findings observed for patients with greater disability in the Australian and Italian studies are likely due to differences in MS populations and study designs. Finally, patient perception of RebiSmart® ease of use and being well informed about the technical features of the device were also associated with higher adherence. A previous study in patients with other chronic disease (asthma and chronic obstructive pulmonary disease) have also reported the importance of being well informed about devices and medication for patients with chronic illness [18].

Limitations of the current study include selection bias towards compliant MS populations participating in the study, which is inherent to studies of this nature. Thus, these findings must be interpreted with caution. This was an exploratory study and the questionnaire will need further validation in additional cohorts of patients. The limited sample size may also have prevented the detection of additional factors potentially influencing adherence. Finally we chose adherence thresholds that were stricter than those usually reported [6, 19, 20], to allow a more equal distribution of patients across categories and a more valid statistical analysis. Indeed, only seven patients in this study had an objective adherence below 80% and this did not allow us to reliably investigate associations with adherence measures inferior to this threshold. While we cannot exclude the possibility that other factors could be associated with low adherence to injections, we believe our data can provide useful information for neurologists and care givers in MS. Our findings are also in-line with more recent publications concerning adherence to injectables at the observational study level [12, 13].

Conclusions

Patient-reported adherence was substantially in line with objective adherence, indicating that the frequently of administration is reported accurately by patients to their neurologists. The adherence to injectable treatments in patients with MS using RebiSmart® was very high. The importance of being adherent to treatments should be particularly stressed in younger and less disabled individuals and all patients should be well informed about their medication and the device they are using.

Additional files

Additional file 1: Neurologist and patient questionnaires. Neurologist questionnaire (Appendix I) used to collect patient demographics and medical history at month 0 and patient questionnaire (Appendix II) used to record subjective adherence at M0 and after a 6-month observational period.

Additional file 2: Series of six figures comparing adherence with age, EDSS score, neurologists' estimations of adherence, ease of administration, patient's perceived relevance of storage and being well informed about RebiSmart® features.

Additional file 3: Table S1. List of individual adverse drug reactions. Details of 15 cases of adverse drug reactions reported by 11 patients.

Abbreviations

ADRs: Adverse drug reactions; EDSS: Expanded disability status scale (EDSS); IFN: Interferon (IFN); IQR: Interquartile range (IQR); M0: Month 0 (M0); M6: 6-month observational period (M6); MS: Multiple sclerosis (MS); RMS: Relapsing remitting MS (RRMS); sc IFN β-1a: Subcutaneous interferon β-1a (sc IFN β-1a); sc: Subcutaneous (sc); tiw: Three times weekly (tiw)

Acknowledgements

Technical set up and data analyses were conducted by impulze GmbH, Zurich, Switzerland and funded by Merck (Schweiz) AG. Medical writing assistance was provided by Juliette Gray of inScience Communications, Chester, UK, and funded by Merck KGaA, Darmstadt, Germany.

Funding

The study and analyses were supported by Merck (Schweiz) AG, an affiliate of Merck KGaA, Darmstadt, Germany.

Authors' contributions

CZ, GD, CG and SM were involved in the conception and coordination of the study, and interpretation of the data. CZ, GD and CG were involved in data collection and statistical analysis. All authors provided input in the development and critical revision of the manuscript. All authors read and approved the final manuscript.

Competing interests

CZ, GD and CG: the Department of Neurology, Regional Hospital Lugano (EOC), Lugano, Switzerland receives financial support from Teva, Merck, Biogen Idec, Bayer Schering, Genzyme and Novartis, and the submitted work is not related to these agreements; SM: employee of Merck (Schweiz) AG, an affiliate of Merck KGaA, Darmstadt, Germany.

Author details
[1]Multiple Sclerosis Center, Neurocenter of Southern Switzerland, Ospedale Regionale di Lugano, Lugano, Switzerland. [2]Merck (Schweiz) AG, Zug, Switzerland. [3]Multiple Sclerosis Center, Neurocenter of Southern Switzerland, Ospedale Regionale di Lugano, Via Tesserete 46, 6903 Lugano, Switzerland.

References
1. Sabaté E. Adherence to long-term therapies: evidence for action. Geneva: World Health Organization; 2003. http://apps.who.int/iris/bitstream/10665/42682/1/9241545992.pdf. Accessed 25 Aug 2016.
2. Viswanathan M, Golin CE, Jones CD, Ashok M, Blalock SJ, Wines RCM, et al. Interventions to improve adherence to self-administered medications for chronic diseases in the united StatesA systematic review. Ann Intern Med. 2012;157(11):785–95. doi:10.7326/0003-4819-157-11-201212040-00538.
3. Al-Sabbagh A, Bennet R, Kozma C, Dickson M, Meletiche D. Medication gaps in diseasemodifying therapy for multiple sclerosis are associated with an increased risk of relapse: findings from a national managed care database. J Neurol. 2008;255(Suppl. 2):S79. doi:10.1007/s00415-008-2001-5.
4. Steinberg SC, Faris RJ, Chang CF, Chan A, Tankersley MA. Impact of adherence to interferons in the treatment of multiple sclerosis: a non-experimental, retrospective, cohort study. Clin Drug Investig. 2010;30(2):89–100. doi:10.2165/11533330-000000000-00000.
5. Menzin J, Caon C, Nichols C, White LA, Friedman M, Pill MW. Narrative review of the literature on adherence to disease-modifying therapies among patients with multiple sclerosis. J Manag Care Pharm. 2013;19(1 Suppl A):S24–40. 10.18553/jmcp.2013.19.s1.S24.
6. Devonshire V, Lapierre Y, Macdonell R, Ramo-Tello C, Patti F, Fontoura P, et al. The global adherence project (GAP): a multicenter observational study on adherence to disease-modifying therapies in patients with relapsing-remitting multiple sclerosis. Eur J Neurol. 2011;18(1):69–77. doi:10.1111/j.1468-1331.2010.03110.x.
7. Hansen K, Schussel K, Kieble M, Werning J, Schulz M, Friis R, et al. Adherence to disease modifying drugs among patients with multiple sclerosis in Germany: a retrospective cohort study. PLoS One. 2015;10(7):e0133279. doi:10.1371/journal.pone.0133279.
8. Depont F, Berenbaum F, Filippi J, Le Maitre M, Nataf H, Paul C, et al. Interventions to improve adherence in patients with immune-mediated inflammatory disorders: a systematic review. PLoS One. 2015;10(12):e0145076. doi:10.1371/journal.pone.0145076.
9. Lugaresi A. RebiSmart (version 1.5) device for multiple sclerosis treatment delivery and adherence. Expert Opin Drug Deliv. 2013;10(2):273–83. doi:10.1517/17425247.2013.746311.
10. Bayas A, Ouallet JC, Kallmann B, Hupperts R, Fulda U, Marhardt K. Adherence to, and effectiveness of, subcutaneous interferon beta-1a administered by RebiSmart(R) in patients with relapsing multiple sclerosis: results of the 1-year, observational SMART study. Expert Opin Drug Deliv. 2015;12(8):1239–50. doi:10.1517/17425247.2015.1057567.
11. Moccia M, Palladino R, Russo C, Massarelli M, Nardone A, Triassi M, et al. How many injections did you miss last month? A simple question to predict interferon beta-1a adherence in multiple sclerosis. Expert Opin Drug Deliv. 2015;12(12):1829–35. doi:10.1517/17425247.2015.1078789.
12. Edo Solsona MD, Monte Boquet E, Casanova Estruch B, Poveda Andres JL. Impact of adherence on subcutaneous interferon beta-1a effectiveness administered by Rebismart(R) in patients with multiple sclerosis. Patient Prefer Adherence. 2017;11:415–21. doi:10.2147/PPA.S127508.
13. Jarvinen E, Multanen J, Atula S. Subcutaneous interferon beta-1a administration by electronic auto-injector is associated with high adherence in patients with relapsing remitting multiple sclerosis in a real-life study. Neurol Int. 2017;9(1):6957. doi:10.4081/ni.2017.6957.
14. Lugaresi A, De Robertis F, Clerico M, Brescia Morra V, Centonze D, Borghesan S, et al. Long-term adherence of patients with relapsing-remitting multiple sclerosis to subcutaneous self-injections of interferon beta-1a using an electronic device: the RIVER study. Expert Opin Drug Deliv. 2016:[Epub ahead of print; doi:10.1517/17425247.2016.1148029.
15. Treadaway K, Cutter G, Salter A, Lynch S, Simsarian J, Corboy J, et al. Factors that influence adherence with disease-modifying therapy in MS. J Neurol. 2009;256(4):568–76. doi:10.1007/s00415-009-0096-y.
16. Jokubaitis VG, Spelman T, Lechner-Scott J, Barnett M, Shaw C, Vucic S, et al. The Australian multiple sclerosis (MS) immunotherapy study: a prospective, multicentre study of drug utilisation using the MSBase platform. PLoS One. 2013;8(3):e59694. doi: 10.1371/journal.pone.0059694.
17. Paolicelli D, Cocco E, Di Lecce V, Direnzo V, Moiola L, Lanzillo R, et al. Exploratory analysis of predictors of patient adherence to subcutaneous interferon beta-1a in multiple sclerosis: TRACER study. Expert Opin Drug Deliv. 2016;13(6):799–805. doi:10.1517/17425247.2016.1158161.
18. Partridge MR, Dal Negro RW, Olivieri D. Understanding patients with asthma and COPD: insights from a European study. Prim Care Respir J. 2011;20(3):315–23. doi:10.4104/pcrj.2011.00056.
19. Puigventos F, Riera M, Delibes C, Penaranda M, de la Fuente L, Boronat A. Adherence to antiretroviral drug therapy. A systematic review. Med Clin (Barc). 2002;119(4):130–7.
20. Ruddy K, Mayer E, Partridge A. Patient adherence and persistence with oral anticancer treatment. CA Cancer J Clin. 2009;59(1):56–66. doi:10.3322/caac.20004.

8

Development and validation of a claims-based measure as an indicator for disease status in patients with multiple sclerosis treated with disease-modifying drugs

Michael Munsell[1], Molly Frean[1], Joseph Menzin[1*] and Amy L. Phillips[2]

Abstract

Background: Administrative healthcare claims data provide a mechanism for assessing and monitoring multiple sclerosis (MS) disease status across large, clinically representative "real-world" populations. The estimation of MS disease status using administrative claims can be a challenge, however, due to a lack of detailed clinical information. Retrospective claims analyses in MS have traditionally used rates of MS relapses to approximate disease status. Healthcare costs may be alternate, broader claims-based indicators of disease activity because costs reflect multiple facets of care of patients with MS, and there is a strong correlation between quality of life of patients with MS and costs of the disease. This study developed, tested, and validated a healthcare cost-based measure to serve as an indicator of overall disease status in patients with MS treated with disease-modifying drugs (DMDs) utilizing administrative claims.

Methods: Using IMS Health Real World Data Adjudicated Claims – US data (January 2006–June 2013), a negative binomial regression predicted annual all-cause medical costs. Coefficients reaching statistical significance ($p < 0.05$) and increasing costs by ≥5% were selected for inclusion into an MS-specific severity score (scale of 0 to 100). Components of the score included rehabilitation services, altered mental state, pain, disability, stiffness, balance disorder, urinary incontinence, numbness, malaise/fatigue, and infections. Coefficient weights represented each predictor's contribution. The predictive model was derived using 50% of a random sample and tested/validated using the remaining 50%.

Results: Average overall predicted annual total medical cost was $11,134 (development sample, $n = 11,384$, vs. $10,528 actual) and $11,303 (validation sample, $n = 11,385$, vs. $10,620 actual). The model had consistent bias (approximately +$600 or +6% of actual costs) for both samples. In the validation sample, mean MS disease status scores were 0.24, 8.95, and 21.77 for low, medium, and high tertiles, respectively. Mean costs were most accurately predicted among less severe patients ($5243 predicted vs. $5233 actual cost for lowest tertile).

Conclusion: The algorithm developed in this study provides an initial step to helping understand and potentially predict cost changes for a commercially insured MS population.

Keywords: Multiple sclerosis, Disease status measure, Retrospective database, Validation, Costs

* Correspondence: jmenzin@bhei.com
[1]Boston Health Economics, Inc., 20 Fox Road, Waltham, MA 02451, USA
Full list of author information is available at the end of the article

Background

Multiple sclerosis (MS) is an inflammatory-mediated, chronic neurodegenerative disease characterized by a range of symptoms including fatigue, impaired motor skills, blurred vision, bladder and bowel dysfunction, and cognitive impairment [1, 2]. The disease has a highly variable prognosis causing early severe disabilities in some patients, but leaving others ambulatory and functional for many years [3, 4]. Comorbidities are also highly prevalent in the MS population, and co-morbid disease is recognized as a critical issue in MS given the breadth of adverse impacts with which it is associated [5]. The identification of patients with varying levels of overall disease status is important to help select patient populations most likely to benefit from interventions and to assess the value and effectiveness of treatments [6].

Administrative healthcare claims data provide a mechanism for assessing and monitoring MS disease status in patients with MS across large, clinically representative "real-world" populations [7–9]. Retrospective claims analyses in MS have traditionally used the rates of MS relapses (defined as MS-related hospitalizations, emergency room [ER] visits, or outpatient visits with pharmacy claims for a corticosteroid) as proxy measures for MS disease status [10–19]. Relapses alone, however, do not appropriately capture changes in disease progression and impairment [20]. For instance, as patients with MS progress over time, the number of relapses appears to decrease, despite worsening health status [20]. The estimation of MS disease status using administrative claims can be a challenge, however, due to a lack of detailed clinical information. Retrospective claims analyses in MS have traditionally used rates of MS relapses to approximate disease status. Furthermore, traditional medical models of impairment and disability in MS provide only an incomplete summary because they omit the consideration of comorbidities, secondary conditions, and health behaviors, which may influence the quality of life and disease burden of patients with MS along with biologic variables [21, 22].

Indicators of disease status that incorporate multiple facets of MS may permit assessment of the health status of the patient at a wider level [13, 23–26]. Healthcare costs may be alternate, broader claims-based indicators of disease activity because costs reflect multiple facets of care of patients with MS, and there is a strong correlation between quality of life of patients with MS and costs of the disease [27, 28]. This study utilized an administrative claims dataset to develop, test, and validate a healthcare costs-based measure to serve as an indicator of disease status in patients with MS treated with disease-modifying drugs (DMDs).

Methods

Data source and patient population

This retrospective database study used IMS Health Real World Data (RWD) Adjudicated Claims – US data from January 1, 2006 to June 30, 2013. The IMS Health RWD Adjudicated Claims – US database includes complete, adjudicated insurance data, including complete inventory of a patient's prescriptions, inpatient hospital, and outpatient medical claims. The database consists primarily of patients with commercial health insurance and can thus under-represent the patients with government-paid health insurance (Medicaid or Medicare) relative to patients with private commercial insurance. The database includes ~150 million patients with a medical benefit, and a subset of 95 million patients with both medical and pharmacy benefits.

Patients were aged 18–64 years, had at least one MS diagnosis claim (International Classification of Diseases, Ninth Revision, Clinical Modification [ICD-9-CM] code: 340.xx), and at least one claim for a DMD between January 1, 2007 and June 30, 2012. The date of the first DMD prescription was designated as the index date. Patients were included if they had continuous eligibility 12 months pre- and post-index. Patients were excluded if they had any indication of pregnancy.

Model development

The data were divided into two samples: an original development sample and a validation/test sample (each comprised 50% of the total patient population). Patients were randomized using the "surveyselect" procedure in Statistical Analysis Software (SAS). A "seed" was set for the randomization process; therefore, the same patients were assigned to the same group every time the analysis was run (i.e., results were therefore replicable). The goal was to create claims-based measures of disease status, one specific to MS and the other focused on general health, using various comorbidity and MS symptom-related codes, as well as additional variables (i.e., sex, age, census region, adherence, newly treated). The general health measure, which uses common Clinical Classification System (CCS) and Charlson criteria, is well-suited for the population as it provides a more complete view of the MS patient's health, and general health concerns can greatly increase costs among the MS population. MS and a general health measures were included in order to ensure the range of inputs that could affect the algorithm were captured. Costs were used as a proxy for disease status. The analysis evaluated healthcare costs using constant US dollars (i.e., costs were adjusted for inflation using the medical care component of the Consumer Price Index).

Multiple steps were implemented to achieve this goal. First, a negative binomial regression analysis was performed to predict all-cause total direct medical costs (excluding DMD costs) during the follow-up period. Regression covariates included 16 MS-related condition indicators (identified by diagnosis codes), 18 CCS codes, and 17 Charlson-Deyo comorbidities. Condition coefficients that reached both statistical ($p \leq 0.05$) and economic (MS condition indicators, ≥5% increase in costs; general condition indicators [CCS and Charlson-Deyo], ≥20% increase in costs) significance were included in two normalized scores: an MS score and a general health score (Table 1). Additional file 1: Table S1 and Additional file 2: Table S2 provide the regression results and details of the MS and general score composition that were obtained in the development of the measures.

Secondly, coefficients included in each score were re-weighted on a scale from 0 to 100, such that weights represented each predictor's relative contribution to disease status, as measured by costs (Table 1). Finally, the original negative binomial regression model was re-evaluated to predict costs as a function of the two scores, together with remaining covariates not included in the models for the MS or general health score. The fit of the two models was compared using Bayesian information criteria (BIC). The analysis demonstrated that the model including the MS and general health score was superior to the full regression model at predicting total direct medical costs (score model BIC: 227,340, full model: 227,508; a BIC difference > 10 demonstrates very strong evidence) [29].

Model validation and testing
As the scores are intended to represent disease status as measured by costs, the MS score, the general health score, and the model combining them were tested and validated in the remaining 50% of the patient population

Table 1 MS and general health score components and points

MS score		General health score	
Parameter	Points	Parameter	Points
Rehabilitation	25.597	Myocardial infarction (Charlson)	20.823
Altered mental state	15.802	Metastatic solid tumor (Charlson)	19.027
Pain	12.946	Any primary malignancy (Charlson)	12.172
Disability	10.000	Drug/device complication (CCS)	10.453
Balance disorder	9.211	Diabetes with chronic complications (Charlson)	8.937
Stiffness	8.651	Hematologic (CCS)	6.251
Urinary incontinence	6.366	Gastrointestinal disease (CCS)	5.891
Numbness	4.779	Psychiatric (CCS)	5.785
Malaise and fatigue	4.271	Rheumatologic (Charlson)	5.424
Infections	2.377	Genitourinary (CCS)	5.238

CCS Clinical Classification System, Charlson Charlson-Deyo comorbidities, MS multiple sclerosis

(validation/test population) by assessing the relationship between the two scores and both the predicted and actual costs.

Patients were divided into separate MS and general health score tertiles (i.e., low, medium, and high disease status based on MS or general health score), and predicted and actual costs were summarized for each tertile. Tertiles were generated by ranking all patients according to their disease status score and then dividing the total population into three equal groups, with group cut-offs defined by score ranking. Patients with tied values were grouped into the same tertile. Tertiles were selected for ease of interpretation and because they effectively presented changes in MS/general disease status scores, as the distribution of patients across tertiles was relatively even. An increase in the proportion of patients with a given condition could be seen in each tertile.

All-cause total direct healthcare cost measures were summarized for each tertile using mean, standard deviation (SD), median, interquartile range, and minimum/maximum. Statistical testing was employed to test the significance of difference in predicted versus actual costs between score groups. Differences between actual and predicted costs were assessed using Wilcoxon–Mann–Whitney tests for both the MS and general health score tertiles. Separate analyses were completed for both MS and general health score tertiles.

Additional validity testing was employed using general measures of model error. The bias and absolute prediction error of the model were calculated for both the original model sample and the remaining 50% validation sample. This exercise was conducted to ensure that model error was consistent when using different patient populations. The equations below were used in the bias mean absolute prediction error (MAPE) analyses. These types of prediction accuracy measures have been used in previous health economic studies (e.g., Austin 2003 compared the accuracy of different regression models used to predict coronary artery bypass graft surgery medical costs) [30].

$$\text{Bias} = (\text{mean of individual predictions}) - (\text{mean of actual observations}).$$
$$= \frac{1}{n}\sum_k \hat{Y}_k - \frac{1}{n}\sum_k Y_k$$
$$\text{MAPE} = \frac{1}{n}\sum_k |\hat{Y}_k - Y_k|$$

Exploration of MS/general health score composition
The proportion of patients with each condition used to calculate the MS and general health score was evaluated for each MS/general health score tertile. This analysis was conducted to determine how disease status factors change as MS/general health score increases.

Results

A total of 11,384 patients (50%) were included in the original development population, and 11,385 patients (50%) were included in the validation/test population.

A breakdown of the number of patients included in each MS and general health score tertile, as well as overall MS/general health scores for each tertile, are shown in Tables 2 and 3.

Mean MS scores were 0.24, 8.95, and 21.77 in the low, medium, and high MS disease status tertiles, respectively. Patients in the low tertile had a median score of 0 and maximum score of 2.38, corresponding to the presence of an infection. Patients who experienced the three condition indicators associated with the highest scores – rehabilitation services, altered mental state, and pain – were all categorized in the highest tertile. Mean general health scores were 0.00, 5.72, and 16.07 for the low, medium, and high tertiles, respectively. No patients in the lowest tertile had any general health score condition indicators, and patients with any of the five condition indicators associated with the greatest score were all grouped in the highest tertile. Average annual predicted and actual costs in the overall population (i.e., not stratified by disease status tertile) for each group are shown in Fig. 1.

Bias was similar in both models, with predicted costs being approximately 6% higher than actual costs. The mean (SD) absolute prediction error was consistent across both populations: $7274 (15,306) in the original

development population and $7387 (17,670) in the validation/test population.

Average annual predicted and actual costs within the validation/test population for the MS score and the general health score disease status tertiles are shown in Table 4.

The model predicted average costs most accurately for patients in the lowest disease status tertiles (bias of 0.2–1.9%; Fig. 2).

A bias of 11.1–12.4% ($2567 for MS score, $2418 for general health score) was recorded in the high disease status tertiles (Fig. 2). Differences in predicted vs. actual costs were significantly different across disease status tertiles for both MS and general health scores ($p < 0.0001$ for all).

Discussion

Overall (i.e., without stratification by disease status tertiles), the average predicted annual direct healthcare cost was $11,134 for the original development sample (vs. $10,528 actual cost) and $11,303 for the validation/test sample (vs. $10,620 actual cost). Therefore, the model had consistent bias (approximately $600, or 6% of actual costs) for both samples. In Austin 2003, other regression-based prediction models had similar degrees of bias [30].

The mean absolute prediction error also remained consistent in both populations (approximately $7000 for

Table 2 MS score and MS score component frequency within the validation/test population

	MS disease status group		
	Low tertile	Medium tertile	High tertile
Patients, n	3902	3801	3682
MS score			
Mean (SD)	0.24 (0.71)	8.95 (2.46)	21.77 (9.23)
Median (IQR)	0.00 (0.00–0.00)	10.00 (9.05–10.00)	19.21 (14.78–23.99)
Minimum	0	4.27	12.92
Maximum	2.38	12.38	91.35
MS score components, n (%)			
Rehabilitation	0	0	135 (3.7)
Altered mental state	0	0	133 (3.6)
Pain	0	0	370 (10.0)
Disability	0	2409 (63.4)	3369 (91.5)
Stiffness	0	4 (0.1)	115 (3.1)
Balance disorder	0	362 (9.5)	1823 (49.5)
Urinary incontinence	0	126 (3.3)	425 (11.5)
Numbness	0	317 (8.3)	1223 (33.2)
Malaise and fatigue	0	686 (18.0)	1892 (51.4)
Infections	388 (9.9)	550 (14.5)	731 (19.9)

IQR interquartile range, *MS* multiple sclerosis, *SD* standard deviation

Table 3 General health score and general health score component frequency within the validation/test population

| | General disease status group | | |
	Low tertile	Medium tertile	High tertile
Patients, n	4400	3426	3559
General health score			
Mean (SD)	0.00 (0.00)	5.72 (0.31)	16.07 (7.22)
Median (IQR)	0.00 (0.00–0.00)	5.78 (5.42–5.89)	12.14 (11.13–17.46)
Minimum	0	5.24	8.94
Maximum	0	6.25	64.82
General health score components, n (%)			
Myocardial infarction	0	0	47 (1.3)
Metastatic solid tumor	0	0	45 (1.3)
Any primary malignancy	0	0	363 (10.2)
Drug/device complication	0	0	658 (18.5)
Diabetes with chronic complications	0	0	159 (4.5)
Hematologic	0	329 (9.6)	1038 (29.2)
Gastrointestinal disease	0	1033 (30.2)	2301 (64.7)
Psychiatric	0	1190 (34.7)	2090 (58.7)
Rheumatologic	0	31 (0.9)	125 (3.5)
Genitourinary	0	843 (24.6)	1876 (52.7)

IQR interquartile range, *MS* multiple sclerosis, *SD* standard deviation

the original development and validation/test samples), demonstrating further validity of the model.

The mean absolute prediction error represents the average deviation of each individual predicted value from the actual value, and is therefore more sensitive to outliers than the measure of bias. However, the magnitude of the absolute prediction error in the analysis is comparable with the predictive cost models from Austin 2003, which resulted in a mean absolute error of approximately $6600 for a dataset with mean actual costs of $17,900 [30].

The slightly higher absolute prediction error in this study is most likely due to the magnitude of outliers from evaluating all-cause total direct medical costs vs. event-specific costs (i.e., maximum actual total cost in the analysis was $1,046,113, while maximum actual surgery-specific cost was $166,461 in Austin 2003 [30]).

On average, the model predicted costs most accurately among patients with lower disease status. Specifically, the model under-predicted costs by an average of $96 for the low MS disease status tertile (mean predicted

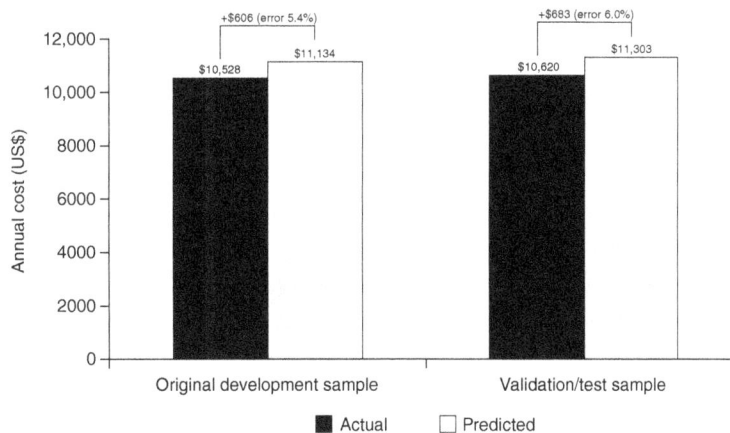

Fig. 1 Mean predicted vs. actual annual all-cause total medical costs for original development and validation/test samples*. *All costs adjusted to 2015 US dollars using the medical care component of the Consumer Price Index

Table 4 Predicted vs. actual costs in the validation/test population, by MS or general health score disease status tertiles[a]

	Disease status tertile		
	Low	Medium	High
MS score			
n	3902	3801	3682
Predicted costs, $			
Mean (SD)	5047 (2867)	8583 (5397)	20,743 (34,041)
Median (IQR)	4269 (3393–5712)	7193 (5359–10,042)	12,941 (8926–21,055)
Minimum	2149	2415	3642
Maximum	55,398	82,177	1,046,113
Actual costs, $			
Mean (SD)	5143 (9204)	8923 (12,770)	18,176 (27,936)
Median (IQR)	2688 (1065–6052)	5344 (2617–10,210)	10,215 (5212–19,976)
Minimum	0	0	0
Maximum	241,470	293,690	499,099
General health, score			
n	4400	3426	3559
Predicted costs, $			
Mean (SD)	5243 (2630)	8202 (4413)	21,781 (34,500)
Median (IQR)	4507 (3471–6260)	7175 (5239–10,019)	13,973 (9567–22,598)
Minimum	2149	2638	3552
Maximum	39,259	73,002	1,046,113
Actual costs, $			
Mean (SD)	5233 (7947)	8455 (10,609)	19,363 (29,432)
Median (IQR)	2950 (1187–6195)	5510 (2686–10,350)	10,725 (5429–21,577)
Minimum	0	0	0
Maximum	133,669	135,713	499,099

IQR interquartile range, *MS* multiple sclerosis, *SD* standard deviation
[a]All costs adjusted to 2015 US dollars using the medical care component of the Consumer Price Index

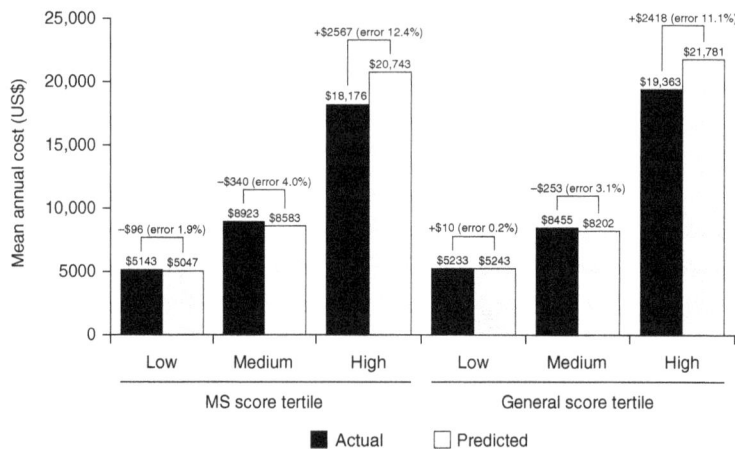

Fig. 2 Mean predicted vs. actual annual all-cause total medical costs and general health score tertile. *MS* multiple sclerosis*. *All costs adjusted to 2015 US dollars using the medical care component of the Consumer Price Index

$5047; mean actual $5143; bias 1.9% of actual) and over-predicted by only $10 for the low general health score tertile (mean predicted $5243; mean actual $5233; bias 0.2% of actual). The difference between predicted and actual cost was approximately $2500 for both the highest MS disease status and general health disease status tertiles (bias 11.1–12.4% of actual). Differences in predicted vs. actual costs were significantly different ($p < 0.0001$) between disease status tertiles. The better prediction in the lowest tertile could be explained by the likely lower amounts of variation in this subpopulation compared with the other subpopulations.

The MS score model predicted annual all-cause total medical costs with acceptable estimations. While there does not appear to be a standard threshold for evaluating the accuracy of predictive cost models (i.e., most publications simply evaluate several different models and comment on relative accuracy by comparing model bias), the predictive model appears to be consistent with other published validated models. The bias of models used to predict coronary artery bypass graft surgery costs in the Austin 2003 publication ranged from 3.5% to 19.1% of the actual cost, with the negative binomial regression resulting in a 5.3% bias (vs. 6% bias in this analysis) [30]. An additional analysis that used a logistic regression to predict stroke treatment costs resulted in a 3% bias (range 0–5% of actual cost, depending on the subgroup analyzed), with the paper concluding that the predictive model's minimal bias directly confirmed its accuracy [31].

There are limitations in this analysis. The ICD-9-CM code for systemic MS does not distinguish between different MS types. Not all indicators of disease status may be captured in all-cause total medical costs as assessed by healthcare claims. Findings could be confounded by cost variations across settings, but relative relationships could be expected to hold. Also, a limited number of patients had very high MS or general health scores (mean disease status scores in the highest tertile did not exceed 25 out of a maximum score of 100 in either condition group). It is, therefore, difficult to evaluate the predictive accuracy of the model at the highest levels of MS disease status that were not present in the database. Finally, there is a possible lack of generalizability of the data given the inherent characteristics of claims databases and sample cohorts. The sample consisted of US patients with commercial claims. US patients with commercial claims are typically younger than 65 years of age, and most likely come from an employed population since they have commercial insurance; therefore, they may have better access to treatment. Also, the magnitude of claims is expected to be different in non-US patients; however, the conditions that are associated with high claims may still be relevant to other countries. Further research in other populations is warranted.

Conclusions

This analysis demonstrated that claims-based measures that incorporate MS-specific as well as general health components can be used as indicators for disease status in patients with MS treated with DMDs. The performance of the predictive model is consistent with other published validated models. Healthcare decision makers and researchers may use these models to better ascertain the disease status of patients with MS. This may help in identifying patients likely to benefit from intervention and help to assess the value and effectiveness of treatments.

Abbreviations
BIC: Bayesian information criteria; *CCS*: Clinical Classification System; *DMD*: Disease-modifying drug; *ER*: Emergency room,; *ICD-9-CM*: International Classification of Diseases, Ninth Revision, Clinical Modification; *IQR*: Interquartile range; *MAPE*: Mean absolute prediction error; *MS*: Multiple sclerosis.; *SAS*: Statistical Analysis Software.; *SD*: Standard deviation.

Acknowledgements
The authors thank Natalie Edwards of Health Services Consulting Corporation, Boxborough, MA, USA (supported by EMD Serono, Inc., Rockland, MA, USA [a business of Merck KGaA, Darmstadt, Germany]) for editorial assistance in drafting the manuscript, collating the comments of authors, and assembling tables and figures.

Funding
This study was supported by EMD Serono, Inc., Rockland, MA, USA (a business of Merck KGaA, Darmstadt, Germany) and Pfizer Inc., New York, NY, USA. EMD Serono, Inc., Rockland, MA, USA also funded editorial assistance in the preparation of this article.

Authors' contributions
MM, MF, and JM were involved in the design of the study, the analysis and interpretation of data, and in writing the manuscript. AP was involved in the design of the study, in the interpretation of data, and in writing the manuscript. All authors read and approved the final manuscript.

Competing interests
MM and JM are employees of Boston Health Economics, Inc., which received funding from EMD Serono, Inc., to conduct the analyses. MF is a former employee of Boston Health Economics, Inc. AP is an employee of EMD Serono, Inc., Rockland, MA, USA (a business of Merck KGaA, Darmstadt, Germany). The authors received no funding for their participation in the writing of the manuscript.

Author details
[1]Boston Health Economics, Inc., 20 Fox Road, Waltham, MA 02451, USA. [2]Health Economics & Outcomes Research, EMD Serono, Inc., One Technology Place, Rockland, MA 02370, USA.

References
1. Compston A, Coles A. Multiple sclerosis. Lancet. 2002;359:1221–31.
2. National Multiple Sclerosis Society. Multiple Sclerosis FAQs. Last updated 2016 [cited 18 Mar 2016]. Available from: http://www.nationalmssociety.org/What-is-MS/MS-FAQ-s
3. Baghizadeh S, Sahraian MA, Beladimoghadam N. Clinical and demographic factors affecting disease severity in patients with multiple sclerosis. Iran J Neurol. 2013;12:1–8.

4. Disanto G, Berlanga AJ, Handel AE, Para AE, Burrell AM, Fries A, et al. Heterogeneity in multiple sclerosis: scratching the surface of a complex disease. Autoimmune Dis. 2010;2011:932351.

5. Marrie RA. Comorbidity in multiple sclerosis: some answers, more questions. Int J MS Care. 2016;18:271–2.

6. Signori A, Schiavetti I, Gallo F, Sormani MP. Subgroups of multiple sclerosis patients with larger treatment benefits: a meta-analysis of randomized trials. Eur J Neurol. 2015;22:960–6.

7. Chrischilles E, Schneider K, Wilwert J, Lessman G, O'Donnell B, Gryzlak B, et al. Beyond comorbidity: expanding the definition and measurement of complexity among older adults using administrative claims data. Med Care. 2014;52(Suppl 3):S75–84.

8. Macaulay D, Sun SX, Sorg RA, Yan SY, De G, Wu EQ, et al. Development and validation of a claims-based prediction model for COPD severity. Respir med. 2013;107:1568–77.

9. Sung SF, Hsieh CY, Kao Yang YH, Lin HJ, Chen CH, Chen YW, et al. Developing a stroke severity index based on administrative data was feasible using data mining techniques. J Clin Epidemiol. 2015;68: 1292–300.

10. Bergvall N, Makin C, Lahoz R, Agashivala N, Pradhan A, Capkun G, et al. Comparative effectiveness of fingolimod versus interferons or glatiramer acetate for relapse rates in multiple sclerosis: a retrospective US claims database analysis. Curr med res Opin. 2013;29:1647–56.

11. Bergvall N, Makin C, Lahoz R, Agashivala N, Pradhan A, Capkun G, et al. Relapse rates in patients with multiple sclerosis switching from interferon to fingolimod or glatiramer acetate: a US claims database study. PLoS One. 2014;9:e88472.

12. Bergvall N, Lahoz R, Reynolds T, Korn JR. Healthcare resource use and relapses with fingolimod versus natalizumab for treating multiple sclerosis: a retrospective US claims database analysis. Curr med res Opin. 2014;30:1461–71.

13. Capkun G, Lahoz R, Verdun E, Song X, Chen W, Korn JR, et al. Expanding the use of administrative claims databases in conducting clinical real-world evidence studies in multiple sclerosis. Curr med res Opin. 2015;31:1029–39.

14. Castelli-Haley J, Oleen-Burkey MA, Lage MJ, Johnson K. Glatiramer acetate and interferon beta-1a for intramuscular administration: a study of outcomes among multiple sclerosis intent-to-treat and persistent-use cohorts. J med Econ. 2010;13:464–71.

15. Halpern R, Agarwal S, Dembek C, Borton L, Lopez-Bresnahan M. Comparison of adherence and persistence among multiple sclerosis patients treated with disease-modifying therapies: a retrospective administrative claims analysis. Patient Prefer Adherence. 2011;5:73–84.

16. Ivanova JI, Bergman RE, Birnbaum HG, Phillips AL, Stewart M, Meletiche DM. Impact of medication adherence to disease-modifying drugs on severe relapse, and direct and indirect costs among employees with multiple sclerosis in the US. J med Econ. 2012;15:601–9.

17. Johnson BH, Bonafede MM, Watson C. Platform therapy compared with natalizumab for multiple sclerosis: relapse rates and time to relapse among propensity score-matched US patients. CNS Drugs. 2015;29:503–10.

18. Kozma CM, Phillips AL, Meletiche DM. Use of an early disease-modifying drug adherence measure to predict future adherence in patients with multiple sclerosis. J Manag Care Spec Pharm. 2014;20:800–7.

19. Tan H, Cai Q, Agarwal S, Stephenson JJ, Kamat S. Impact of adherence to disease-modifying therapies on clinical and economic outcomes among patients with multiple sclerosis. Adv Ther. 2011;28:51–61.

20. Goldman MD, Motl RW, Rudick RA. Possible clinical outcome measures for clinical trials in patients with multiple sclerosis. Ther adv Neurol Disord. 2010;3:229–39.

21. Marrie RA, Hanwell H. General health issues in multiple sclerosis: comorbidities, secondary conditions, and health behaviors. Continuum (Minneap Minn). 2013;19:1046–57.

22. Mitchell AJ, Benito-Leon J, Gonzalez JM, Rivera-Navarro J. Quality of life and its assessment in multiple sclerosis: integrating physical and psychological components of wellbeing. Lancet Neurol. 2005;4:556–66.

23. Bueno AM, Sayao AL, Yousefi M, Devonshire V, Traboulsee A, Tremlett H. Health-related quality of life in patients with longstanding 'benign multiple sclerosis'. Mult Scler Relat Disord. 2015;4:31–8.

24. Kalincik T, Cutter G, Spelman T, Jokubaitis V, Havrdova E, Horakova D, et al. Defining reliable disability outcomes in multiple sclerosis. Brain. 2015;138: 3287–98.

25. Uitdehaag BM. Clinical outcome measures in multiple sclerosis. Handb Clin Neurol. 2014;122:393–404.

26. Zhang J, Waubant E, Cutter G, Wolinsky J, Leppert D. Composite end points to assess delay of disability progression by MS treatments. Mult Scler. 2014; 20:1494–501.

27. Henriksson F, Fredrikson S, Masterman T, Jonsson B. Costs, quality of life and disease severity in multiple sclerosis: a cross-sectional study in Sweden. Eur J Neurol. 2001;8:27–35.

28. Kobelt G, Berg J, Lindgren P, Fredrikson S, Jonsson B. Costs and quality of life of patients with multiple sclerosis in Europe. J Neurol Neurosurg Psychiatry. 2006;77:918–26.

29. Raftery AE. Bayesian model selection in social research. Sociol Methodol. 1995;25:111–63.

30. Austin PC, Ghali WA, Tu JV. A comparison of several regression models for analysing cost of CABG surgery. Stat med. 2003;22:2799–815.

31. Caro JJ, Huybrechts KF, Kelley HE. Predicting treatment costs after acute ischemic stroke on the basis of patient characteristics at presentation and early dysfunction. Stroke. 2001;32:100–6.

9

Cognitive rehabilitation and mindfulness in multiple sclerosis (REMIND-MS)

Ilse M. Nauta[1*], Anne E. M. Speckens[2], Roy P. C. Kessels[3,4], Jeroen J. G. Geurts[5], Vincent de Groot[6], Bernard M. J. Uitdehaag[1], Luciano Fasotti[3,7] and Brigit A. de Jong[1]

Abstract

Background: Cognitive problems frequently occur in patients with multiple sclerosis (MS) and profoundly affect their quality of life. So far, the best cognitive treatment options for MS patients are a matter of debate. Therefore, this study aims to investigate the effectiveness of two promising non-pharmacological treatments: cognitive rehabilitation therapy (CRT) and mindfulness-based cognitive therapy (MBCT). Furthermore, this study aims to gain additional knowledge about the aetiology of cognitive problems among MS patients, since this may help to develop and guide effective cognitive treatments.

Methods/design: In a dual-centre, single-blind randomised controlled trial (RCT), 120 MS patients will be randomised into one of three parallel groups: CRT, MBCT or enhanced treatment as usual (ETAU). Both CRT and MBCT consist of a structured 9-week program. ETAU consists of one appointment with an MS specialist nurse. Measurements will be performed at baseline, post-intervention and 6 months after the interventions. The primary outcome measure is the level of subjective cognitive complaints. Secondary outcome measures are objective cognitive function, functional brain network measures (using magnetoencephalography), psychological symptoms, well-being, quality of life and daily life functioning.

Discussion: To our knowledge, this will be the first RCT that investigates the effect of MBCT on cognitive function among MS patients. In addition, studying the effect of CRT on cognitive function may provide direction to the contradictory evidence that is currently available. This study will also provide information on changes in functional brain networks in relation to cognitive function. To conclude, this study may help to understand and treat cognitive problems among MS patients.

Keywords: Multiple sclerosis, Cognition, Cognitive rehabilitation therapy, Mindfulness-based cognitive therapy, Brain networks, Randomised controlled trial

* Correspondence: i.nauta1@vumc.nl
[1]Department of Neurology, Amsterdam Neuroscience, MS Center Amsterdam, VU University Medical Center, PO Box 7057, 1007 MB Amsterdam, the Netherlands
Full list of author information is available at the end of the article

Background

Multiple sclerosis (MS) is a chronic disease of the central nervous system, which leads to physical, neuropsychiatric and cognitive problems. Cognitive problems are commonly reported by MS patients, with prevalence rates of objective cognitive deficits varying between 43 and 70% [1]. The most frequently affected cognitive domains are information processing speed, memory, attention, visuospatial processing and executive function. These objective cognitive deficits (i.e. assessed with cognitive tests) only show a weak relation with the cognitive complaints reported by MS patients themselves [2, 3]. Despite this weak relation, subjectively experienced cognitive problems are arguably as important as objective cognitive deficits, since they may reflect the burden of cognitive problems in daily life.

The impact of cognitive problems on daily life can be extensive given the relatively young age of disease onset. Problems in social relations and work participation are likely to occur, consequently negatively affecting the quality of life of MS patients [1, 4]. This highlights the need for effective cognitive treatment options for MS patients. To develop and guide effective cognitive treatments, knowledge about the aetiology of objective and subjective cognitive problems is essential.

Aetiology of cognitive problems

The aetiology of objective and subjective cognitive problems in MS is complex and not completely understood. Objective cognitive deficits in MS patients have been linked to cortical, deep grey matter and white matter damage [5, 6]. Researchers have argued that this widespread pathology may result in a disruption of the connectivity between brain regions, which in turn may result in cognitive decline [7]. Changes in brain networks are indeed present in MS patients: studies have reported changes in functional connectivity [7] and a loss of hierarchal structure [8], which both related to reduced objective cognitive performance in MS patients.

Whereas the aetiology of objective cognitive deficits is widely studied, studies focusing on the aetiology of subjective cognitive complaints are rare. Since subjective and objective cognitive problems correlate weakly [2, 3], their aetiology might be different [9]. One recent study found that subjectively experienced cognitive problems could not be explained by brain pathology, but no measures of brain networks were included [9]. To date, the study of brain networks and their relation to objective and subjective cognitive function among MS patients is still in its infancy. Additional well-designed studies are needed to unravel the aetiology of objective and subjective cognitive problems in MS.

Treatment of cognitive problems

The best cognitive treatment options for MS patients are still a matter of debate [10]. A promising non-pharmacological treatment option is cognitive rehabilitation therapy (CRT) [10]. CRT entails the learning of new cognitive strategies aimed at compensating for cognitive problems. The use of these strategies shows positive effects on cognitive function among stroke and brain injury patients [11]. There is also some evidence for positive effects of CRT on cognitive function among MS patients. However, no final conclusion on the effectiveness of CRT can be established due to contradictory findings [12, 13]. These contradictory findings may be explained by small sample sizes, heterogeneous interventions across studies and methodological limitations (e.g. biased selection) [12, 13].

A second promising non-pharmacological treatment option is mindfulness-based cognitive therapy (MBCT) [14]. MBCT entails mindfulness training combined with elements of cognitive behavioural therapy. There is preliminary evidence that mindfulness-based interventions positively affect cognitive function in healthy individuals [14, 15] and they may even influence brain structures and functions that are involved in cognitive function [14, 16, 17]. In MS patients, positive effects of mindfulness-based interventions on psychological symptoms have been found [18–20], and a recent pilot study reported some positive effects of mindfulness on objective cognitive function [19]. To our knowledge, no other studies have investigated the effect of mindfulness-based interventions on cognitive function among MS patients. In summary, well-designed studies are necessary to investigate the effect of MBCT and CRT on cognitive function among patients with MS.

The REMIND-MS study

The REMIND-MS study is a randomised controlled trial (RCT) that investigates the effect of CRT and MBCT on subjective and objective cognitive function in MS patients. Additionally, resting-state magnetoencephalography (MEG) data will be obtained to gain additional knowledge about the aetiology of subjective and objective cognitive problems with respect to functional brain networks, and to unravel if cognitive improvements after both interventions are associated with functional brain network changes.

Objectives

This study primarily aims to examine the effectiveness of CRT and MBCT on subjectively experienced cognitive problems among MS patients. We hypothesise that both CRT and MBCT positively affect subjective cognitive function compared to enhanced treatment as usual (ETAU). We also expect positive effects on the secondary outcome measures objective cognitive function, functional brain network measures, psychological symptoms, well-being, quality of life and daily life functioning. Additionally, we will evaluate in an exploratory way whether there are differences in intervention effects between CRT and MBCT.

Secondary study objectives are:

1) to explore the role of functional brain network measures (using MEG) in subjective and objective cognitive problems, and to evaluate whether there are differences in functional brain network measures between these types of cognitive problems;
2) to explore the role of functional brain network measures as possible mediators in the effect of the interventions;
3) to evaluate whether alterations in objective cognitive function, functional brain network measures, psychological symptoms, well-being, quality of life and daily life functioning are mediating factors that determine subjective cognitive function;
4) to evaluate which factors determine whether a patient is likely to benefit from one of the therapies, such disease severity, severity of cognitive problems and mood at baseline, or gender.

Methods-design
Design
The REMIND-MS study is a dual-centre, single-blind RCT with three parallel groups: CRT, MBCT and ETAU. All interventions last nine weeks in total. Measurements take place at baseline, post-intervention and after a 6-month follow-up period. The full trial design is summarised in Fig. 1.

Setting
Selection and measurements take place at the VU University Medical Center in Amsterdam, the Netherlands. Part of the measurements, that is, the self-report questionnaires, can be completed by the participants at home. The interventions take place at two centres in the Netherlands: VU University Medical Center in Amsterdam and Klimmendaal Rehabilitation Center in Arnhem.

Participants
Recruitment and consent
Participants are recruited through the participating centres (VU University Medical Center and Klimmendaal Rehabilitation Center), the 'VUmc MS Center Amsterdam' website and MS patient associations. All potentially eligible participants who express interest in the study are provided with written trial information, which contains information about the rationale, purpose and personal implications of the study. The information sheet also includes contact details of the trial coordinator and of an independent medical doctor who is not part of the research team, who can both be contacted for additional information. After sufficient time for consideration, potential participants who are still interested to participate are invited by the trial coordinator to sign the informed consent form. After signing the informed consent form, it will be checked whether the participants are fully eligible.

On the informed consent form, participants have the option to give permission for an informant to be contacted. If permission is given, an informant of the participants will also receive written information and an informed consent form, as informants will be asked to complete one questionnaire at three time-points (see outcome measures). On the informed consent form, participants and their informants also have the option to give permission for using their data for other research, for sharing their data with researchers outside of the European Union and to be contacted again for follow-up research.

Inclusion criteria
Participants are eligible to participate if they meet the following criteria: (1) between 18 and 65 years of age, (2) confirmed diagnosis of MS according to the McDonald 2010 criteria [21], (3) a minimum score of 23 on the Multiple Sclerosis Neuropsychological Questionnaire – Patient version (MSNQ-P), which measures subjective cognitive complaints [22].

Exclusion criteria
Participants who meet any of the following criteria are excluded from participation: (1) psychosis, (2) suicidal ideation, (3) an inability to speak or read Dutch, (4) previous experience with a similar intervention (e.g. a comparable cognitive rehabilitation training or mindfulness training), (5) physical or cognitive disabilities, comorbidities or treatments that would interfere too much with the interventions to enrol in this study (to be evaluated on an individual level). The reasons for excluding participants who express interest in the study will be accurately documented.

Sample size calculation
Mixed model analyses will be applied with three measurements comparing two groups (MBCT vs. ETAU, CRT vs. ETAU). There are no previous studies with MS patients that investigated the effect of CRT or MBCT on the primary outcome measure, the Cognitive Failure Questionnaire (CFQ) [23]. Based on a previous RCT using a comparable outcome measure, a medium effect size can be expected [24, 25]. With an alpha of .05, a power of .80, an intra-class correlation of .06, and 33 participants per group, a minimal difference of 0.62 SD can be detected between two groups. Taking into account drop-out and loss to follow-up, we intend to recruit 40 MS patients per group.

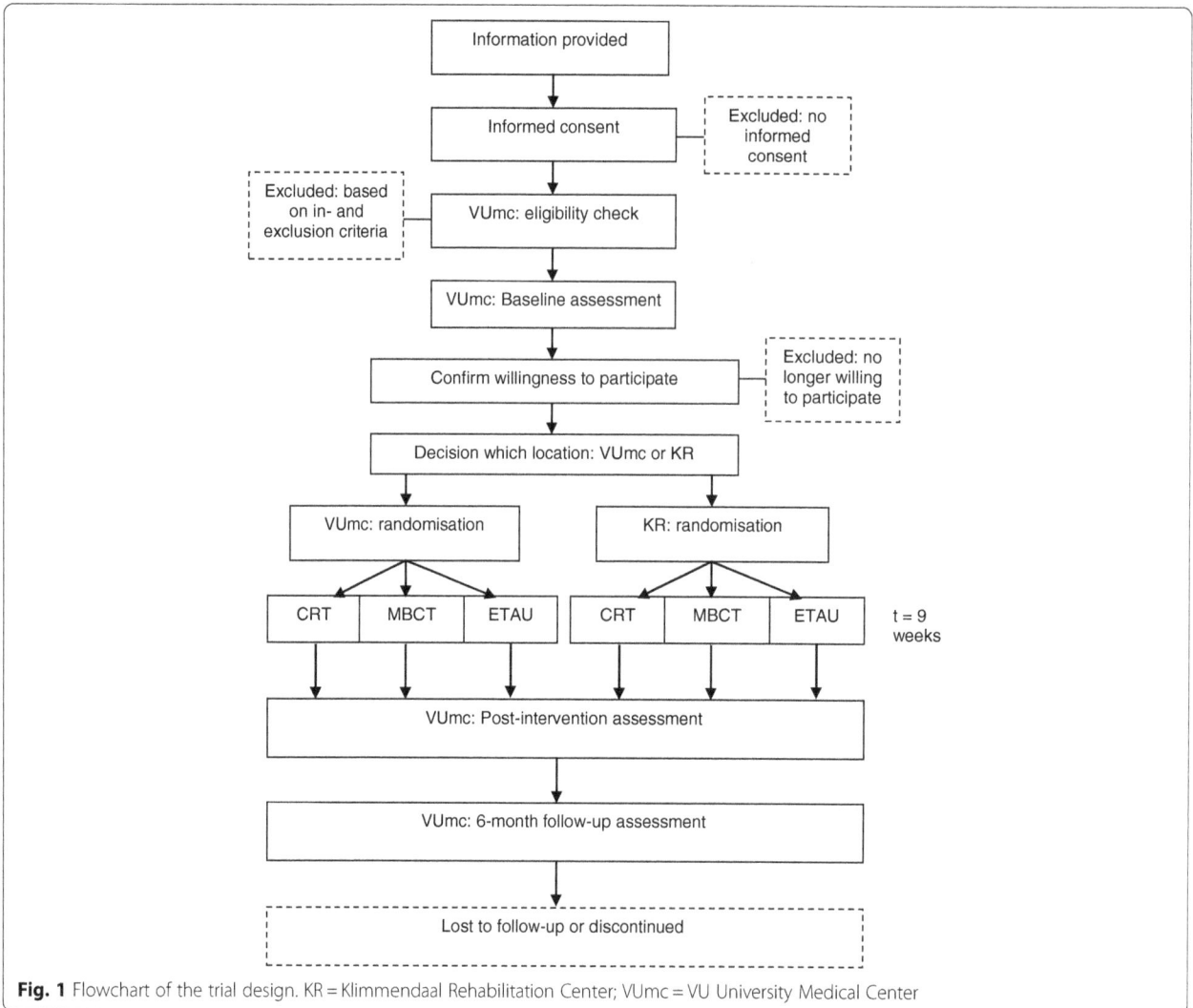

Fig. 1 Flowchart of the trial design. KR = Klimmendaal Rehabilitation Center; VUmc = VU University Medical Center

Interventions

All interventions last nine weeks. The CRT consists of nine 2.5-h group sessions, MBCT of eight 2.5-h group sessions and one 'silent day', and enhanced treatment as usual (ETAU) of one individual appointment within the 9-week period. For CRT and MBCT, the optimal group size was determined based on previous experiences. Groups will consist of a maximum of 6 people in the CRT group and a maximum of 10 people in the MBCT group. Professionally trained psychologists will guide the CRT sessions, certified mindfulness trainers will teach the MBCT sessions and MS specialist nurses will have appointments with participants from the ETAU group. All trainers will be instructed and supervised by the same specialists. The interventions will be provided in a standardised manner using a written protocol. The trainers are instructed not to disclose treatment information to trainers from another treatment arm. All participants will receive an information brochure on MS and cognition.

Cognitive rehabilitation therapy (CRT)

The CRT protocol focuses on the following cognitive domains: speed of information processing, memory, executive function and mental fatigue. Cognitive impairments will be treated by a combination of compensatory strategy training and psycho-education. The proposed strategies are based on MS-tailored variants of evidence-based treatments that have been developed in CRT research with brain-injured subjects. Treatment of problems in information processing speed will be based on 'Time Pressure Management' [26, 27], memory on 'Training Memory strategies' [28], executive function on a 'Multifaceted Treatment for Executive Dysfunction' [29, 30] and mental fatigue on 'Cognitive and Graded Activity Training' [31, 32]. These four treatments are incorporated in the protocol as described by Geusgens, Baars-Elsinga, Visser-Meily and van Heugten [33]. In addition to cognitive strategy training, CRT focuses on emotional and behavioural changes, and grief resolution. Grief resolution will be included by explaining the stages of bereavement and by discussing the loss of physical independence, mobility, cognitive ability and emotional control on self-esteem and future perspective. The participants will receive homework assignments aimed at identifying their own cognitive problems and at applying the learned strategies in daily life situation. These homework assignments will take 30 to 45 min a day, 6 days per week.

Mindfulness based cognitive therapy (MBCT)

The MBCT protocol is primarily based on the MBCT program by Segal, Williams and Teasdale [34]. MBCT is an intervention in which aspects of mindfulness meditation are combined with aspects of cognitive behavioural therapy. MBCT focuses on increasing awareness of the present moment. To achieve this, participants will be trained in both self-regulation of attention and non-judgmental awareness of moment-to-moment experience. Patients will become more aware of their emotions, thoughts and behaviours and will learn to use more adaptive behaviour to respond to their symptoms. The program will be adapted to the MS patients in terms of tailoring psycho-educative elements to themes relevant to the MS patient (e.g. cognitive problems) and modified movement exercises (for patients suffering from physical impairments). Participants will receive guided mindfulness meditation exercises of 30 to 45 min, 6 days per week, for home practice and a reader with home practice instructions and background information. All therapists will fulfil the advanced criteria of the Association of Mindfulness Based Teachers in the Netherlands and Flanders, which are in concordance with those of the UK Mindfulness-Based Teacher Trainer Network [35].

Enhanced treatment as usual (ETAU)

Enhanced treatment as usual (ETAU) entails an appointment with an MS specialist nurse in addition to usual care. The appointment will focus on psycho-education. More specifically, the MS specialist nurse will provide the participants with information on the frequently affected cognitive domains in MS and their relation to brain pathology. This will occur in a standardised manner.

Teacher ratings

CRT and MBCT sessions will be recorded on video to evaluate teacher competence and protocol adherence. These video recordings will solely be used for the purpose of trainer evaluation, and the camera will be directed at the trainer. For the CRT sessions, adherence to the protocol will be checked using a checklist. For the MBCT sessions, the Mindfulness-Based Interventions - Teachers Assessment Criteria [36] will be used.

Adherence

For all groups, attendance to the sessions will be documented. For the CRT group, adherence to homework assignments will be checked and evaluated during each visit of the treatment period. For the MBCT group, adherence will be assessed during the entire treatment period with a calendar on which participants fill out whether they adhere to both formal (e.g. the sitting meditation) and informal (e.g. 3-min breathing space) mindfulness exercises.

Replacement and follow-up of withdrawn participants

Participants can leave the study at any time for any reason without any consequences. Follow-up measurements will still be scheduled if the participant is willing and able to participate in follow-up measurements. There will be no replacement of individual participants after withdrawal. If a high rate of participants drops out during the study, more participants will be included in the study. These participants will be randomly allocated to one of three parallel groups using the randomisation and minimisation procedure as described under 'randomisation and blinding'.

Relevant concomitant care and interventions

During the intervention period and the 6-months follow-up period, patients are asked not to follow an intervention outside this study that focuses on mindfulness or cognition, and to keep their level of care constant during this period when possible. Naturally, usual care should continue, as do new treatment options when the health situation of the patient changes.

Demographic and patient characteristics

At baseline, the following demographic characteristics are collected: age, gender, work status and education. In addition, the following clinical characteristics will be noted: comorbid condition as defined by the Cumulative Illness Rating Scale (CIRS) [37], subtype of MS, year of diagnosis, disease duration and MS disability as defined by the Expanded Disability Status Scale (EDSS) [38]. If an EDSS score is not available, or if this score has been determined more than three months ago, a new EDSS score will be gathered at baseline. The use of medication will be noted at each assessment. Health care consumption will be measured with a questionnaire on healthcare utilisation and productivity losses in patients with a psychiatric disorder (TIC-P) [39] and will be administered at each measurement. Table 1 presents an overview of the demographic and patient characteristics that will be collected at each assessment.

Outcome measures

All outcome measures will be administered at each assessment: at baseline, post-intervention and 6-months follow-up (see Table 1).

Table 1 Overview of outcome measures per assessment

Assessment	Baseline	Post-intervention	Follow-up
Demographic characteristics	X		
Medical history (e.g. MS subtype)	X		
Use of medication	X	X	X
Expanded Disability Status Scale (EDSS)	X		
Health care consumption	X	X	X
Questionnaires measuring subjective cognitive complaints, psychological symptoms, quality of life, well-being and daily life functioning	X	X	X
Neuropsychological assessment	X	X	X
Magnetoencephalography (MEG)	X	X	X
Qualitative data to improve the interventions		X	

Primary outcome measure

The primary outcome measure is the level of subjective cognitive complaints and is measured with the CFQ [23]. Subjective cognitive complaints in terms of executive function will be measured with the Behaviour Rating Inventory of Executive Function – Adult Version (BRIEF-A) [40]. The BRIEF-A consists of a self- and an informant report version.

Secondary outcome measures

Cognitive function A test battery based on the Minimal Assessment of Cognitive Function in MS (MACFIMS) will be used [41]. Verbal learning and memory is assessed with the Dutch version of the California Verbal learning Test (CVLT) [42]. Spatial learning and memory are measured with the Brief Visuospatial Memory Test-Revised (BVMT-R) [43]. Visual-spatial abilities are measured with the Benton Judgment of Line Orientation Test (JLO) [44]. Visual processing speed and working memory are measured with the Symbol Digit Modalities Test (SDMT) [45]. Verbal fluency and memory retrieval are assessed with the Controlled Oral Word Association Test (COWAT) [46]. Higher executive function is measured with the Delis-Kaplan Executive Function System sorting test (D-KEFS) free sorting condition [47]. Selective attention and response inhibition are measured with the Stroop Colour-Word Test [48]. When available, parallel versions of tests will be administered for repeated assessment to account for material-specific learning effects.

Functional brain networks Resting-state MEG data will be recorded using a 306-channel whole-head MEG system (Elekta Neuromag Inc., Helsinki, Finland) in a magnetically shielded room (Vacuumschmelze GmbH, Hanau, Germany) at the VU University Medical Center. Magnetic fields will be recorded during resting state (i.e. a no-task, eyes-closed condition). Pre-processing of data and removal of noise will be done on Linux computers

with available scripts [49]. The MEG data will be used to determine resting-state functional connectivity and brain network organisation. To study functional connectivity, synchronisation measures will be computed, such as the phase-lag index [7, 50]. To study brain network organisation, tools from modern network theory will be applied to the entire network and a subset of the network (i.e. the minimum spanning tree (MST)) [8, 50]. Measures such as degree, clustering coefficient and path length will be computed, as well as MST-network derived measures, such as betweenness centrality, tree hierarchy and eccentricity. There will be an emphasis on node centrality measures to identify the 'hubs' (i.e. highly connected nodes) of the network [51]. Since the field of modern network science is constantly developing, the best methods and measures will be selected once the study is completed.

Psychological symptoms Depression and anxiety are measured with the Hospital Anxiety and Depression Scale (HADS) [52]. The level of fatigue is measured with the Checklist Individual Strength-20-r (CIS-20-r) [53]. The tendency to ruminate when being sad or depressed is measured with the subscale 'brooding' of the Dutch Ruminative Response Scale (RRS-NL) [54].

Quality of life Health-related quality of life is measured with the Multiple Sclerosis Quality of Life Questionnaire (MSQoL-54) [55].

Well-being Emotional, psychological and social well-being is measured with the Mental Health Continuum-Short Form (MHC-SF) [56]. The ability to be mindful, that is, non-judgmental awareness of moment-to-moment experience, is measured with the Five Facets of the Mindfulness Questionnaire short form (FFMQ-SF) [57]. Self-compassion, that is, the ability to act with compassion towards oneself in difficult times, is measured with the short form of the Self-Compassion Scale (SCS-SF) [58].

Daily life functioning Participation in society is measured with the Utrecht Scale for Evaluation of Rehabilitation – Participation (USER-P) [59]. Goal Attainment Scaling (GAS) is used to determine the effect of the treatment on personalised goals in daily situations [60].

Randomisation and blinding
Following baseline assessment, participants will be randomly allocated to one of three treatment arms (MBCT, CRT or ETAU). First, the location of the intervention will be determined based on the patient's living location and preference. For each location, randomisation will be performed in variable blocks of 6 and 9, and with an 1:1:1 allocation ratio. A minimisation program will be used to ensure balance between all groups. Minimisation will be performed on three factors: (1) subjective cognitive function, (2) age and (3) gender. Weighting is equal for each factor. The minimisation program will be constructed before the start of the study by an independent scientific programmer. The randomisation procedure will be performed by a researcher who is not involved in administering any outcome measure. Outcome measurements will be administered by assessors who are blind to treatment assignment, but this blinding is not feasible with regard to participants and therapists. Prior to each post-measurement, participants will be reminded not to disclose their group allocation to the assessor.

Data management
The collected data will be labelled with a participant identification code. The name and other identifiers of the participant will be removed from the data. The link between the participant identification code and the names of the participants will be kept separately. An electronic case report form is developed according to the guidelines of Good Clinical Practice (GCP) to document the data collected in the study. This case report form will include demographic and clinical characteristics, and all outcomes of the study parameters. The data will be treated confidentially and will only be available to the trial coordinator and principal investigator. Other investigators can only get access to the data for the purpose of research and with permission of the principal investigator. The data gathered in this study will be protected in accordance with the Dutch Personal Data Protection Act and the Medical Treatment Contracts Act.

Statistical analysis
Descriptive statistics
Data on demographic and clinical characteristics will be summarised in a table. For adherence and other feasibility indicators, frequencies and percentages will be calculated. Satisfaction with the program will be summarised in qualitative descriptions. Differences between groups (CRT vs. ETAU, MBCT vs. ETAU, CRT vs. MBCT, drop-outs vs. treatment completers) in demographic and clinical characteristics and outcome measurements at baseline are analysed using independent samples t-tests (normally distributed continuous outcome variables), Mann-Whitney U tests (skewed continuous outcome variables) and Pearson's chi-square tests (categorical outcome variables).

Primary and secondary objectives
To evaluate the effectiveness of the interventions, mixed-model analyses will be performed for the primary and secondary outcome measurements with time (baseline, post-intervention, follow-up) as a within subjects factor and condition (CRT vs. ETAU, MBCT vs. ETAU, and exploratory: CRT vs. MBCT) as a between-subjects factor. These analyses will be performed using an intention-to-treat approach, including all randomised participants regardless of adherence and measurement completion. Secondarily, per-protocol analyses will be performed for further exploration of the intervention effects.

To evaluate the secondary study aims, mediation and moderation analyses [61] will be performed to evaluate whether alterations in functional brain networks play a role in the effect of the interventions. In addition, cross-sectional associations between functional brain networks and cognitive function (subjective and objective) will be analysed using Pearson's correlation and linear regression analyses. To evaluate whether alterations in secondary study parameters are mediating factors that determine subjective cognitive function, mediation analyses [61] and linear regression analyses will be performed. Finally, logistic and linear regression models will be performed to evaluate which factors determine whether a patient is likely to benefit from one of the therapies.

For all analyses, confounding variables will be inserted, such as age and education. Bonferroni corrections will be applied to correct for multiple comparisons within each objective.

Monitoring and harms
An independent monitor, the Clinical Research Bureau (CRB) of the VU University Medical Center, will monitor the data of this study according to GCP. The CRB will check the following aspects of the participants: (1) informed consents, (2) source data verification, (3) the reported (serious) adverse events ((S)AEs). Considering the nature of this study, SAEs are not expected. All AEs that are reported spontaneously by the participant or observed by the research staff or therapists will be recorded. All SAEs will be reported by the investigator to the sponsor, and the sponsor will inform the accredited Medical Ethics Committee (MEC).

Discussion

The best treatment options for cognitive problems in MS patients are still a matter of debate. This study will therefore investigate the effect of two promising non-pharmacological treatments: MBCT and CRT. To our knowledge, this will be the first RCT that investigates the effect of MBCT on cognitive function among MS patients. In addition, studying the effect of CRT on cognitive function may provide direction to the contradictory evidence that is currently available [12, 13]. If these treatments appear to be effective, we will investigate which factors predict this beneficial effect. These prognostic factors may lead towards tailored treatments for MS patients who suffer from cognitive problems.

An important strength of our study is that we use functional brain network measures, such as functional connectivity and nodal centrality, as an outcome variable. These measures may help to explain treatment effects and may provide information on whether network deterioration can be halted. Additionally, if functional brain network measures at baseline predict treatment outcomes, network analyses can be used as a prognostic factor. We will also relate functional brain network measures to objective and subjective cognitive problems in MS, which may help to understand the overlap and distinctiveness between these types of cognitive problems.

In summary, this study may help to unravel and treat cognitive problems among MS patients.

Abbreviations

AE: Adverse event; BRIEF-A: Behaviour Rating Inventory of Executive Function – Adult Version; BVMT-R: Brief visuospatial memory test-revised; CFQ: Cognitive failure questionnaire; CIRS: Cumulative illness rating scale; CIS-20-r: Checklist individual strength-20-r; COWAT: Controlled oral word association test; CRB: Clinical Research Bureau; CRT: Cognitive rehabilitation therapy; CVLT: California verbal learning test; CWO: Scientific Research Committee; D-KEFS: Delis-Kaplan Executive Function System sorting test; EDSS: Expanded disability status scale; ETAU: Enhanced treatment as usual; FFMQ-SF: Five facets of mindfulness questionnaire short form; GAS: Goal attainment scale; GCP: Good clinical practice; HADS: Hospital anxiety and depression scale; JLO: Judgment of line orientation test; KR: Klimmendaal Rehabilitation Center; MBCT: Mindfulness-based cognitive therapy; MEC: Medical Ethics Committee; MEG: Magnetoencephalography; MHC-SF: Mental Health Continuum-Short Form; MS: Multiple sclerosis; MSNQ-P: Multiple Sclerosis Neuropsychological Questionnaire – Patient version; MSQoL-54: Multiple sclerosis quality of life questionnaire; MST: Minimum spanning tree; RCT: Randomised controlled trial; REMIND-MS: Cognitive Rehabilitation and Mindfulness in Multiple Sclerosis; RRS-NL: Dutch Ruminative Response Scale; SAE: Serious adverse event; SCS-SF: Short form of the self-compassion scale; SDMT: Symbol digit modalities test; TIC-P: Questionnaire on healthcare utilisation and productivity losses in patients with a psychiatric disorder; USER-P: Utrecht Scale for Evaluation of Rehabilitation – Participation; VUmc: VU University Medical Center

Acknowledgements

We would like to thank the Dutch MS Research Foundation for funding our project.

Funding

This investigator-initiated trial is funded by the Dutch MS Research Foundation (project number 15–911). The funder had no influence on the design of the protocol, and will not have any impact on data generation, statistical analyses or writing of the final manuscript.

Dissemination policy

When the data collection is completed, the total data set will be analysed and the results will be published in scientific journals and presented at (inter)national scientific meetings. A summary of the results will be released to the participants of this study. The identity of the participants will not be disclosed in any of these publication forms. The researchers of this study will attempt to reduce the time between the completion of data collection and the release of the study results.

Authorship

The principal investigator will justify the names for authorship. Individuals who fulfil authorship criteria will be an author on the manuscripts.

Ancillary and post-trial care

At the end of the study, participants can take part in one of the other interventions of the study. The REMIND-MS study does not provide additional care outside these interventions.

Authors' contributions

BAJ initiated the study, applied for funding and is the principal investigator. IMN is the study coordinator, drafted this manuscript and will perform the data collection. BAJ, LF, AEMS, RPCK, JJGG, VG and BMJU were involved in the conception and design of the study. LF contributed his CRT expertise to the study protocol development and the CRT intervention protocol, and he will train and supervise the CRT therapists. AEMS contributed her mindfulness expertise to the study protocol development and the MBCT intervention protocol, and she will train and supervise the MBCT therapists. RPCK made important statistical contributions. All authors provided feedback on drafts of this paper and read and approved the final manuscript.

Competing interests

The authors declare to have no competing interests.

Author details

[1]Department of Neurology, Amsterdam Neuroscience, MS Center Amsterdam, VU University Medical Center, PO Box 7057, 1007 MB Amsterdam, the Netherlands. [2]Department of Psychiatry, Radboud University Medical Center, PO Box 9101, 6500 HB Nijmegen, the Netherlands. [3]Donders Institute for Brain, Cognition and Behaviour, Radboud University, PO Box 9101, 6500 HB Nijmegen, the Netherlands. [4]Department of Medical Psychology, Radboud University Medical Center, PO Box 9101, 6500 HB Nijmegen, the Netherlands. [5]Department of Anatomy and Neurosciences, Amsterdam Neuroscience, MS Center Amsterdam, VU University Medical Center, PO Box 7057, 1007 MB Amsterdam, the Netherlands. [6]Department of Rehabilitation Medicine, MS Center Amsterdam, VU University Medical Center, PO Box 7057, 1007 MB Amsterdam, the Netherlands. [7]Klimmendaal Rehabilitation Center, PO Box 9044, 6800 CG Arnhem, the Netherlands.

References

1.   Chiaravalloti ND, DeLuca J. Cognitive impairment in multiple sclerosis. Lancet Neurol. 2008;7(12):1139–51.
2.   Benedict RH, Munschauer F, Linn R, Miller C, Murphy E, Foley F, et al. Screening for multiple sclerosis cognitive impairment using a self-administered 15-item questionnaire. Mult Scler. 2003;9(1):95–101.
3.   Kinsinger SW, Lattie E, Mohr DC. Relationship between depression, fatigue, subjective cognitive impairment, and objective neuropsychological functioning in patients with multiple sclerosis. Neuropsychology. 2010;24(5):573–80.
4.   Wynia K, Middel B, van Dijk JP, De Keyser JH, Reijneveld SA. The impact of disabilities on quality of life in people with multiple sclerosis. Mult Scler. 2008;14(7):972–80.

5.   DeLuca GC, Yates RL, Beale H, Morrow SA. Cognitive impairment in multiple sclerosis: clinical, radiologic and pathologic insights. Brain Pathol. 2015; 25(1):79–98.

6.   Rocca MA, Amato MP, De Stefano N, Enzinger C, Geurts JJ, Penner IK, et al. Clinical and imaging assessment of cognitive dysfunction in multiple sclerosis. Lancet Neurol. 2015;14(3):302–17.

7.   Tewarie P, Schoonheim MM, Stam CJ, van der Meer ML, van Dijk BW, Barkhof F, et al. Cognitive and clinical dysfunction, altered MEG resting-state networks and thalamic atrophy in multiple sclerosis. PLoS One. 2013;8(7):e69318.

8.   Tewarie P, Hillebrand A, Schoonheim MM, van Dijk BW, Geurts JJ, Barkhof F, et al. Functional brain network analysis using minimum spanning trees in multiple sclerosis: an MEG source-space study. NeuroImage. 2014;88:308–18.

9.   Hulst HE, Gehring K, Uitdehaag BM, Visser LH, Polman CH, Barkhof F, et al. Indicators for cognitive performance and subjective cognitive complaints in multiple sclerosis: a role for advanced MRI? Mult Scler. 2014;20(8):1131–4.

10. Lovera J, Kovner B. Cognitive impairment in multiple sclerosis. Curr Neurol Neurosci Rep. 2012;12(5):618–27.

11. Cicerone KD, Langenbahn DM, Braden C, Malec JF, Kalmar K, Fraas M, et al. Evidence-based cognitive rehabilitation: updated review of the literature from 2003 through 2008. Arch Phys Med Rehabil. 2011;92(4):519–30.

12. Mitolo M, Venneri A, Wilkinson ID, Sharrack B. Cognitive rehabilitation in multiple sclerosis: a systematic review. J Neurol Sci. 2015;354(1–2):1–9.

13. Rosti-Otajarvi EM, Hamalainen PI. Neuropsychological rehabilitation for multiple sclerosis. Cochrane Database Syst Rev. 2014;2:CD009131.

14. Tang YY, Holzel BK, Posner MI. The neuroscience of mindfulness meditation. Nat Rev Neurosci. 2015;16(4):213–25.

15. Chiesa A, Calati R, Serretti A. Does mindfulness training improve cognitive abilities? A systematic review of neuropsychological findings. Clin Psychol Rev. 2011;31(3):449–64.

16. Fox KC, Nijeboer S, Dixon ML, Floman JL, Ellamil M, Rumak SP, et al. Is meditation associated with altered brain structure? A systematic review and meta-analysis of morphometric neuroimaging in meditation practitioners. Neurosci Biobehav Rev. 2014;43:48–73.

17. Tomasino B, Chiesa A, Fabbro F. Disentangling the neural mechanisms involved in Hinduism- and Buddhism-related meditations. Brain Cogn. 2014;90:32–40.

18. Bogosian A, Chadwick P, Windgassen S, Norton S, McCrone P, Mosweu I, et al. Distress improves after mindfulness training for progressive MS: a pilot randomised trial. Mult Scler. 2015;21(9):1184–94.

19. Blankespoor RJ, Schellekens MPJ, Vos SH, Speckens AEM, de Jong BA. The effectiveness of mindfulness-based stress reduction on psychological distress and cognitive functioning in patients with multiple sclerosis: a pilot study. Mindfulness. 2017; doi:10.1007/s12671-017-0701-6.

20. Grossman P, Kappos L, Gensicke H, D'Souza M, Mohr DC, Penner IK, et al. MS quality of life, depression, and fatigue improve after mindfulness training: a randomized trial. Neurology. 2010;75(13):1141–9.

21. Polman CH, Reingold SC, Banwell B, Clanet M, Cohen JA, Filippi M, et al. Diagnostic criteria for multiple sclerosis: 2010 revisions to the McDonald criteria. Ann Neurol. 2011;69(2):292–302.

22. Sonder JM, Mokkink LB, van der Linden FA, Polman CH, Uitdehaag BM. Validation and interpretation of the Dutch version of the multiple sclerosis neuropsychological screening questionnaire. J Neurol Sci. 2012;320(1–2):91–6.

23. Merckelbach H, Muris P, Nijman H, de Jong PJ. Self-reported cognitive failures and neurotic symptomatology. Pers Indiv Differ. 1996;20(6):715–24.

24. Mantynen A, Rosti-Otajarvi E, Koivisto K, Lilja A, Huhtala H, Hamalainen P. Neuropsychological rehabilitation does not improve cognitive performance but reduces perceived cognitive deficits in patients with multiple sclerosis: a randomised, controlled, multi-centre trial. Mult Scler. 2014;20(1):99–107.

25. Rosti-Otajarvi E, Mantynen A, Koivisto K, Huhtala H, Hamalainen P. Neuropsychological rehabilitation has beneficial effects on perceived cognitive deficits in multiple sclerosis during nine-month follow-up. J Neurol Sci. 2013;334(1–2):154–60.

26. Fasotti L, Kovacs F, Eling PATM, Brouwer WH. Time pressure management as a compensatory strategy training after closed head injury. Neuropsychol Rehabil. 2000;10(1):47–65.

27. Winkens I, Van Heugten CM, Wade DT, Fasotti L. Training patients in time pressure management, a cognitive strategy for mental slowness. Clin Rehabil. 2009;23(1):79–90.

28. van Kessel M, Fasotti L, Berg I, van Hout M, Wekking E. Training geheugenstrategieën. Amsterdam: Boom Uitgevers; 2010.

29. Boelen DH, Spikman JM, Fasotti L. Rehabilitation of executive disorders after brain injury: are interventions effective? J Neuropsychol. 2011;5(Pt 1):73–113.

30. Spikman JM, Boelen DH, Lamberts KF, Brouwer WH, Fasotti L. Effects of a multifaceted treatment program for executive dysfunction after acquired brain injury on indications of executive functioning in daily life. J Int Neuropsychol Soc. 2010;16(1):118–29.

31. Zedlitz AM, Fasotti L, Geurts AC. Post-stroke fatigue: a treatment protocol that is being evaluated. Clin Rehabil. 2011;25(6):487–500.

32. Zedlitz AM, Rietveld TC, Geurts AC, Fasotti L. Cognitive and graded activity training can alleviate persistent fatigue after stroke: a randomized, controlled trial. Stroke. 2012;43(4):1046–51.

33. Geusgens C, Baars-Elsinga A, Visser-Meily A, van Heugten C. Niet Rennen maar Plannen: Trends Service in kommunikatie B.V.; 2012.

34. Segal ZV, Williams JMG, Teasdale JD. Mindfulness-based cognitive therapy for depression. second ed. New York: The Guilford Press; 2013.

35. Good practice guidelines for teaching mindfulness-based courses. UK Mindfulness-Based Teacher Trainer Network. 2011. http://mindfulnessteachersuk. org.uk/pdf/teacher-guidelines.pdf. Accessed 1 June 2017.

36. Crane RS, Kuyken W, Williams JM, Hastings RP, Cooper L, Fennell MJ. Competence in teaching mindfulness-based courses: concepts, development and assessment. Mindfulness (N Y). 2012;3(1):76–84.

37. Miller MD, Paradis CF, Houck PR, Mazumdar S, Stack JA, Rifai AH, et al. Rating chronic medical illness burden in Geropsychiatric practice and research - application of the cumulative illness rating-scale. Psychiatry Res. 1992;41(3):237–48.

38. Kurtzke JF. Rating neurologic impairment in multiple sclerosis: an expanded disability status scale (EDSS). Neurology. 1983;33(11):1444–52.

39. Bouwmans C, Jong KD, Timman R, Zijlstra-Vlasveld M, Van d, Feltz-Cornelis C, Tan SS, et al. Feasibility, reliability and validity of a questionnaire on healthcare consumption and productivity loss in patients with a psychiatric disorder (TiC-P). BMC Health Serv Res. 2013;13

40. Roth RM, Isquith PK, Gioia GA, Widows M. Development of the Behavior Rating Inventory of Executive Function-Adult version. Arch Clin Neuropsych. 2005;20(7):906.

41. Benedict RH, Cookfair D, Gavett R, Gunther M, Munschauer F, Garg N, et al. Validity of the minimal assessment of cognitive function in multiple sclerosis (MACFIMS). J Int Neuropsychol Soc. 2006;12(4):549–58.

42. Mulder JL, Dekker R, Dekker DH. Verbale Leer- & Geheugen test: Handleiding [Verbal Learning & Memory Test: manual]. Lisse, the Netherlands: Swets & Zeitlinger; 1996.

43. Benedict RHB, Schretlen D, Groninger L, Dobraski M, Shpritz B. Revision of the brief visuospatial memory test: studies of normal performance, reliability, and validity. Psychol Assessment. 1996;8(2):145–53.

44. Benton AL, Hamsher KD, Varney NR, Spreen O. Judgment of line orientation. New York: Oxford University Press; 1983.

45. Smith A. Symbol digit modality test (SDMT): manual (revised). Los Angeles. Psychol Serv. 1982;

46. Benton LA, Hamsher KD, Sivan AB. Controlled oral word association test. Multilingual aphasia examination. 3 ed. Iowa City, IA: AJA; 1994.

47. Delis DC, Kaplan E, Kramer JH. The delis-Kaplan executive function system: Examiner's manual. San Antonio: The Psychological Corporation; 2001.

48. Hammes JGW. The STROOP color-word test: manual. Amsterdam: Swets and Zeitlinger; 1973.

49. Hillebrand A, Barnes GR, Bosboom JL, Berendse HW, Stam CJ. Frequency-dependent functional connectivity within resting-state networks: an atlas-based MEG beamformer solution. NeuroImage. 2012;59(4):3909–21.

50. Stam CJ, van Straaten ECW. The organization of physiological brain networks. Clin Neurophysiol. 2012;123(6):1067–87.

51. Stam CJ. Modern network science of neurological disorders. Nat Rev Neurosci. 2014;15(10):683–95.

52. Zigmond AS, Snaith RP. The hospital anxiety and depression scale. Acta Psychiat. Scandinavica. 1983;67(6):361–70.

53. Vercoulen JHMM, Alberts M, Bleijenberg G. De checklist individuele spankracht (CIS). Gedragstherapie. 1999;32:131–6.

54. Raes F, Hermans D, Eelen P. Kort instrumenteel De Nederlandstalige versie van de Ruminative Response Scale (RRS-NL) en de Rumination on Sadness Scale (RSS-NL). Gedragstherapie. 2003;36(2):97–104.

55. Vickrey BG, Hays RD, Harooni R, Myers LW, Ellison GWA. Health-related quality-of-life measure for multiple-sclerosis. Qual Life Res. 1995;4(3):187–206.

56. Lamers SMA, Westerhof GJ, Bohlmeijer ET, ten Klooster PM, Keyes CLM. Evaluating the psychometric properties of the mental health continuum-short form (MHC-SF). J Clin Psychol. 2011;67(1):99–110.

57. Bohlmeijer E, ten Klooster PM, Fledderus M, Veehof M, Baer R. Psychometric properties of the five facet mindfulness questionnaire in depressed adults and development of a short form. Assessment 2011;18(3):308–320.

58. Raes F, Pommier E, Neff KD, Van Gucht D. Construction and factorial validation of a short form of the self-compassion scale. Clin Psychol Psychot 2011;18(3):250–255.

59. Post MWM, van der Zee CH, Hennink J, Schafrat CG, Visser-Meily JMA, van Berlekom SB. Validity of the Utrecht scale for evaluation of rehabilitation-participation. Disabil Rehabil. 2012;34(6):478–85.

60. Kiresuk TJ, Sherman RE. Goal attainment scaling - general method for evaluating comprehensive community mental health programs. Community Ment Hlt J. 1968;4(6):443–53.

61. Holmbeck GN. Toward terminological, conceptual, and statistical clarity in the study of mediators and moderators: examples from the child-clinical and pediatric psychology literatures. J Consult Clin Psychol. 1997;65(4):599–610.

10

Patient-reported questionnaires in MS rehabilitation: responsiveness and minimal important difference of the multiple sclerosis questionnaire for physiotherapists (MSQPT)

Nico Arie van der Maas

Abstract

Background: The Multiple Sclerosis Questionnaire for Physical Therapists (MSQPT) is a patient-rated outcome questionnaire for evaluating the rehabilitation of persons with multiple sclerosis (MS). Responsiveness was evaluated, and minimal important difference (MID) estimates were calculated to provide thresholds for clinical change for four items, three sections and the total score of the MSQPT.

Methods: This multicentre study used a combined distribution- and anchor-based approach with multiple anchors and multiple rating of change questions. Responsiveness was evaluated using effect size, standardized response mean (SRM), modified SRM and relative efficiency. For distribution-based MID estimates, 0.2 and 0.33 standard deviations (SD), standard error of measurement (SEM) and minimal detectable change were used. Triangulation of anchor- and distribution-based MID estimates provided a range of MID values for each of the four items, the three sections and the total score of the MSQPT. The MID values were tested for their sensitivity and specificity for amelioration and deterioration for each of the four items, the three sections and the total score of the MSQPT. The MID values of each item and section and of the total score with the best sensitivity and specificity were selected as thresholds for clinical change.
The outcome measures were the MSQPT, Hamburg Quality of Life Questionnaire for Multiple Sclerosis (HAQUAMS), rating of change questionnaires, Expanded Disability Status Scale, 6-metre timed walking test, Berg Balance Scale and 6-minute walking test.

Results: The effect size ranged from 0.46 to 1.49. The SRM data showed comparable results. The modified SRM ranged from 0.00 to 0.60. Anchor-based MID estimates were very low and were comparable with SD- and SEM-based estimates. The MSQPT was more responsive than the HAQUAMS in detecting improvement but less responsive in finding deterioration. The best MID estimates of the items, sections and total score, expressed in percentage of their maximum score, were between 5.4% (activity) and 22% (item 10) change for improvement and between 5.7% (total score) and 22% (item 10) change for deterioration.

Conclusions: The MSQPT is a responsive questionnaire with an adequate MID that may be used as threshold for change during rehabilitation of MS patients.

Keywords: Multiple sclerosis, Rehabilitation, Physical therapy, Patient outcome assessment, Questionnaires, Responsiveness

Correspondence: ipforschung@sunrise.ch
Institut für Physiotherapieforschung, Lindenweg 48, 2503 Biel, Switzerland

Background

Many individuals with multiple sclerosis (MS) undergo physical therapy. Because MS cannot be cured, physical therapy focuses on preserving and increasing quality of life. The effects of treatment on the quality of life of MS patients should be measured at all relevant levels defined by the World Health Organization in the International Classification of Functioning, Disability and Health: body functions and structures, activities and participation. Patient Rated Outcome (PRO) instruments, such as the Short Form Health Survey (SF-36), the Multiple Sclerosis Impact Scale (MSIS-29) or the Hamburg Quality of Life Questionnaire in Multiple Sclerosis (HAQUAMS), can measure the influence of MS on the quality of life. However, these questionnaires do not focus specifically on the goals of physiotherapy or the effects of physiotherapeutic treatment. To enable an appropriate assessment of treatment-related improvement in chronic diseases, such as MS, and be applicable even for MS patients with slow progression, the questionnaire should be able to measure small changes in activity and participation. Furthermore, the questionnaire should contain sufficient items related to activities and participation that are important for the daily life of MS patients and that can be influenced by physiotherapy.

The Multiple Sclerosis Questionnaire for Physiotherapists (MSQPT) is a German patient-reported outcome measure (see Additional files 1 and 2) that was designed as an aid for physiotherapists to assess the course of treatment in MS patients. The MSQPT has 34 items that are related to physiotherapeutic treatment and are relevant for activities and participation that can be influenced by physiotherapy. They describe different aspects of the impact of MS on patient daily life and the impact of physiotherapeutic treatment [1, 2].

The answers are given on a 9- or 10-point scale. The former is a symmetric, bipolar, Likert-like scale that may be treated as an interval scale [3, 4], as stated and discussed in [1]. Three items (8b, 9a and 9b) have a 10-point interval scale.

Table 1 shows the range of scores of three sections of the MSQPT, the total score of the MSQPT and four reliable items. The three sections were identified by factor analysis [1]. They consist of activity-associated, participation-associated and balance items and were labelled as the activity, participation and balance sections, respectively [1]. The three sections of Table 1 and the total score of the MSQPT are reliable (Table 2). The criterion validity of the MSQPT, using the SF-36 and HAQUAMS as criteria, is high [1]. The MSQPT also fulfils additional demands for assessments (comparability, economy, usefulness and acceptance) [1, 2].

The responsiveness of the MSQPT, i.e., its ability to measure change over time, has not yet been evaluated. Moreover, it is not yet clear how to interpret changes in MSQPT scores of the four items and sections of the MSQPT. This represents an important issue for using this tool in daily practice, as it is critical to estimate the minimal change that translates into real change (improvement or deterioration) in persons with MS.

The responsiveness (i.e., the ability to measure change over time) and interpretation of PRO measures have been topics of debate for many years. No established method exists to date, but there is a growing consensus regarding suitable approaches [5].

The anchor-based approach assigns patients to subgroups based on the degree of change (none, small, large); specifically, the change in the score given by the PRO instrument (PRO score) is compared with external evidence of change (real change), such as patient-based global rating of change questions. The change in PRO score for the patient subgroup reporting a small change represents an anchor-based estimate of the minimal important difference (MID) [6].

The distribution-based approach uses various statistical measures based on the distribution of the PRO

Table 1 Description of relevant items and sections of the Multiple Sclerosis Questionnaire for Physiotherapists

Item/Section	Description	Range of scores
4	I can take a shower by myself.	1–9
8a	How far can you walk on flat ground without sitting down?	1–9
8b	How long can you walk on flat ground without sitting down?	1–10
10	I can get in and out of the car by myself.	1–9
Activity section (14 items)	Dressing, bathing, standing, walking, climbing stairs, getting in and out of a car, using public transport, strenuous activities, writing, spasticity	14–128
Participation section (11 items)	Feeling rested, vitality, physical strength, fatigue, being active, adaption of activities, resilience, family life, going on a trip, fear of the consequences of MS	11–199
Balance section (2 items)	Taking a shower, balance	2–18
Total score (34 items)	Activity, participation and balance sections; global rating of change; brushing teeth, pain, sensitivity, bladder control, defecation; goals in life.	34–308

Table 2 Reliability of 4 items, all 3 sections and the total score of the Multiple Sclerosis Questionnaire for Physiotherapists [1]

Section	Reliability (Pearson's r)
Taking a shower	0.90
How far can you walk?	0.95
How long can you walk?	0.89
Getting in and out of a car	0.80
Activity section	0.93
Participation section	0.77
Balance section	0.84
Total score	0.87

scores in a given sample [7–9]. Distribution-based MID estimates can be calculated based on the standard deviation (SD) [5, 6, 10–12], standard error of measurement (SEM) [6, 13] or minimal detectable change (MDC) for the 90% (MDC_{90}) and 95% (MDC_{95}) confidence intervals [6]. When small effects are expected, the SEM is estimated as the standard deviation of PRO scores multiplied by the square root of the difference between one and the intraclass correlation reliability coefficient [13]. By combining the distributional and reliability components, SEM takes into consideration that some of the observed change may be caused by random measurement errors. Thus, the SEM measures response stability. Wyrwich et al. [13] stated that the one-SEM criterion can be applied to detect intra-individual change using health-related quality-of-life instruments.

The MDC represents another statistical estimate of the smallest change that can be detected by an instrument and is calculated as the product of SEM, the square root of 2 and 1.96 or 1.26 for MDC_{95} and MDC_{90}, respectively. The MDC gives the smallest amount of change beyond random error for a certain level of confidence. It is always higher than SEM because it is calculated as SEM multiplied by the square root of 2 and 1.96 or 1.26.

The anchor-based and distribution-based MID estimates represent different concepts of establishing a value for minimal change. The anchor-based concept uses external clinical information from the patient or clinician to express minimal change. The distributional method relies solely on statistical calculations and does not directly inform about minimal clinical change. Both Revicki [5] and Turner [6] recommended the use of both concepts to establish an MID, giving more weight to the anchor-based MID estimate and using the distribution-based estimates as benchmarks. Turner et al. [6] showed that 0.5 and one SEM come closest to the anchor-based estimates and that the MDC cannot replace an anchor-based MID.

The effect size (ES) measures the change caused by an intervention as the difference between the mean scores obtained during the pre- and post-intervention assessments divided by the SD of the baseline scores. ES values of 0.2, 0.5 and 0.8 indicate small, medium and large changes, respectively. The standardized response mean (SRM) is considered a more informative measure than the ES, as it uses the SD of change in scores between assessments (instead of the SD at baseline) in the denominator, taking the variability of change into account. The modified SRM (MSRM) uses the same numerator as the ES and SRM, but the denominator is the SD of change in scores between assessments calculated only for those individuals who are identified as stable based on independent external information, typically provided in the form of a rating of change question during the post-intervention assessment. The MSRM provides us with an estimate of the inherent variability of changes recorded by the PRO instrument, with lower scores indicating lower variability [7].

Further information on the responsiveness of a PRO instrument can be obtained using the relative efficiency method, which compares the responsiveness of two PRO instruments. The relative efficiency is calculated as the square of the ratio of the t-statistics for the two instruments being compared, thus revealing which instrument is more responsive in a given survey population.

The purpose of this study was to evaluate the responsiveness of the German MSQPT and to establish reasonable estimates of MID in order to provide practical guidelines on how to interpret changes in MSQPT scores.

Methods

We used a longitudinal multicentre design with a convenience sample. Eleven private practices and two physiotherapy departments of hospitals in Switzerland participated in this study. The physical therapists of each participant institution recruited the patients.

Inclusion criteria

We included patients who were diagnosed with MS according to the McDonald criteria, undergoing physiotherapeutic treatment for MS, older than 18 years, able to read the MSQPT, native German speakers and given an Expanded Disability Status Scale (EDSS) score of ≤6.5.

Exclusion criteria

Patients were excluded if they presented acute exacerbation of MS, any condition that made them bedridden, distinct fatigue that made it impossible to concentrate for ≥2 h or grave cognitive change (judged by the treating physical therapist).

The execution of the testing was standardized using a study manual with detailed instructions. The two testers were experienced in using the MSQPT and HAQUAMS, as they were testers in the validation study for the MSQPT [1]. They were familiarized with the study manual and were trained by experts in physical testing for evaluating the patients in a standardized manner, as instructed in the study manual.

Outcome measures

The anchor-based approach usually measures change by employing one global rating of change question with a symmetrical scale of 7 to 15 points [14]. Depending on the width of this scale, a change of one or two points may represent a minimal change. However, anchor-based estimates are always flawed with the uncertainty of the value indicating global change (real change). The wide range of symptoms experienced by MS patients can make it especially difficult to assess the extent of change on one global rating scale [14]. For example, when asking whether the patient generally feels better or worse, we might not register an amelioration in walking if, at the same time, the pain worsened. One should always ask oneself whether a single question assessing the global change is sufficiently sensitive. We used several patient-based and therapist-based questions to rate the change in order to obtain a clearer view of real change in the patients. The questions assessing change described issues relevant to the physiotherapeutic treatment, such as pain, fatigue, walking and balance, as well as therapeutic goals, such as improved activity and participation, which lie at the core of MSQPT. By formulating the questions in this way, we ensure that we are comparing similar constructs (various items and sections of MSQPT vs. questions rating global change). Furthermore, a more detailed rating system, assessing various symptoms separately, may also serve to ensure that the comparison is relevant [5, 15–17]. However, this implies the use of a multiple rating approach, which results in a range of MID estimates [5, 14].

The detailed questions on global rating of change were provided on two different questionnaires considering two different perspectives: that of the patient and that of the treating therapist. These two questionnaires differed only regarding phrasing of the questions, not regarding the matter being asked. Each questionnaire had 9 rating of change questions that concerned general health status, balance, walking ability, arm function, fatigue, pain, activity level, social participation and general impairment due to MS. The first question for the patient was: "Compared to the situation before the first testing, how would you describe your general health now"? The other 8 questions were similarly phrased, varying the topic as listed above. Furthermore, each question had a 9-level scale, similar to the one in the MSQPT, with the extremes "much worse" and "much better", and the middle level being "the same".

The HAQUAMS is a reliable, valid and responsive instrument [18, 19]. It is a German self-rated quality of life questionnaire developed for use in an MS population. In the MSQPT validation study [1], the HAQUAMS showed good correlations with the main groups of the MSQPT.

The patients were evaluated using the following physical tests: the 6-Metre Timed-Walking Test (6MTWT), 6-Minute-Walk Test (6MWT) and Berg Balance Scale (BBS). The 6MTWT and 6MWT were standardized using a static start, and patients were asked to walk at a comfortable, usual speed [8, 20, 21] to ensure safety, as many tests were executed in the confined space of private practices. A 20% change was used as the threshold for change [21–24].

The BBS was standardized using a conservative protocol, in which the lowest of two levels was given in cases of uncertainty. Each test was demonstrated to the patients by the testers during its testing session, in agreement with the test manual. A 7-point change in BBS was the limit used for real change [25].

Procedures

To compare the study population with those of former studies in Switzerland [1, 26] and assess the representativeness of the population, we recorded age, gender, type of MS and disease duration since diagnosis of the patients at baseline. Furthermore, patients were allocated to groups according to their score in the EDSS at baseline. The tests were executed in the following order: MSQPT, 6MTWT, BBS, HAQUAMS, patient rating of change questionnaire and 6MWT. Patients were allowed to have a break at any time, and the break times were recorded. The treating therapist filled out the rating of change questionnaire during or after the testing session, without any contact with the patient.

The usefulness of the MSQPT may be different for the different treatment situations in Switzerland. Both long-term and short-term treatments were included in order to evaluate whether the MSQPT is useful for all treatment situations. I considered long-term patients to be those who were in physiotherapeutic treatment for one year or more. These patients may show little change over time, and advancement of quality of life is central for treatment. The long-term patients were tested twice, once at baseline and once 6 months later. Short-term patients were considered those who underwent 9–27 treatment sessions. These patients were tested at baseline and after 3–4 months or at the end of the treatment period if the latter period was shorter.

All patients were in a non-standardized physiotherapeutic treatment. The treatment was individually tailored depending on the presented symptoms, and the goals for each therapy were determined by the patient and therapist together.

Data analysis

The full dataset was subjected to analysis. No subgroup analyses for short- and long-term patients were executed for this analysis. The responsiveness of the MSQPT was assessed using ES and SRM for patients with change and using MSRM for patients without change in the results. I computed the relative efficiency between the MSQPT and the HAQUAMS scores for amelioration and deterioration. The t-statistics of the items and sections of the MSQPT were used in the numerator, and the t-statistics of the groups of the HAQUAMS were used in the denominator. A relative efficiency of >1 indicated that the MSQPT was more responsive than the HAQUAMS, whereas a relative efficiency of <1 indicated the opposite.

A combined distribution- and anchor-based approach was used to establish an MID. For the distribution-based MID estimates, 0.2^*SD, 0.33^*SD, SEM and the MDC were calculated for the 90% and 95% confidence intervals (MDC_{90} and MDC_{95}, respectively). Although 0.5^*SD is the best choice for SD [6, 11, 12], it is equivalent to 1 SEM [12] or greater [6] and therefore does not contribute additional information. Thus, 0.2^*SD was chosen, as is often used [5, 10], and 0.33^*SD was used for comparable reasons, as the MID of the HAQUAMS was based on 0.33^*SD [11]. They represent the lowest distribution-based MIDs in this study.

For anchor-based estimates, it is important that there be a reasonable correlation between baseline and final testing [5, 27, 28]. I calculated the correlation coefficients to assess whether this requirement was fulfilled. The anchor-based values were considered reasonably correlated and were used in the evaluation when the coefficient was ≥0.30 [1]. Furthermore, in this analysis, I considered only global rating of change questions for items, sections or total scores of the MSQPT that had a similar content to the global rating of change questions. Table 3 shows the linking between items, sections and total score and the global rating of change questions with similar content. This linking will be used for MSRM (using anchor-based information for no change) and anchor-based MID estimates.

The anchor-based MIDs for the 4 items, 3 sections and the total score were determined using the global ratings of change in the rating of change questionnaires. Changes of one or two levels in the global rating of change questions were classified as minimal differences. For all patients exhibiting a one- or two-level change, the average change

of the items and sections of the MSQPT between baseline and final testing was computed.

The anchor- and distribution-based MIDs present a range of MID estimates for each item, each section and the total score. I expressed all distribution- and anchor-based estimates of MID in integer numbers, rounding the MID to the next higher number, because the answer scales of the MSQPT correspond to integer numbers.

To narrow the range of all calculated MIDs to possibly one value, the sensitivity and specificity statistics of all the MID scores were used.

The sensitivity described the agreement regarding change for each item and section between the assessments and the true change rate given by the global rating of change. The specificity described the agreement regarding no change for each item and section between the assessments and the absence of change as measured by the global rating of change. Thus, the sensitivity and specificity for amelioration and deterioration were calculated for each MID of the items, sections and total score based on the global ratings of change given by the patients and therapists.

The best MID was defined as the MID with the best values of sensitivity and specificity. The best MID for an item of MSQPT was obtained by choosing the MID out of the whole range of integer MIDs of that item that had the highest sensitivity and specificity values for the global ratings of change that had similar content. If two values had a similar range of sensitivity and specificity, the lower value was chosen as the best MID. In addition, the sensitivity and specificity based on the patients' rating of change questions were given more weight than those based on the therapist rating. The same method was used for the sections and total score.

Finally, the best MIDs for the 4 items of Table 1 and for the balance section were compared with real changes as seen in physical tests.

In the discussion, I examine the method and the value of the findings.

When benchmarking the best MID with anchor- and distribution-based values, I follow the recommendations [5, 6], giving the anchor-based approach more weight. It will be assumed that the anchor-based estimate will be

Table 3 Linking of items, sections and total score to global rating of change questions

Global rating of change questions	Items, section and total score of MSQPT							
	M4	M8a	M8b	M10	Activity	Participation	Balance	Total score
Global health					*	*		*
Balance	*	*	*	*			*	
Walking	*	*	*	*				
Participation					*	*		*
Impairment					*	*		*

M4 taking a shower, *M8a* walking distance, *M8b* walking time, *M10* taking a shower, * displaying similar content of similar value to the SEM [6, 13]. As the 0.5 SD might be similar to SEM [6, 12], the 0.2 and 0.33 SD might be lower, and the MDC will be higher than SEM. In addition, other characteristics can be taken into account, such as the distribution of scores (floor and ceiling effects) and reliability [7]. If an item has a ceiling effect, it is hard to show improvement. Furthermore, a low MID is more plausible for a very highly reliable item or section than when the reliability is low.

Results

Demographic data

Sixty-one patients from thirteen test locations were included in the study. All patients provided informed consent. However, due to a new and serious diagnosis, one patient in long-term treatment decided not to continue in the study.

Of the 60 remaining patients, 25 in long-term treatment and 35 in short-term treatment finished the study. Moreover, 53 patients were treated in private practice, while 7 were treated in a hospital setting.

The population of the study has almost the same percentage of women and range of age as the validation study of the MSQPT [1] and as the Multiple Sclerosis and Rehabilitation, Care- and Health Services study (MARCH), the Swiss contribution to the international research programme to close gaps in the knowledge of the living conditions of persons with MS [26] (Table 4). The main difference is that in this study, the average age, the mean age of male patients and the percentage of patients over 60 years old were slightly higher, while the percentage of patients between 40 and 60 years old was slightly lower. I concluded that the sample has a population comparable to the validation study of the MSQPT and to the MARCH study of Switzerland and is plausibly representative of the Swiss MS population.

Percentage of missing data

The MSQPT and HAQUAMS had very low rates of missing data (0.13 and 0.47%, respectively). Moreover, the patient rating of change question in the MSQPT and HAQUAMS did not exhibit missing data. The therapist rating of change questionnaire had a 5.4% missing data rate. The patient rating of change questionnaire was completed by 77% of the patients. Statistics were calculated excluding patients with missing data from the corresponding dataset.

Evaluation of responsiveness

The distribution-based estimates of the ES and SRM are shown in Table 5 for data with negative change items (deterioration) and positive change items (improvement) between baseline and final testing scores. The ES showed low deterioration for the activity section items (−0.46), medium for the M4 item (getting in and out of a car, −0.67), the participation section items (−0.64) and total score (−0.58) and high deterioration for the other items. Regarding improvement, except for item M10, which exhibited a high ES (1.49), most ES values were similar to the deterioration items. Each SRM was higher than its corresponding ES except for M4.

The group of people without change, as identified using the global rating of change questions, was used for the evaluation of MSRM, which should be as low as possible. Table 6 shows the MSRM for each item of Table 1, each section and the total score (rows) based on the different global ratings of change for both patient and therapist answers (lines). The number of patients who were without change was different for each global rating of change question. The MSRMs were generally low except for Item M4. The activity section exhibited the highest MSRM among the sections.

Tables 7 and 8 show the relative efficiency between the MSQPT and HAQUAMS scores. The data of Table 7 show that the MSQPT total score seems to be as responsive as the HAQUAMS total score for showing

Table 4 Demographic data of the MARCH study, the validation study of the MSQPT and the current study

Demographic data	MARCH study Switzerland all data	MARCH study Switzerland physical therapy	Validation study MSQPT	Responsiveness and MID study MSQPT
Percent women	63	58	63	65
Mean age	50.2 (±11.9)	51.2 (±11.4)	51.7 (±10.4)	53.3 (±11.4)
Mean age women	49.8	52	50.8	52.6 (±12.5)
Mean age men	50.1	49.5	53.3	54.5 (±9.0)
Min-max age	16–79	26–79	29–84	23–77
Percent 40–60 years	60	60	62	53
Percent ≥ 60 years	22	21	24	30
N	185	113	141	60
Mean years of illness	13	Not available	15	18 (±9.7)

Table 5 Responsiveness of questionnaire items and sections with respect to physiotherapy-related deterioration and improvement in patients

		M4	M8a	M8b	M10	Activity	Participation	Balance	Total Score
Deterioration	n	3	19	19	6	32	28	18	29
	ES	−2.84	−0.91	−1.03	−0.67	−0.46	−0.64	−1.00	−0.58
	SRM	−1.23	−3.09	−2.57	−1.12	−0.82	−1.21	−1.27	−0.96
Improvement	n	1	16	17	5	22	28	19	31
	ES	*	1.02	0.80	1.49	0.49	0.75	1.04	0.57
	SRM	*	1.92	2.20	1.41	1.38	1.48	1.68	1.29

ES effect size, *SRM* standardized response mean, *M4* showering, *M8a* walking distance, *M8b* walking time, *M10* getting in and out of the car
*Not computable (n = 1)

improvement. The participation section of the MSQPT was better at indicating improvement than each HAQUAMS section. In contrast, the activity section of the MSQPT was much less efficient in showing improvement than the corresponding HAQUAMS sections. When improvement in walking was compared, item M8a of the MSQPT ("How far can you walk without a rest"?) was more responsive than the mobility factors of the lower limb in the HAQUAMS, while in the same comparison, the M8b of the MSQPT (walking time) was less responsive.

The MSQPT total score was more effective in demonstrating deterioration than the HAQUAMS total score (Table 8). Furthermore, regarding deterioration, the MSQPT participation section was clearly more responsive than any HAQUAMS score. The MSQPT activity section showed deterioration with similar efficiency to that of the mobility sections but less efficient than the total score of the HAQUAMS. Both mobility items of

the MSQPT were more responsive than the lower limb mobility section of the HAQUAMS.

Estimates for MID

Table 9 shows the distribution-based estimates for MID. There was a considerable difference regarding the use of SD, SEM or MDC statistics, with the first two resulting in much lower values than those obtained using the MDC. Regarding the MSQPT, the distribution-based MID estimates of item M4 were 1 or 2. The other MID estimates were between 1 and 3 for items M8a, M8b and M10; between 4 and 19 for the activity section; between 3 and 22 for the participation section; between 1 and 5 for the balance section; and between 7 and 45 for the total score.

Before calculating the anchor-based MID estimates, I tested whether the items and sections exhibited a minimum and substantial correlation between baseline and target score. All correlation coefficients except that for

Table 6 Modified standardized response mean for multiple sclerosis patients identified as stable based on questions assessing the global rating of change

Item, section and total score of the MSQPT	M4	M8a	M8b	M10	Activity	Participation	Balance	Total score
Global rating of change questions								
Perspective of the patient								
Global change	*	*	*	*	0.15	0.00	*	0.03
Balance	0.27	−0.04	0.12	0.10	*	*	0.03	*
Walking	**	−0.04	0.17	0.10	*	*	*	*
Participation	*	*	*	*	0.12	0.00	*	0.03
Disability	*	*	*	*	0.14	0.00	*	0.03
Perspective of the therapist								
Global change	*	*	*	*	0.12	0.00	*	0.03
Balance	0.60	−0.05	0.13	0.06	*	*	0.04	*
Walking	0.26	−0.05	0.11	0.07	*	*	*	*
Participation	*	*	*	*	0.12	0.00	*	0.03
Disability	*	*	*	*	0.14	0.00	*	0.03

M4 taking a shower, *M8a* walking distance, *M8b* walking time, *M10* getting in and out of the car, * not applicable, ** not computable

Table 7 Relative efficiency between the MSQPT and the HAQUAMS with respect to improvement

| HAQUAMS | MSQPT | | | | |
	M8a Walking distance	M8b Walking time	Activity	Participation	Total score MSQPT
Fatigue/thinking	*	*	*	1.28	*
Lower limb mobility	1.48	0.84	0.37	1.07	0.70
Upper limb mobility	*	*	0.36	1.05	0.68
Social functioning	*	*	*	1.35	*
Mood	*	*	0.51	1.47	0.96
Total score HAQUAMS	*	*	0.52	1.51	0.98

MSQPT Multiple Sclerosis Questionnaire for Physiotherapists, *HAQUAMS* Hamburg Quality of Life Questionnaire in Multiple Sclerosis. Only the combinations for which the correlation is >0.4 are shown. *These sections do not assess similar aspects

item M10 fulfilled the minimum requirement of $r = 0.30$, with r of 0.57–0.84, $p < 0.0001$. For this reason, item M10 was excluded from the anchor-based MID calculations.

Table 10 shows the anchor-based MID. These results represent the average change between baseline and final testing, using the MSQPT sections and items, for MS patients with deterioration or improvement that were identified by the rating of change questionnaires as having a change level of 1 or 2. The table shows the pairs of items and sections that seemed to exhibit a meaningful relationship as described in Table 3.

The MID estimates of the activity section were between 2 and 13, those of the participation section were between 2 and 11, those of the activity section were between 1 and 2 and those of the total score were between 2 and 25. The estimates for the items were all well below 1, the lowest possible score for the MSQPT items.

Sensitivity and specificity were assessed for the whole range of MID described in Tables 9 and 10. All MIDs were rounded to the next integer number. Table 11 shows the MIDs for deterioration and amelioration for the items. The best MID (in bold), presenting the best sensitivity and specificity, and the sensitivity and specificity for the next level of the item are shown. As outlined in the method section, if 2 levels showed similar values, the lower MID was chosen as the best MID. Those sensitivity and specificity values were used and shown if the

data for at least 4 persons were available. Values were used in the description of the results if and only if an item (or section) had a similar content to a rating of change question (see Tables 9 and 10, column 2). Both the perspective of the patient and the perspective of the therapist were used.

The integer MID for item M4 ranged from 1 to 2. There were not enough data ($n < 4$) for calculating more than one level change in the item. The best MID for improvement and for deterioration of item M4 was set at one.

The Walking items had an integer MID range of 1–3. The items had a similar level for the sensitivity and specificity of the one- or two-level change in the item. Only the sensitivity for a two-level deterioration for item 8b showed one clear higher value (0.83) than a one-level change. The best MID was set at one level of change.

Only distribution-based MID estimates were available for item 10, with an integer range from 1 to 3. A three-level change could not be calculated for item M10 ($n < 4$). Because the sensitivity for deterioration with a 2-level MID was generally higher than for level one, the MID was set at a two-level change.

Table 12 shows (similar to Table 11) sensitivity and specificity values of the best MIDs of the sections and total score and the adjacent available values.

The activity section displays integer anchor- and distribution-based MID estimates ranging from 3 to 19.

Table 8 Relative efficiency between the MSQPT and the HAQUAMS with respect to deterioration

| HAQUAMS | MSQPT | | | | |
	M8a Walking distance	M8b Walking time	Activity	Participation	Total score MSQPT
Fatigue/thinking	*	*	*	2.24	*
Lower limb mobility	1.48	3.83	0.92	2.46	1.75
Upper limb mobility	*	*	0.95	2.53	1.80
Social functioning	*	*	*	1.84	*
Mood	*	*	0.69	1.85	1.32
Total score HAQUAMS	*	*	0.66	1.76	1.25

MSQPT Multiple Sclerosis Questionnaire for Physiotherapists, *HAQUAMS* Hamburg Quality of Life Questionnaire in Multiple Sclerosis. Only the combinations for which the correlation is >0.4 are shown. *These sections do not assess similar aspects

Table 9 Distribution-based estimates of the minimal important difference

	M4	M8a	M8b	M10	Activity	Participation	Balance	Total score
0.2*SD	0.25	0.30	0.33	0.18	3.31	2.68	0.52	6.20
0.33*SD	0.41	0.51	0.56	0.30	5.52	4.46	0.86	10.33
SEM	0.67	0.81	0.85	0.77	6.64	7.66	1.70	15.93
MDC$_{95}$	1.87	2.24	2.39	2.13	18.40	21.23	4.70	44.16
MDC$_{90}$	1.57	1.89	1.98	1.80	15.49	17.87	3.96	37.17

SD standard deviation, *SEM* standard error of measurement, *MDC$_{90}$* minimal detectable change of the 90% confidence interval, *MDC$_{95}$* minimal detectable change of the 95% confidence interval, *M4* taking a shower, *M8a* walking distance, *M8b* walking time, *M10* getting in and out of the car

Of the available values for improvement, 7 levels of change provide the best MID, with higher sensitivity and specificity than 6 levels and similar sensitivity and specificity. The best MID for improvement was set at 7 levels. Because the sensitivity values for 11 were generally higher than for a 10-level change, the best MID for deterioration was set at 11 levels.

The participation section, with an integer range of MID estimates between 2 and 22, had a best MID of 17 for both deterioration and amelioration based on the sensitivity levels. The sensitivity for amelioration was based on only the therapist perspective for global change because other ratings had n < 4. For deterioration, a 17-

level change generally represents more high values than a 15-level change.

The range of 1–5 levels of change for the MID of the balance section is a wide range for a section that consists of two items. There was a clear choice for a three-level best MID for deterioration based on the sensitivity results. The choice of a best MID for amelioration was difficult to make as all three levels were similar. The best MID level was set at two and will be discussed later.

The total score range for MID was 3–45. The sensitivity for improvement was the basis for the choice of a best MID of 20. The values of the MID for deterioration did not show a clear picture. Sensitivity for global health

Table 10 Anchor-based estimates of the minimal important difference predicting change with respect to deterioration and improvement

Global rating of change questions	Item/Section of the MSQPT						
	M4	M8a	M8b	Activity	Participation	Balance	Total score
Therapist, global rating, deterioration (35)	*	*	*	−3.09	−3.40	*	−9.09
Therapist global rating, improvement (18)	*	*	*	3.00	2.00	*	7.78
Patient, global rating, deterioration (41)	*	*	*	−2.17	−1.71	*	−5.02
Patient, global rating, improvement (12)	*	*	*	3.63	1.17	*	4.96
Therapist, walking rating, deterioration (41)		−0.46	−0.37	*	*	*	*
Therapist, walking rating, improvement (12)		0.58	0.08	*	*	*	*
Patient, walking rating, deterioration (15)		−0.13	−0.53	*	*	*	*
Patient, walking rating, improvement (6)		0.67	0.67	*	*	*	*
Therapist, balance rating, deterioration (30)	−0.27	−0.50	−0.47	*	*	−1.00	*
Therapist, balance rating, improvement (18)	0.22	0.28	0.06	*	*	0.17	*
Patient, balance rating, deterioration (9)	−0.11	−0.22	−0.67	*	*	−1.78	*
Patient, balance rating, improvement	**	**	**	**	**	**	**
Patient, participation rating, deterioration (8)	*	*	*	−1.71	4.86	*	−6.86
Patient, participation rating, improvement (6)	*	*	*	4.00	2.00	*	14.57
Therapist participation rating, deterioration (7)	*	*	*	−7.63	−11.00	*	−21.88
Therapist participation rating, improvement (7)	*	*	*	5.67	5.00	*	16.50
Patient, impairment rating, deterioration (12)	*	*	*	−12.20	−2.80	*	−24.40
Patient, impairment rating, improvement (9)	*	*	*	2.00	−3.00	*	2.20
Therapist, impairment rating, deterioration (5)	*	*	*	−6.08	−1.42	*	−10.42
Therapist, impairment rating, improvement (5)	*	*	*	2.22	3.33	*	2.33

M4 taking a shower, *M8a* walking distance, *M8b* walking time; () displays the number of cases; *rating and section are not relevantly related; **not computable

Table 11 Sensitivity and specificity of the estimates for minimal important difference (MID) for 4 items

Item	Global rating questions used	MID improvement	Specificity	Sensitivity	MID deterioration	Specificity	Sensitivity
M4	Balance, Arm function	*1*	0.52–0.81	*	*1*	0.52–0.81	0.20–0.67
		2	*	*	2	*	*
M8a	Walking, Balance	*1*	0.40–0.71	0.1–0.25	*1*	0.45–0.71	0.36–0.67
		2	0.47–0.69	0.1–0.3	2	0.40–0.68	*
M8b	Walking, Balance	*1*	0.47–0.65	**	*1*	0.47–0.65	0.32–0.53
		2	0.42–0.70	0.0–0.5	2	0.43–0.70	0.36–0.83
M10	Walking, Balance	1	0.41–0.74	0.00–0.33	1	0.41–0.74	0.36–0.60
		2	0.43–0.74	*	*2*	0.4–0.80	0.67–0.8
		3	*	*	3	*	*

M4 taking a shower, *M8A* walking distance, *M8B* walking time, *M10* getting in and out of the car; *n<4; **not computable, *** no values available. Italic numbers represent the best MID

was highest (0.78) for an MID of 16 from the patient perspective but highest (0.75) for 22 from the therapist perspective. To select a best MID of 16 would contradict the higher values for participation and impairment from the therapist view for 22. A best MID of 18 for deterioration was the most balanced choice.

The best MIDs of the items and of the balance section were compared with the results of the physical tests. A 20% change was used as a threshold for change for the 6MTWT and 6MWT, and a 7-point change was used for real change in the BBS.

Only the specificity for the best MID was calculated against the real change of the physical tests because few patients exhibited change in the physical tests. The results are shown in Table 13. The MID values of the items showed a high specificity for the physical tests BBS and 6MWT and slightly lower specificity for the 6MTWT. The balance section showed a high specificity for the BBS and a clearly lower specificity for the walking tests.

Discussion

The main finding of the present study is that the MSQPT is a responsive questionnaire. The proposed PRO score thresholds associated with minimal change are low, indicating the high responsiveness of the MSQPT.

Based on the ES and SRM, the MSQPT can measure change. Moreover, when MS patients did not experience change (as determined by questions assessing the global rating of change), the MSQPT hardly showed any change, and the MSRM values were low.

The HAQUAMS is a reliable, valid and responsive instrument [11, 18] that showed good overlap with the main sections of the MSQPT [1]. The relative efficiency of the MSQPT over the HAQUAMS in this cohort relied on the improved ability of the MSQPT participation section to detect change; however, the HAQUAMS proved better than the MSQPT activity section at detecting improvement. The total score of the MSQPT seems to be more suitable than that of the HAQUAMS for

Table 12 Sensitivity and specificity of estimates for minimal important difference (MID) for the sections and total score of the MSQPT

Section	Global rating questions used	MID improvement	Specificity	Sensitivity	MID deterioration	Specificity	Sensitivity
Activity	Global health, Impairment, Walking	6	0.25–0.65	0.10–0.67	10	0.36–0.72	0.39–0.70
		7	0.29–0.86	0.12–0.75	*11*	0.44–0.78	0.33–0.78
		8	0.28–0.86	0.13–0.75	25	0.42–0.72	*
Participation	Global health, Impairment, Participation	16	0.47–0.90	0.50	15	0.44–0.9	0.22–0.78
		17	0.45–0.88	0.67	*17*	0.43–0.91	0.40–0.80
		20	0.45–0.89	0.50	22	*	*
Balance	Balance	1	0.46, 0.69	0.13, 0.15	2	0.42, 0.69	0.42, 0.42
		2	0.48, 0.68	0.10, 0.21	*3*	0.49, 0.72	0.5, 0.67
		3	0.49–0.71	0.13, 0.25	4	*	*
Total score	Global health, Participation Impairment	16	0.44–0.97	0.11–0.66	16	0.26–0.65	0.17–0.68
		20	0.47–0.95	0.14–0.80	*18*	0.29–0.65	0.21–0.67
		25	0.47–0.95	0.20–0.80	22	0.29–0.64	0.25–0.75

*n<4; **not computable. Italic numbers represent the best MID

Table 13 Specificity of the best MID of relevant items in relation to the physical tests

	6MTWT	BBS	6MWT
M4 (*1)	0.79 (7.6, 3.6, 4.2–26.2)	0.92 (49, 5.1, 33–56)	0.81 (238, 75.0, 65–462)
M8a (*1)	0.82 (8.0, 3.7, 4.6–22.4)	0.94 (49, 4.3, 38–56)	0.92 (228, 89.2, 96–462)
M8b (*1)	0.83 (7.1, 3.3, 4.0–22.4)	0.98 (50, 5.2, 33–56)	0.90 (254, 78.9, 114–462)
M10 (*2)	0.66 (8.4, 5.5, 3.0–46.0)	0.98 (48, 6.1, 25–56)	0.82 (223, 88.0, 34–462)
Balance (*2,3)	0.66 (7.5, 3.8, 4.2–24.8)	0.95 (49, 4.8, 33–56)	0.64 (229, 77.3, 60–462)

6MTWT 6-metre timed walking test (mean, SD and range in seconds), *BBS* Berg Balance Scale (mean, SD and range in points), *6MWT* 6-minute walking test (mean, SD and range in metre), *M4* taking a shower, *M8a* walking distance, *M8b* walking time, *M10* getting in and out of the car; * the best thresholds for the minimal important difference

detecting deterioration. Similarly, the MSQPT items related to walking were more responsive than the HAQUAMS items on mobility of the lower limb. When comparing the responsiveness between measures, one must take into account that although the sections are related, they do not assess exactly the same phenomena. In this context, the MSQPT can measure change and does so as efficiently as the HAQUAMS.

The MDC estimates for MID were generally higher than the other estimates because MDC is based on SD and SEM but also considers the confidence interval. The SD and SEM were more similar to the anchor-based estimates, with MID for all studied items being lower than 1, which is the lowest possible integer MID. The MDC values were much higher, as was expected above.

The best MID was identified based on the sensitivity and specificity of the various MID estimates found in this study. Most values for specificity were high, and not all values for sensitivity could be calculated. Considering that the physical test suggested little change, we may conclude that this population was rather stable.

Furthermore, there was a clear difference between the perspective of the therapists and that of the patients, which indicates that using only therapist-based global ratings may lead to different conclusions than using patient-based global ratings. Future research should thus consider the choice of anchor.

The best MID estimates were all well lower than the highest MDC estimates but higher than most anchor-based estimates. In this study population, the procedure for establishing a clinically relevant MID seemed to offer a best MID close to anchor-based MIDs that rely on external evidence of change and that lie within the upper and lower limits set by the distribution-based approach, which relies solely on statistics of the distribution of changes in PRO scores. The value and credibility of the best MID are further discussed in detail, weighing the existing evidence regarding the value of the items and sections included in the questionnaire and the results of the present survey, to reach a comprehensive conclusion.

Unlike the anchor-based estimates, distribution-based estimates provide a simple way of expressing change in a standardized statistic; however, such metrics are criticized

as being only theoretical indicators, with no physical meaning [5]. Thus, MIDs estimated using only distribution-based metrics may not indicate a clinically meaningful minimal change. Combining both approaches may give an extensive overview of the ability of a PRO measure to detect change, but it also results in a wide range of possible MID estimates. When choosing a suitable MID out of a range of estimates to be used as a clinical threshold indicating change, the highest weight was given to the anchor-based estimates assessed from the patient's perspective [5, 6].

The database for estimating the anchor-based MID derived from M4 (ability to shower independently) is small. First, many patients rated the maximum score, which indicates that the patient rating for minimal balance improvement (anchor estimate) was absent. For the same reason, the ES for improvement could not be calculated. The ES for deterioration was high (though based on only $n = 3$ measurements), indicating a high responsiveness. The few anchor-based MIDs (for deterioration and amelioration) as well as the SDs and SEMs were well below one. Considering that SEM may be close to the anchor-based estimate [7, 8], it seems appropriate to take a 1-point change as the estimate of MID. The very high reliability of this item supports this choice. The 1-point MID for deterioration had a sensitivity of 0.6 and a specificity of 0.52 based on the balance-related global rating (which is relevant to M4) and 0.92 based on the BBS. However, because the high MSRM that did not indicate a small MID and the database for this 1-point MID was small, further research should clarify the MID threshold for this item.

The items concerning walking (M8a and M8b) had similar content and showed similar results. They had high responsiveness, with high ES for deterioration (−0.91 and −1.03, respectively) and improvement (1.02 and 0.8, respectively), and low MSRM for MS patients who did not show change following physiotherapy (0.03–0.05 and 0.11–0.17, respectively). The anchor-based MIDs for walking were also quite low and under 1. The fact that the SDs and SEMs were low and that these items were also highly reliable [1] and more suitable for detecting change compared to the HAQUAMS questions regarding lower limb mobility, suggests that it is appropriate to consider a 1-point change as the clinically relevant MID threshold. Only the MDCs (1.89–2.39) suggest that the MID might be higher.

Regarding the walking-related item M8a and the patient perspective for Walking, there was a sensitivity of 0.20 for improvement and a better sensitivity of 0.5 (M8b: 0.53) for deterioration. The specificity values were 0.50–0.53 for both M8a and M8b. A higher specificity (0.82–0.98) was found with respect to the physical tests (BBS, TWT and 6MWT).

An anchor-based estimate was not calculated for item 10. The given MID was mainly computed from the distribution-based statistics. The medium ES for deterioration (–0.67), low MSRM (0.04–0.13) and low MIDs (only the $MDC_{95} > 2$) suggests that a 2-point change is a reasonable threshold for a clinically relevant MID.

The activity section provided moderate ES (–0.46 and 0.49 for deterioration and improvement, respectively) and low MSRM (0.12–0.15), showing that this section is responsive. The best MIDs were 11 for deterioration and 7 for improvement. The SD and SEM estimates were lower than 7, and the integer MDC values were 16 and 19. The anchor-based MID estimates for deterioration were 3.09 to 6.08 (therapist-based) and 2.17–12.2 (patient-based). The best MID of 11 for deterioration was close to the upper limit of the anchor- and patient-based MID, higher than SEM and lower than the MDC. Weighting anchor-based MID estimates more heavily, 11 was a more conservative value. It had a sensitivity of 0.50 (specificity of 0.48), calculated from the patient-based ratings of global health, and a specificity of 0.7–0.8 for impairment.

The anchor-based estimates for improvement were 2.22–5.67 (therapist-based) and 2.00–4.00 (patient-based). A best MID of 7, equal to the SEM, was over the upper limit of all anchor-based MID estimates but much lower than the MDC values. The best MID of 7 was more reflective of an anchor-based estimate and was a reasonable, but considering MDC, also an optimistic choice, which requires further evaluation. It had a sensitivity of 0.75 (specificity of 0.57) calculated from the patient-based ratings of global health and a specificity of 0.70–0.89 for impairment.

The participation section also showed high responsiveness, with moderate ES (–0.64 and 0.75 for deterioration and improvement, respectively) and very low MSRM (0.00). The best MID was 17 for both deterioration and improvement. The distribution-based benchmarks SD and SEM were below 9, and the MDCs were 18 and 22. The anchor-based estimates for deterioration were quite low, ranging from 1.42 to 11, and those for amelioration ranged from 1.17 to 5. Based on anchor-based MID and SEM, a lower best MID than 17 could be expected.

However, it is important to note that the patient rating for worsening participation was positive, while the patient rating for improvement of impairment was negative. This might be explained by the fact that the participation section had items that were indirectly related to participation and therefore was not identical to participation as rated by the patients. Change in these items may have caused this phenomenon. These two values should be viewed with caution. Furthermore, the sensitivity was based on few values that were mainly therapist-based. Additionally, the participation section had a reliability of 0.77 [1] that did not speak in favour of a low MID. Because of these reasons, an MID of 17 seems to be a reasonable estimate for the clinically relevant threshold. The sensitivity for deterioration was 0.8 for participation rating from the perspective of the therapist, while its specificity for participation was 0.91 (therapist) and 0.76 (patient). The sensitivity for amelioration was based on only the global change of health question (0.8, therapist perspective). Its specificities for participation were 0.88 (therapist) and 0.65 (patient).

The balance section showed high responsiveness, with high ES (–1.00 and 1.04 for deterioration and improvement, respectively) and very low MSRM (0.03 and 0.04). The best MIDs for improvement (2 points) and deterioration (3 points) were considerably higher than the anchor-based estimates (–1.78 and 0.17, respectively) and SEM (1.70) but lower than the MDCs (3.96 and 4.70, respectively). Taking into account that these MIDs have high specificity with respect to the BBS (0.95) and sufficient test-retest reliability (0.84) [1], these MID thresholds are well justified.

The total score of the MSQPT was responsive to change, with medium ES (–0.58 and 0.57 for deterioration and improvement, respectively) and very low MSRM (0.03). The best MID for deterioration (improvement) was 18 (resp. 20). The distribution-based benchmarks were 6.20 and 10.33 for SD, 15.93 for SEM and 37.17 and 44.16 for the MDCs. The anchor-based MIDs for deterioration ranged from 5.2 (patient perspective, global rating) to 24.4 (patient perspective, impairment rating). This MID was higher than SEM, SD and the anchor-based MID except for impairment. Because the total score had a reliability of 0.87 [9], this low best MID appears to be an anchor-based, reasonable but optimistic estimate for the clinically relevant threshold. It had a sensitivity of 0.67 and a specificity of 0.3 for global health (both patient perspective). The anchor-based MIDs for amelioration ranged from 2.20 to 16.60. The upper limit was similar to SEM, higher than SD and much lower than the MDC. The MID also seems to be an anchor-based, reasonable and optimistic MID. It had a sensitivity of 0.60 and a specificity of 0.47 for global health (both patient perspective).

These proposed MIDs had very different absolute sizes. If we set them in relation to the maximum value of each item and section for which the MID was proposed and calculate the percentage of change, we can better appreciate their value. Table 14 shows these percentages of change.

The proposed MIDs could detect from 5.4% (activity section) to 22% change with respect to improvement and from 5.7% (total score) to 22% change with respect to deterioration. These MIDs are low, and most of them are more anchor- than distribution based.

The MSQPT was validated against the SF-36 and the HAQUAMS, another German PRO instrument specially tailored for MS patients. The MSQPT performed similarly to the HAQUAMS against the SF-36 [1]. In the present study, the MSQPT showed comparable responsiveness (relative efficiency) in relation to the HAQUAMS. MSQPT may detect small changes based on a 9- and 10-point answer scale, which is very important for the evaluation of the effect of physiotherapeutic treatment. These psychometric qualities make the MSQPT a very promising PRO instrument for the evaluation of outcomes of physiotherapy in MS patients.

This study uses a mixed population of which all persons were in short- or long-term treatment, and no predefined intervention was used. The focus of this study was the evaluation of responsiveness in a broad spectrum of therapy because the MSQPT is used in this way. The population of this sample was rather stable. To further evaluate the value of the proposed MID, a comparison of persons without treatment versus persons in treatment may bring important insights into the performance of the MID, especially if the population with treatment shows considerable change.

Study limitations

The present study is limited in the following aspects. The study population, although representative, was relatively small and rather stable. It is not clear how the proposed MIDs will fare in a population exhibiting a higher degree of change and especially higher improvement. Some sensitivity values could not be calculated or were based on small numbers. The approach of using rating of change questions for the global ratings gave a range of sensitivity and specificity values that were not fully coherent; thus, the choice of the best MIDs based on a range of sensitivity and specificity values was partly arbitrary. Only 77% of the patients filled out the questionnaire regarding global rating of change.

Conclusions

The present study showed that the MSQPT is responsive and can detect physiotherapy-induced changes in MS patients. The proposed MIDs are reasonable estimates that may be used in daily practice as clinical thresholds indicating change. Further research in an MS population exhibiting considerable change is needed to provide more data to understand how the proposed thresholds perform in detecting change.

Abbreviations

6MTWT: 6-metre timed walking test; 6MWT: 6-minute walk test; BBS: Berg balance scale; EDSS: Expanded disability status scale; ES: Effect size; HAQUAMS: Hamburg quality of life questionnaire for multiple sclerosis; MARCH: Multiple sclerosis and rehabilitation, care- and health services; MDC: Minimal detectable change; MDC$_{90}$: Minimal detectable change for the 90% confidence interval; MDC$_{95}$: Minimal detectable change for the 90% confidence interval; MID: Minimal important difference; MS: Multiple sclerosis; MSIS-29: Multiple sclerosis impact scale; MSQPT: Multiple sclerosis questionnaire for physical therapists; MSRM: Modified standardized response mean; PRO: Patient rated outcome; SD: Standard deviation; SEM: Standard error of measurement; SF-36: Short form health survey; SRM: Standardized response mean

Acknowledgements

The author is grateful for the support of many members of the physiotherapy group specialized in MS and all the MS patients participating in the study. The author thanks Regula Steinlin Egli and Ursula Biland-Thommen for their support in executing the survey. This article was edited by Editage.

Funding

This study was funded by grants from the Swiss Multiple Sclerosis Society and from Physioswiss.

Author's contributions

The author is solely responsible for the study and the manuscript.

Competing interests

The author declares that there are no competing interests.

References

1. Van der Maas NA, Biland-Thommen U, Grillo JT. Die Valididität, Reliabilität und Akzeptanz des Multiple Sclerosis Questionnaire for Physiotherapists (MSQPT). Physioscience. 2010;5:135–42.
2. Van der Maas NA, Steinlin Egli R. Evaluation des subjektiven Gesundheitszustandes von MS-Patienten in physiotherapeutischer Behandlung: Multiple Sclerosis Questionnaire for Physiotherapists®(MSQPT®). In: Schädler S et al., editors. Assessments in der rehabilitation, band 1: neurologie. 3rd ed. Bern: Verlag Hans Huber; 2012. p. 532–9.

Table 14 Best MID in percentage of maximum value

Item/Section	Improvement		Deterioration	
	Best MID	Best MID in %	Best MID	Best MID in %
M4	1	11%	1	11%
M8a and M8b	1	10%	1	10%
M10	2	22%	2	22%
Activity	7	5.4%	11	8.6%
Participation	17	17.2%	17	17.2%
Balance	2	11%	3	16.6%
Total score	20	6.3%	18	5.7%

M4 taking a shower, *M8a* walking distance, *M8b* walking time, *M10* getting in and out of the car

3. Bortz J, Döring N. Forschungsmethoden und evaluation für human- und sozialwissenschaftler. 3rd ed. Berlin Heidelberg New York: Springer; 2003. p. 180–1.

4. Wirtz M, Caspar F. Beurteilerübereinstimmung und Beurteilerreliabilität. Göttingen Bern Toronto Seattle: Hogrefe-Verlag; 2002. p. 123–7.

5. Revicki D, Hays RD, et al. Recommended methods for determining responsiveness and minimally important differences for patient-reported outcomes. J Clin Epidemiol. 2008;61(2):102–9.

6. Turner D, Schünemann HJ, et al. The minimal detectable change cannot reliably replace the minimal important difference. J Clin Epidemiol. 2010; 63(1):28–36.

7. Fitzpatrick R, Davey C, et al. Evaluating patient-based outcome measures for use in clinical trials. Health Technol Assess. 1998;2(14):i–iv. 1-74.

8. Baert I, Freeman J, et al. Responsiveness and clinically meaningful improvement, according to disability level, of five walking measures after rehabilitation in multiple sclerosis: a European multicenter study. Neurorehabil Neural Repair. 2014;28(7):621–31.

9. De Groot V, Beckerman H, et al. The usefulness of evaluative outcome measures in patients with multiple sclerosis. Brain. 2006;129(Pt10):2648–59.

10. Fayers PM, Hays RD. Don't middle your MIDs: regression to the mean shrinks estimates of minimally important differences. Qual Life Res. 2014;23(1):1–4.

11. Gold SM, Schulz H, et al. Responsiveness of patient-based and external rating scales in multiple sclerosis: head-to-head comparison in three clinical settings. J Neurol Sci. 2010;290(1–2):102–6.

12. Norman, et al. Interpretation of changes in health-related quality of Life; the remarkable universality of half a standard deviation. Med Care. 2003;41(5): 582–92.

13. Wyrwich KW, Tierney WM, Wolinsky FD. Further evidence supporting an SEM-based criterion for identifying meaningful intra-individual changes in health-related quality of life. J Clin Epidemiol. 1999;52(9):861–73.

14. Wyrwich KW, Norquist JM, et al. Methods for interpreting change over time in patient-reported outcome measures. Qual Life Res. 2013;22:475–83.

15. Middel B, van Sonderen E. Statistical significant change versus relevant or important change in (quasi) experimental design: some conceptual and methodological problems in estimating magnitude of intervention-related change in health services research. Int J Integr Care. 2002;2:e15.

16. Tang A, Eng JJ, Rand D. Relationship between perceived and measured changes in walking after stroke. J Neurol Phys Ther. 2012;36(3):115–21.

17. Middel B, de Greef M, et al. Why do not we ask patients with coronary disease directly how much they have changed after treatment? J Cardiopulm Rehabil. 2002;22(1):47–52.

18. Gold SM, Heesen C, et al. Disease specific quality of life instruments in multiple sclerosis: validation of the Hamburg Quality of Life Questionnaire in Multiple Sclerosis (HAQUAMS). Mult Scler. 2001;7(2):119–30.

19. Wright JG. The minimal important difference: Who's to say what is important? J Clin Epidemiol. 1996;49(11):1221–2.

20. Gijbels D, Dalgas U, et al. Which walking capacity tests to use in multiple sclerosis? A multicentre study providing the basis for a core set. Mult Scler. 2012;18(3):364–71.

21. Feys P, Gijbels D, et al. Effect of time of day on walking capacity and self-reported fatigue in persons with multiple sclerosis: a multi-center trial. Mult Scler. 2012;18(3):351–7.

22. Learmonth YC, Dlugonski DD, et al. The reliability, precision and clinically meaningful change of walking assessments in multiple sclerosis. Mult Scler. 2013;19(13):1784–91.

23. Schwid SR, Goodman AD, et al. Quantitative functional measures in MS: what is a reliable change? Neurology. 2002;58(8):1294–6.

24. Kragt JJ, van der Linden FA, et al. Clinical impact of 20% worsening on timed 25-foot walk and 9-hole peg test in multiple sclerosis. Mult Scler. 2006;12(5):594–8.

25. Tyson SF, Connel LA. How to measure balance in clinical practice. A systematic review of the psychometrics and clinical utility of measures of balance activity for neurological conditions. Clin Rehabil. 2009;23(9):824–40.

26. Latzel G, Fischbacher Schrobiltgen E. Multiple Sklerose in der Schweiz. In: Die Lebensbedingungen von MS-Betroffenen und die finanziellen Folgen ihrer Krankheit. Zürich: Schweizerische MS-Gesellschaft Zürich; 2001.

27. Schmitt JS, Di Fabio RP. Reliable change and minimum important difference (MID) proportions facilitated group responsiveness comparisons using individual threshold criteria. J Clin Epidemiol. 2004;57(10):1008–18.

28. Hays RD, Woolley JM. The concept of clinically meaningful difference in health-related quality-of-life research. Pharmacoeconomics. 2000;18(5):419–23.

11

Subjective and objective assessment of physical activity in multiple sclerosis and their relation to health-related quality of life

Theresa Krüger[1†], Janina R. Behrens[1,2†], Anuschka Grobelny[1], Karen Otte[4], Sebastian Mansow-Model[4], Bastian Kayser[4], Judith Bellmann-Strobl[1,2], Alexander U. Brandt[1,2], Friedemann Paul[1,2,3] and Tanja Schmitz-Hübsch[1*]

Abstract

Background: Physical activity (PA) is frequently restricted in people with multiple sclerosis (PwMS) and aiming to enhance PA is considered beneficial in this population. We here aimed to explore two standard methods (subjective plus objective) to assess PA reduction in PwMS and to describe the relation of PA to health-related quality of life (hrQoL).

Methods: PA was objectively measured over a 7-day period in 26 PwMS (EDSS 1.5–6.0) and 30 matched healthy controls (HC) using SenseWear mini® armband (SWAmini) and reported as step count, mean total and activity related energy expenditure (EE) as well as time spent in PA of different intensities. Measures of EE were also derived from self-assessment with IPAQ (International Physical Activity Questionnaire) long version, which additionally yielded information on the context of PA and a classification into subjects' PA levels. To explore the convergence between both types of assessment, IPAQ categories (low, moderate, high) were related to selected PA parameters from objective assessment using ANOVA. Group differences and associated effect sizes for all PA parameters as well as their relation to clinical and hrQoL measures were determined.

Results: Both, SWAmini and IPAQ assessment, captured differences in PA between PwMS and HC. IPAQ categories fit well with common cut-offs for step count ($p = 0.002$) and mean METs ($p = 0.004$) to determine PA levels with objective devices. Correlations between specifically matched pairs of IPAQ and SWAmini parameters ranged between r .288 and r .507. Concerning hrQoL, the lower limb mobility subscore was related to four PA measures, while a relation with patients' report of general contentment was only seen for one.

Conclusions: Both methods of assessment seem applicable in PwMS and able to describe reductions in daily PA at group level. Whether they can be used to track individual effects of interventions to enhance PA levels needs further exploration. The relation of PA measures with hrQoL seen with lower limb mobility suggests lower limb function not only as a major target for intervention to increase PA but also as a possible surrogate for PA changes.

Keywords: Physical activity, Accelerometry, IPAQ, Multiple sclerosis, Quality of life

* Correspondence: Tanja.schmitz-huebsch@charite.de
[†]Equal contributors
[1]NeuroCure Clinical Research Center, Clinical Neuroimmunology Group,
Charité – Universitätsmedizin Berlin, Charitéplatz 1, 10117 Berlin, Germany
Full list of author information is available at the end of the article

Background

A low level of physical activity (PA) is a known risk factor for health outcomes and effects on disease outcomes have been described in several conditions [1–3].

Also in people with multiple sclerosis (PwMS), aiming to enhance PA is considered beneficial [4]. Like in other chronic disorders, PA assessment may serve as a marker of disability status [5] with different aims: on the one hand to select individuals that may benefit from intervention and to track effects of behavioral interventions and on the other hand to investigate how and which functional changes translate into real-life activity [6].

We here use the term PA according to the classic definition as "all muscle activity exerted by an individual resulting in energy expenditure (EE) above resting EE" [7]. Thus, the intensity of PA is usually expressed in multitudes of individual resting EE, designated as metabolic equivalent of task (MET, unit of work/ kg body weight/ hour), with estimates assigned to different types of PA [8–10]. According to their assigned MET, PA is usually categorized as low, moderate or vigorous activity (LPA, MPA, VPA). In contrast, daily step count or time spent walking specifically refer to locomotor activity which can take on different intensities, e.g. depending on walking speed or inclination. General levels of PA are most often described as step count, total daily EE, activity related EE or time of the day spent active/ inactive as defined by MET thresholds.

The different methods used to assess PA capture different aspects and have their specific limitations [10–13]. The International Physical Activity Questionnaire (IPAQ) [14] is a standardized self-rating questionnaire based on recall over the previous week.

Several portable activity monitors have become available for objective PA assessment [3, 10, 12, 15–17]. Accuracy of the multi-sensor device SenseWear Pro was acceptable in PwMS [18] against indirect calorimetry as standard, while - to our knowledge - the successor SWAmini with reportedly improved performance [19–21] has not been applied in PwMS. We therefore aim to explore its applicability in this population and convergence of results with those obtained from subjective assessment (IPAQ long version). From previous reports we expect lower levels of daily PA to be associated with more severe symptoms of MS and reduced health-related quality of life (hrQoL). By correlation of PA measures with an MS-specific quality of life questionnaire, we aim to define which aspects of MS-related functional impairment relate most closely to decline in daily PA level in PwMS.

Methods

Study participants

Study participants were enrolled at a university MS referral center. Inclusion criteria for all participants were: age 18–65 years, no cardiovascular disease, orthopedic or other conditions thought to affect motor performance or daily activity and additionally for healthy controls (HC) without neurological diagnosis: no impairment of gait or balance evident at testing. Further inclusion criteria for PwMS were: MS diagnosis according to McDonald Criteria 2010 [22], EDSS between 0 and 6, no relapses for at least 30 days prior to study visit, no other neurologic comorbidity. The study was approved by the local ethics committee of the Charité - Universitätsmedizin Berlin (EA1/321/14) and conducted in conformity with the Declaration of Helsinki in its currently applicable form. All participants gave written informed consent.

Objective assessment of daily PA with SWAmini

We used the physical activity monitor SenseWear® Armband and Software Development Kit Version 8.1.1.30 (SenseWear Model Mini, MF-SW; BodyMedia®, Inc. Pittsburgh, Pennsylvania, USA). Subjects were instructed to wear the SWAmini over 7 days (including the weekend) throughout the day and to take the sensor off during night rest and for any water activity. The monitor was placed at the middle of the triceps brachii muscle (left arm) according to the user manual [23]. The device reports individual wearing times that served to prove subjects' compliance.

SWAmini reports physical activity as accelerometrically derived step count and as estimates of individual EE from 1-min epochs of recording based on algorithmic integration of multi-sensor data incorporating subject's age, sex and body size. EE is reported as total MET per recording time (mean METs) and activity related EE (active METs). One MET represents estimated resting EE and by convention equals 1 kcal/ kg body weight/h. The intensity of PA within each epoch is classified according to MET cut-offs of 1.5–3 for light PA (LPA), MET 3 – 6 for moderate PA (MPA), MET 6–9 for vigorous PA (VPA) and MET > 9 for very vigorous PA (VVPA). Duration of PA per intensity is reported in min/hour, calculated as SWAmini output per day divided by individual daily wearing time, MPA and VPA values were combined into MVPA for some analyses. A list of parameters is available as Additional file 1: Table S1.

To account for possible difference in PA behavior between weekdays and weekend, a weighted mean was calculated as follows:

$$\frac{(\text{parameter mean weekend} \times 2) + (\text{parameter mean weekday} \times 5)}{7}$$

For comparison with IPAQ data, activity-related EE was given in MET*min/day calculated as SWAmini mean active METs times duration of all MET > 3 activity per day. Similarly, SWAmini MPA and VPA duration in min/hour were transformed into min/day by multiplication with the mean daily hours of wearing time.

Subjective assessment of daily PA with IPAQ long version

We used the German (Austrian) translation of the IPAQ long version [14] that reports the amount and intensity of patients' PA by recall of the past 7 days. The questionnaire was applied in paper-pencil form after the week of SWA-mini recording and thus, IPAQ data refer to the same time span as SWAmini recordings.

After application of data cleaning rules according to the scoring manual [24] IPAQ results were coded, first, as time per day spent in PA of different intensity, i.e. time spent walking (IPAQ Walking duration), time spent in moderate (IPAQ MPA duration) or vigorous PA (IPAQ VPA duration), that can be summed to total duration of daily PA (IPAQ Total duration). Data are usually presented as min/week that we transformed into min/day for comparison with SWAmini data. As the MET-value of 3.3 assigned for walking in the IPAQ [14] is above the MET-threshold for MPA in the SWAmini, we computed a combined parameter from IPAQ Walking duration + IPAQ MPA duration for comparison. Second, results were rendered as estimates of active EE by multiplication of duration of activity with predefined MET values given in MET*min/week that we transformed into MET*min/day for comparison with SWAmini. Third, both the duration and intensity of PA were coded separately in four ADL domains: work, active transportation, domestic/yard and leisure/sports that were reported as EE per domain in % of total active EE. Fourth, we applied the scoring rules to classify individuals into the IPAQ categories of low, moderate and high PA level.

In sum, IPAQ long form yielded three main outcomes: 1) the activity related EE as well as time spent for walking, MPA and VPA, 2) the distribution of EE in the four different ADL domains and 3) a three-step classification of PA level. In addition, we derived information on occupational status out of IPAQ results.

Clinical severity and health-related Quality of Life

In PwMS, a neurological examination with the Expanded Disability Status Scale (EDSS) scoring [25] was performed prior to SWAmini assessment. The Hamburg Quality of Life Questionnaire in Multiple Sclerosis (HAQUAMS version 10.0) was applied in paper form in its German version (HALEMS) [26, 27]. It consists of 44 items, 28 of which contribute to the total score between 1 (unimpaired) and 5 (very much impaired) as the mean of the following six subscores: fatigue, thinking, mobility lower limb, mobility upper limb, communication and mood. We added a sensory (items 4 and 5) and bladder/bowel (items 26–28) subscore, as we assumed these may impact on subjects' daily PA. As a general measure of overall contentment in life – irrespective of any disease specific impairment – we included item 43 (score 1–5) into analysis.

Statistical analysis

Differences between groups (HC and PwMS) regarding sex and occupational status were calculated using the $\chi2$-test while independent sample t-tests were applied with regard to age, height, weight and BMI and SWAmini parameters. Differences of SWAmini parameter means between weekdays and weekends were explored by paired t-test, separately for each group. Group differences for SWAmini parameters were also expressed as effect sizes (Cohen's d) calculated as mean between-group difference divided by the standard deviation in HC. Between-group differences regarding IPAQ parameters of duration and EE were explored using Mann–Whitney-U-tests. The proportions of IPAQ Total EE spent in the four domains work, transportation, domestic and leisure as well as the distribution of subjects into IPAQ categories of low, moderate and high PA level was compared between groups with $\chi2$-test.

We used Spearman rank correlation for IPAQ data, EDSS and HAQUAMS total and subscores. To relate SWAmini parameters step count and mean METs to the IPAQ categories of low, moderate and high PA level, we applied ANOVA with Bonferroni post-hoc testing, while EDSS scores were related to the IPAQ categories with Jonckheere-Terpstra-Test.

All analyses relating SWAmini to IPAQ as well as inter-correlations of SWAmini parameters (presented as Additional files 1, 2, 3 and 4) were performed for the whole group, while correlations with EDSS and HAQUAMS were only analyzed in PwMS.

Statistical analysis was performed with SPSS version 22 (IBM, Armonk, NY, USA). All tests were two-tailed, significance was assumed when $p < 0.05$. No alpha-error correction for multiple testing was applied in this exploratory study.

Results

Study cohort and data cleaning

From November 2014 to August 2015, 29 PwMS and 30 gender- and age-matched HC were included into the study. Three PwMS were excluded because of incorrect use of the SWAmini (2) or missing SWAmini-data (1). IPAQ data were missing in one HC, and data of one PwMS were excluded in the data cleaning process (>960 min of daily activity time). Truncation of IPAQ active time according to the IPAQ manual had to be applied in 5 subjects (3 HC and 2 PwMS). Data in HAQUAMS item 43 (contentment) were missing in one PwMS. Thus, analyses refer to 26 PwMS and 30 HC (Table 1), while analyses comprising IPAQ data refer to 26 PwMS and 29 HC. A higher rate of unemployment was noted among PwMS that seemed related to higher EDSS (Table 1, Additional file 3: Figure S1).

Table 1 Cohort overview – demographic and clinical data per subject group

		HC	PwMS	p-value
Subjects	N	30	26	
	Relapsing MS		18	
	Progressive MS		8 (7 SPMS; 1 PPMS)	
Sex	Male /female	10 /20	10 /16	.783
Occupational status	without employment/ working	6/23	14/12	.013*
Age (years)	Mean (±SD)	49.7 (±8.3)	50.9 (±5.2)	.522
BMI	Mean (±SD)	25.3 (±3.9)	26.0 (±3.5)	.474
Height (m)	Mean (±SD)	1.70 (±7.4)	1.71 (±6.6)	.398
Weight (kg)	Mean (±SD)	73.8 (±13.7)	76.8 (±12.9)	.588
EDSS	Median (Min-Max)	.	4.0 (1.5–6.0)	

Independent sample t-test was used for between-group comparison of age, BMI, weight and height and χ2-test was used to compare sex and occupational status. Please note that IPAQ-data and thus occupational status from 1 HC is missing. *denotes significance at level <0.05

SWAmini: objectively assessed daily PA

Only small differences between parameter means from weekend and weekday were seen in HC with 0.15 lower active METs ($p = 0.049$) on weekends. No difference was seen for any parameter in PwMS between weekend/ weekday. Therefore, all further SWAmini analyses refer to a weighted mean.

Between-group differences - that is, HC performing better than PwMS - were observed in all parameters except light PA ($p < 0.01$, Table 2). Highest effect sizes (Cohen's d ≥ 0.85) were seen with step count, mean and active METs, while other parameters yielded effect sizes between 0.63 and 0.75 (Table 2).

As expected from the observed between-group differences, the correlations of SWAmini parameters with EDSS were not significant for time spent in light activities, but pointed to a decrease of higher intensity PA with higher EDSS (Fig. 1), reflected in decreased step count (r –0.534, $p = 0.005$), mean METs (r –0.411, $p = 0.037$), MPA and MVPA (r –0.477, $p = 0.014$ and r –0.451, $p = 0.021$). The lack of correlation with VPA and active METs (r –0.327, $p = 0.103$ and r –0.175, $p = 0.394$) is likely due to the generally low amount of VPA in this group with no VPA recorded in 6 of 26 PwMS (Table 2).

IPAQ: subjectively assessed daily PA

Concerning the proportional distribution of IPAQ total EE into ADL domains, a trend for group differences was noted ($p = 0.089$, Table 2) with a tendency of PwMS to spend a smaller part of their daily total EE in active transportation/work but a larger part in leisure and domestic activities (Table 2). This suggests active transportation as a work-related activity.

Second, we explored group differences in total durations of PA irrespective of their contextual domain (Walking, MPA, VPA, MVPA and Total PA duration). PwMS reported less time spent in moderate PA (MWU; MPA $p = 0.010$ and MVPA $p = 0.016$), while no significant differences were seen for walking, vigorous PA, total PA duration as well as total activity-related EE (Table 2). It should be noted for interpretation that as with SWAmini, a considerable number of subjects reported no vigorous (14 HC and 17 PwMS) or even moderate activities (6 HC and 14 PwMS). Similar to SWAmini, reduced PA in PwMS was associated with higher EDSS scores (Fig. 2) for IPAQ Total duration (r –0.752, $p < 0.001$), IPAQ Total EE (r –0.572, $p = 0.003$), IPAQ Walking duration (r –0.462; $p = 0.020$,) MPA duration (r –0.469, $p = 0.018$), VPA duration and MVPA duration (r –0.428, $p = 0.033$ and r –0.424, $p = 0.035$).

Third, we compared the distribution of subjects into the three IPAQ categories of low – moderate – high PA level between groups (Fig. 3a). There was a tendency of HC to be more frequently classified as moderate or high PA level and less frequently as low PA level compared to PwMS (X^2 test, $p = 0.150$, Fig. 3a). EDSS scores differed across the IPAQ PA levels with higher EDSS scores in PwMS assigned as low activity level and low EDSS of 3 in the one highly active MS subject (Jonckheere-Terpstra test; $p = 0.027$; Fig. 3b).

SWAmini and IPAQ: associations between subjectively and objectively assessed daily PA

For testing convergence of both methods we correlated three matching pairs of PA parameters (Additional file 4: Figure S2). The combined parameter moderate PA and walking duration from the IPAQ showed a remarkable association with moderate PA assessed with SWAmini (IPAQ MPA + Walking duration and SWAmini MPA Spearman r .507, $p < 0.001$); subjectively assessed total EE was associated with respective active EE assessed with SWAmini (IPAQ Total EE and SWAmini active EE r .336, $p = 0.013$) and subjective duration of vigorous

Table 2 Amount and intensity of daily physical activity in HC and PwMS assessed with wearable device (SWAmini) reported as weighted mean (± SD) and subjective assessment with IPAQ long version reported as median (interquartile range) from a 7-day period

		Healthy controls N = 30	PwMS N = 26	p-value	Cohen's d
Objective (SWAmini)	Step count (steps/hour)	563.45 (±155.90)	430.66 (±171.68)	**.004**	0.85
	Mean METs (mean/day)	1.77 (±.28)	1.53 (±.16)	**<.001**	0.86
	Active METs (mean/day)	4.41 (±.59)	3.90 (±.46)	**.001**	0.86
	Total EE (kcal/hour)	387.40 (±237.40)	214.08 (±194.20)	**.004**	0.73
	Active EE (kcal/hour)	118.13 (±110.65)	37.89 (±41.73)	**.001**	0.75
	Active EE (MET*min/day)	410.79 (±257.07)	217.70 (±116.19)	**.001**	0.75
	LPA (min/hour)	2.98 (±2.47)	3.90 (±3.27)	.249	0.37
	MPA (min/hour)	5.38 (±2.63)	3.73 (±1.80)	**.008**	0.63
	MVPA (min/hour)	6.23 (±3.21)	3.91 (±1.93)	**.002**	0.72
	VPA (min/hour)	.844 (±.927) *3	.176 (±.403) *6	**.001**	0.72
	VVPA (min/hour)	.148 (±.426) *21	.001 (±.002) *25	.084	0.35
	Full days worn (days/period)	7.23 (±1.36)	7.81 (±1.77)	.220	-
	Mean daily wearing time (hours/day)	15.38 (±1.73)	14.29 (±1.58)	.017	-
Self-perceived (IPAQ)	Walking duration (min/day)	27.86 (45.71) *2	34.29 (71.14) *2	.664	
	MPA duration (min/day)	51.43 (91.79) *6	0.00 (53.57) *14	**.010**	
	MVPA duration (min/day)	68.19 (101.79) *6	0.00 (60.00) *13	**.016**	
	VPA duration (min/day)	2.86 (25.71) *14	0.00 (17.14) *17	.259	
	Total duration (min/day)	108.57 (120.36)	81.43 (135.00)	.327	
	Total EE (MET*min/day)	516.57 (502.04)	501.14 (596.44)	.440	
	Work EE (mean % of total EE and interquartile range)	19.12% (31.22) *8, 6 unemployed	12.66% (17.34) *5, 14 unemployed	.089	
	Transportation EE (mean % of total EE and interquartile range)	34.41% (43.38) *2	28.42% (40.53) *2		
	Domestic EE (mean % of total EE and interquartile range)	24.93% (22.43) *2	28.34% (33.76) *3		
	Leisure EE (mean % of total EE and interquartile range)	21.54% (28.70) *4	30.58% (36.59) *2		
	IPAQ category (n and % of group):			.150	
	Low	5 (17.2%)	10 (40.0%)		
	Moderate	21 (72.4%)	14 (56.0%)		
	High	3 (10.3%)	1 (4.0%)		

Subjects were instructed to wear SWAmini during the waking day excluding water activities. *P*-values for between-group differences of SWAmini parameters refer to t-tests. IPAQ-data (comprising 29 HC and 25 PwMS) were compared between groups using Mann–Whitney-*U*-test, except for χ2-test used to compare the distribution of subjects into different IPAQ physical activity levels and the percentages of total EE spent in different activity domains. Please note that percentage values in IPAQ work EE were set to a value of 0 for unemployed subjects. Numbers of subjects per group that were not assigned any activity for MPA/VPA/VVPA are given with asterisk; these individuals were assigned a value of 0 for the calculation of means

activities duration was related to the corresponding objectively assessed parameter (IPAQ VPA duration and SWAmini VPA duration r .288, $p = 0.035$). Interestingly, of the nine subjects with objectively no vigorous activities (3 HC, 6 PwMS), eight (3 HC, 5 PwMS) reported also no vigorous activities with IPAQ, while vice versa, in subjects with no self-perceived vigorous PA between 0–28 min/day were recorded with SWAmini.

In the second approach, we related the three IPAQ categories of PA level to those SWAmini parameters that have been proposed as classification criteria for individual activity level: total daily step count and mean METs. As expected, both parameters increased from low to moderate to high IPAQ activity level (ANOVA $p = 0.002$ for step count per day, $p = 0.004$ for mean METs per day, Fig. 3c and d). Post-hoc analyses

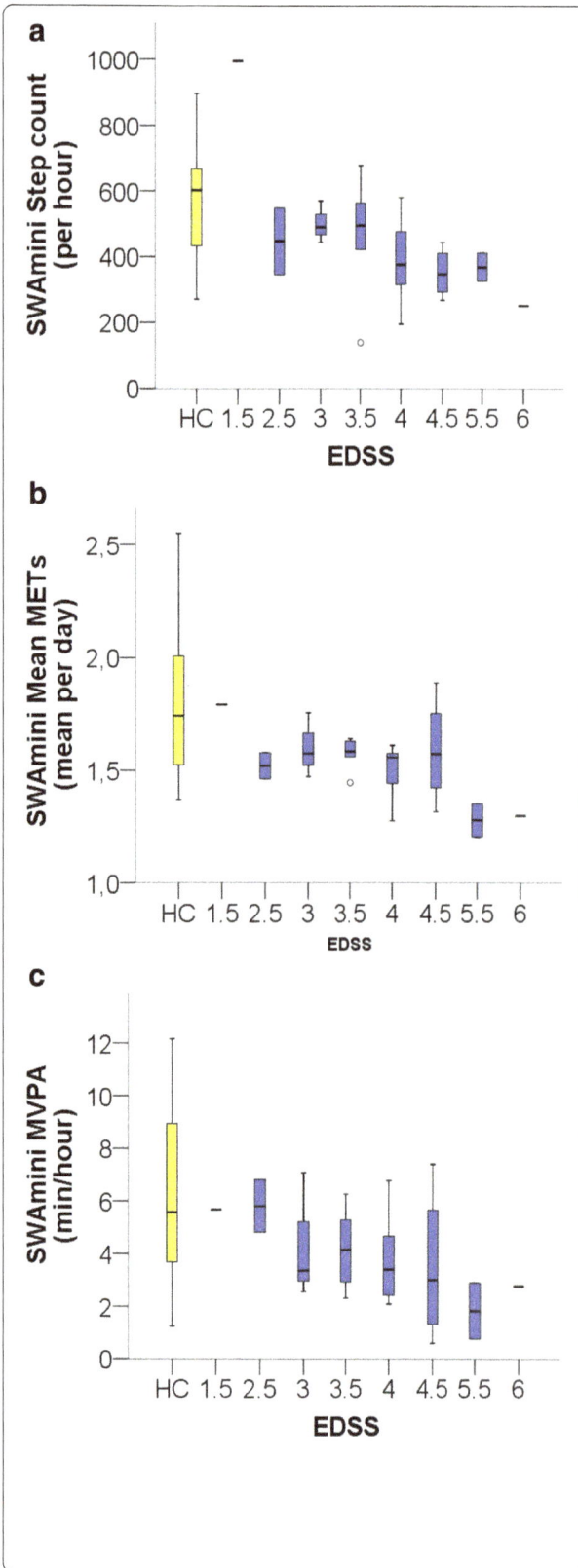

Fig. 1 Selected activity parameters from SWAmini related to EDSS score. **a** Steps per day, **b** Mean METs and **c** MVPA. Results of HCs are depicted in *yellow* for reference, all PwMS results are depicted in *dark blue*. *Lines* refer to median, *boxes* to interquartile range and whiskers to maximum and minimum excluding outliers (outlier defined as > 1.5 IQR of upper or lower quartile)

indicated a better differentiation between high and moderate PA level by step count and between moderate and low PA level by mean METs (Fig. 3c and d).

HAQUAMS: the impact of MS on quality of life related to daily PA

The distribution of HAQUAMS total and subscores were found as expected from other MS cohorts of similar disease stage without major floor or ceiling effects (Tables 3 and 4). HAQUAMS total had a median of 2.20 (range from 1.20 to 3.39) and the median of the single item 43 (global contentment) was 2.00 (range from 1 to 4) with only two subjects scoring category 1 or 4, respectively. Lower EDSS scores were strongly associated with better self-perceived hrQoL in the subscores mobility lower limb (r 0.590, $p = 0.002$), mobility upper limb (r 0.479, $p = 0.013$) and global contentment (r 0.445, $p = 0.026$), but not with other subscores or HAQUAMS total.

When we explored the relation of HAQUAMS total and subscores with the amount of daily PA from both, objective and subjective assessment, correlations of moderate magnitude were seen with HAQUAMS subscore mobility lower limb for four PA parameters: step count, moderate PA assessed objectively and subjectively as well as subjective vigorous PA (Tables 3 and 4), all pointing to higher PA levels being associated with better self-perceived lower limb function. In addition, vigorous PA assessed with SWAmini showed moderate correlation to HAQUAMS pain/sensory subscore (Tables 3 and 4). In contrast, PA parameters were not related to HAQUAMS total or global contentment, except for its moderate correlation with IPAQ Total EE. This argues against a genuine impact of perceived hrQoL on daily PA or vice versa, although correlation analyses are surely limited by small sample size. Considering this, trends seen for the correlation of HAQUAMS contentment with IPAQ Total duration, SWAmini active METs and vigorous PA as well as HAQUAMS total with SWAmini moderate PA and of HAQUAMS fatigue subscore with IPAQ moderate/vigorous PA and SWAmini mean METs and light PA deserve further investigation.

Discussion

The amount of daily physical activity was reduced in PwMS compared to HC. This was expected from previous reports [28–30] as well as from the theoretical conceptualization of PA as the behavioral correlate of disability in MS [31, 32]. Given that the vast majority of evidence on PA in PwMS is

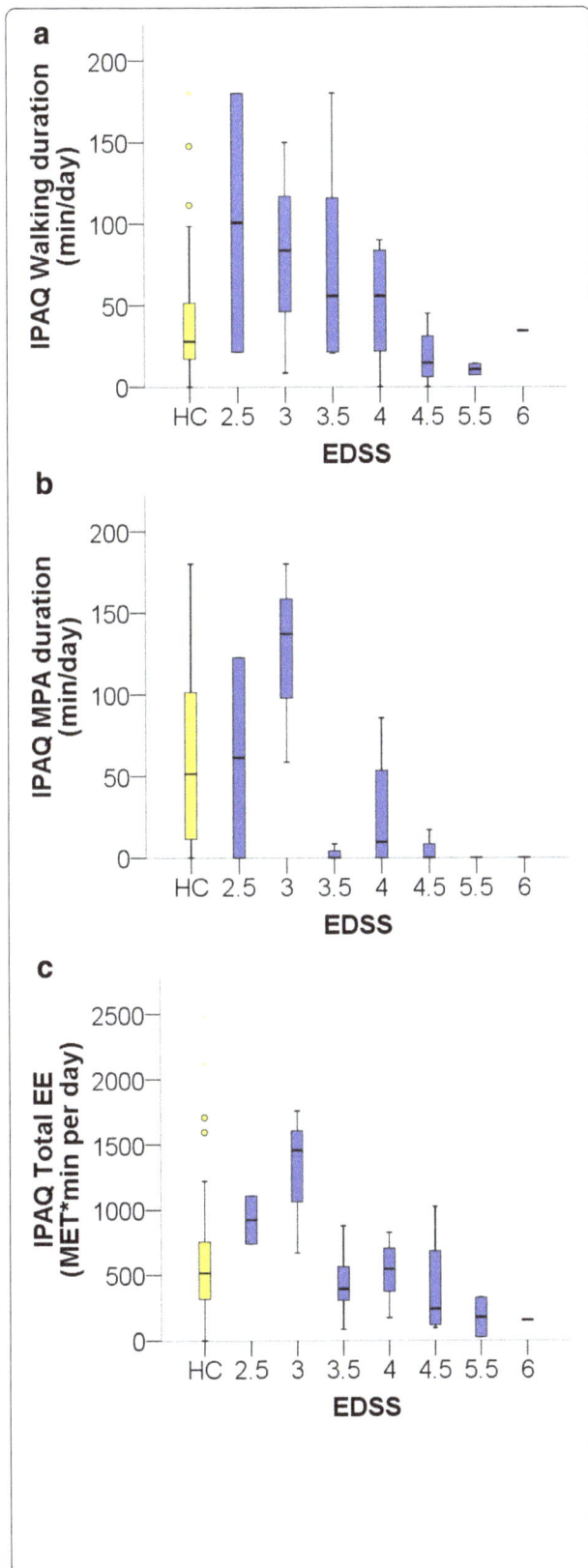

Fig. 2 Selected activity parameters from IPAQ related to EDSS score. **a** Walking duration, **b** MPA duration and **c** Total EE. Results of HCs are depicted in *yellow* for reference, all PwMS results are depicted in *blue*. *Lines, boxes, whiskers* as in Fig. 2. Please note that the one subject with EDSS 1.5 was excluded in the data cleaning process according to the IPAQ manual

from US cohorts, this is also the first confirmatory study in German MS subjects.

When measured objectively with SWAmini, group differences were seen for all parameters except light PA and were most pronounced for higher intensities, indicating the generally lower participation of PwMS in strenuous physical activities. The three most distinctive parameters were step count, mean METs and active METs. This supports the description of changes in PA as (1) reduction in global walking mobility and (2) reduced activity-related EE [7, 33, 34].

Effect sizes ranged from 0.63 to 0.86, which is comparable to previous reports of large MS cohorts [28, 35–37].

While daily step counts were similar to reports using other devices [36, 38, 39], the mean duration of MVPA activities observed in this study was higher than reported from US cohorts (MVPA < 23.5 and < 33.8 min/day in PwMS and HC) [35, 36] but lower than in other non-diseased populations [40]. Besides different recruitment bias and assessment devices, differences in activity lifestyle may also contribute.

An exploratory analysis of parameter inter-correlations (Additional file 2: Table S2) revealed that mean METs were most tightly associated with MVPA, active METs most strongly related to the amount of vigorous PA while step count showed only moderate correlations to both, mean METs and MVPA. Its lack of association with active METs and vigorous PA indicates that locomotor activity is predominantly performed within the low to moderate intensity segments.

This underlines that step count and EE capture complementary aspects of PA: subjects with gait or balance impairment may walk similar distances as HC but at lower speed (lower intensity) or – conversely - walk less efficiently, thus increasing the energy expended per step, which has indeed been shown in PwMS [41, 42].

Although our cohort included rather physically active PwMS, we observed a generally low amount of vigorous activities in PwMS with only one subject performing very vigorous PA, which impeded statistical comparison for this parameter. Concerning light activities, our results imply that this activity segment represents inevitable ADL activities, performed to a similar extent by HC and PwMS. It should further be noted that the group differences in PA relate to a segment of only about 10 min per hour, while both groups spend the largest part of their wake-time physically inactive. According to

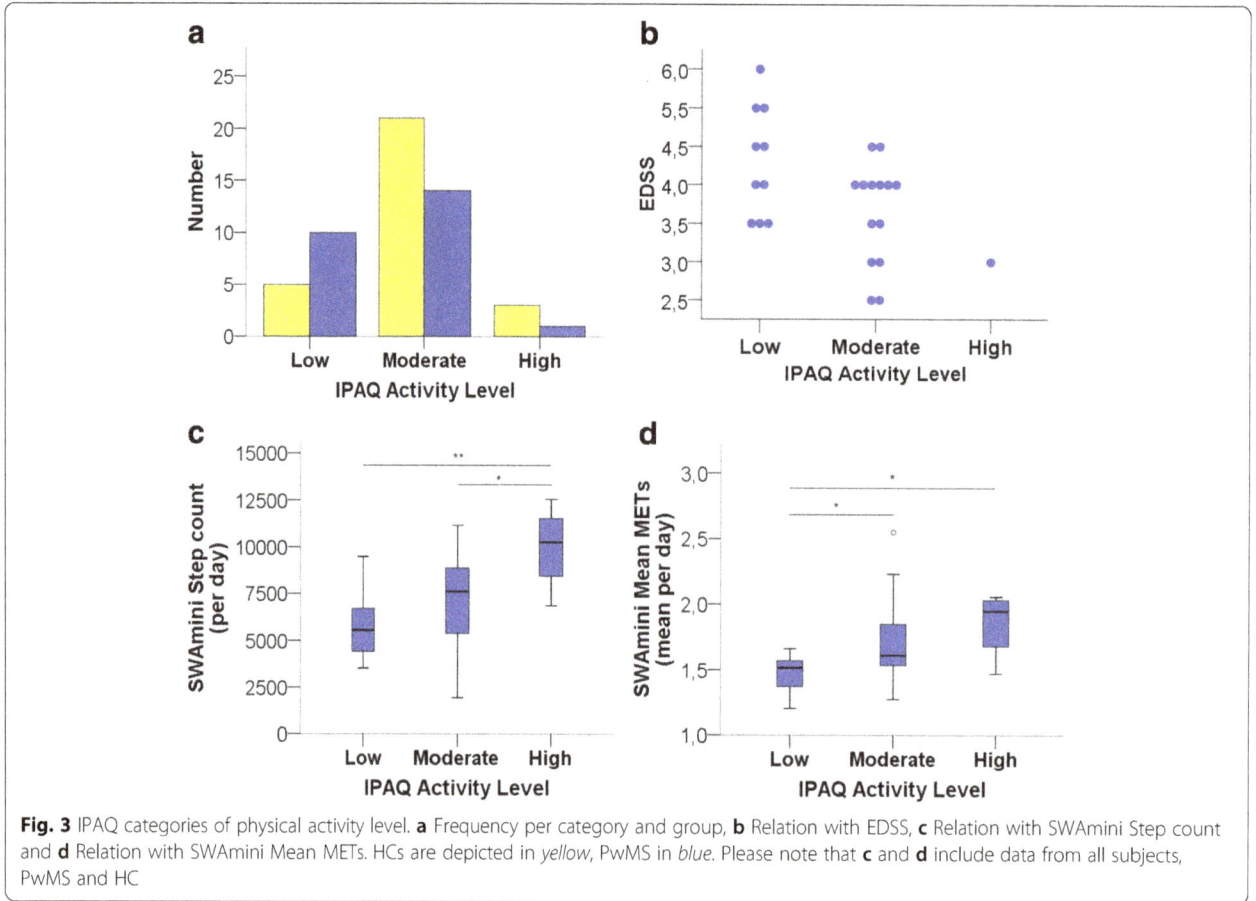

Fig. 3 IPAQ categories of physical activity level. **a** Frequency per category and group, **b** Relation with EDSS, **c** Relation with SWAmini Step count and **d** Relation with SWAmini Mean METs. HCs are depicted in *yellow*, PwMS in *blue*. Please note that **c** and **d** include data from all subjects, PwMS and HC

Table 3 Results of HAQUAMS total and susbcores reported as median (variance) and range in 26 PwMS and their association with daily physical activity according to SWAmini parameters (Spearman correlations)

HAQUAMS parameter	Median (variance)	Min-Max	SWAmini											
			Step count per hour		Mean METs		Active METs		LPA		MPA		VPA	
			rho	p	rho	p	rho	p	rho	p	rho	p	rho	P
Fatigue	2.61 (.866)	1.00–4.25	−.136	.509	−.369	.064	−.156	.446	.350	.080	−.244	.230	−.233	.253
Thinking	2.75 (.980)	1.00–4.50	−.061	.768	−.109	.595	−.186	.364	.124	.547	−.065	.754	−.187	.361
Mobility lower limb	2.13 (.672)	1.00–3.75	**−.442**	**.024**	−.222	.275	−.064	.755	−.069	.738	**−.439**	**.025**	−.310	.123
Mobility upper limb	1.30 (.300)	1.00–3.40	−.178	.385	−.004	.985	.054	.795	−.030	.884	−.267	.188	.000	.999
Communication	2.00 (.561)	1.17–3.83	−.114	.579	−.098	.633	−.083	.689	−.040	.845	−.053	.797	−.006	.975
Mood	2.50 (.716)	1.40–4.60	−.034	.868	−.067	.745	−.202	.322	.128	.533	−.313	.120	−.128	.533
Pain/Sensory	2.00 (.600)	1.00–3.50	.145	.480	−.083	.686	−.232	.255	−.066	.749	.206	.313	**−.473**	**.015**
Bowel/Bladder	1.67 (.549)	1.00–3.33	.000	.999	−.023	.913	.099	.631	−.134	.515	−.127	.538	.090	.662
Contentment	2.00 (.427)	1.00–4.00	−.060	.776	−.026	.903	−.372	.067	−.144	.492	−.161	.442	−.365	.073
Total	2.20 (.299)	1.20–3.39	−.227	.264	−.262	.196	−.212	.298	.130	.528	−.368	.065	−.257	.205

Pain/sensory and bowel/bladder were included in addition to published HAQUAMS subscores. Contentment refers to a single-item question. Significant results at level of <0.05 are given in bold

Table 4 Results of HAQUAMS total and susbcores reported as median (variance) and range in 26 PwMS and their association with daily physical activity according to selected IPAQ

HAQUAMS parameter	Median (variance)	Min-Max	IPAQ Duration (min/day)								EE (MET*min/day)	
			Walking		MPA		VPA		Total		Total	
			rho	p	rho	p	rho	p	rho	p	rho	p
Fatigue	2.61 (.866)	1.00–4.25	.190	.364	−.340	.097	−.390	.054	−.053	.803	−.150	.475
Thinking	2.75 (.980)	1.00–4.50	.133	.527	−.227	.276	−.164	.433	−.055	.793	−.016	.939
Mobility lower limb	2.13 (.672)	1.00–3.75	−.107	.610	**−.413**	**.040**	**−.441**	**.027**	−.274	.185	−.221	.289
Mobility upper limb	1.30 (.300)	1.00–3.40	−.151	.471	−.210	.315	−.171	.413	−.326	.112	−.342	.095
Communication	2.00 (.561)	1.17–3.83	−.074	.725	−.201	.336	−.289	.160	−.180	.390	−.160	.444
Mood	2.50 (.716)	1.40–4.60	−.039	.855	.087	.678	−.073	.728	.044	.836	−.028	.895
Pain/Sensory	2.00 (.600)	1.00–3.50	.344	.092	.012	.955	.099	.639	.091	.664	−.016	.939
Bowel/Bladder	1.67 (.549)	1.00–3.33	.048	.818	.132	.528	.092	.663	.226	.227	.249	.229
Contentment	2.00 (.427)	1.00–4.00	−.253	.233	−.110	.610	−.221	.299	−.360	.084	**−.489**	**.015**
Total	2.20 (.299)	1.20–3.39	−.030	.887	−.219	.294	−.294	.154	−.143	.495	−.084	.690

Pain/sensory and bowel/bladder were included in addition to published HAQUAMS subscores. Contentment refers to a single-item question. Significant results at level of <0.05 are given in bold

the MET definition of light PA, this may comprise low-intensity locomotor activity as well as sedentary time except sleeping which explains the seeming discrepancy to reports of increased sedentary time in PwMS [43, 44]. The effect of occupational status on PA was somewhat unexpected in its direction (tendency to even larger weekend – weekday difference in unemployed subjects) and small effect size, as others reported employment as a relevant factor for PA among PwMS [5, 35, 44, 45], however, in much larger cohorts. From our observation of a lower proportion of PwMS employed (Table 1), that even seems to decrease with higher EDSS scores (Additional file 3: Figure S1), we conclude that effects of occupational status and MS progression on daily PA may be difficult to distinguish or even counteract each other.

Group differences in PA could also be detected with the subjective IPAQ long form and were observed for the amount of MPA and MVPA, but not for the time spent walking. Convergent to SWAmini data, PwMS perceive themselves as (and according to SWAmini "are") less engaged in higher intensity physical activities at group level. This is remarkable given the small group size and previous reports on a tendency for unfit (otherwise healthy) individuals to overestimate their participation in MVPA activities by up to 37% [46]. The questionnaire was easily applicable in our cohort and data exclusion or truncation rules had to be applied at similar rates in HC and PwMS.

With respect to IPAQ walking, it has to be considered, however, that IPAQ data refer only to reported bouts of over 10 min, although most locomotor activity, i.e. steps accumulated during the day, is likely to occur in shorter bouts. When relating results from subjective to objective

assessment, we therefore subsumed reported walking activity within moderate PA.

The observed convergence for this matched parameter pair (r .507) was higher than expected from previous results obtained with other means of objective and subjective PA assessment in PwMS [36, 39, 47–49]. Similarly, the relation of IPAQ PA levels to selected SWAmini PA parameters roughly converge with commonly used cut-offs to detect low and highly active lifestyles by step count or mean METs (step count low level < 5000 steps/day, moderate level 5000–7500 steps/day and high level > 7500 steps/day; mean METs: very low level < 1.2 METs, low level 1.2–1.4 METs, moderate level 1.4–1.6 METs and high level > 1.7 METs) [23, 38]. This supports the validity of this easily applicable classification, e.g. for screening purposes. The trend seen for group difference (p = 0.15) is likely due to small sample size. Only one person with MS was classified as highly active, probably due to high IPAQ Walking durations despite a not specifically high step count around 7000/day and mean METs of 1.5.

This part of analysis further suggested that step count rather differentiates high from moderate PA levels, which may apply early in disease, while mean METs (related tightly to MVPA) is more suited to distinguish between moderate and low PA level. This further implies that increase in PA is mediated by different types of activity according to PA levels and that different PA parameters may be suited to monitor MS populations of different symptom severity.

Another aspect of IPAQ with relevance for intervention design is the context of PA. From our data, it seems unlikely that increases of PA in PwMS will be added as leisure/sports activity, whereas supporting active transportation or integrate PA into subjects' lifestyle [50, 51] seem more appropriate. In this respect, it is worth reconsidering and exploring the role of occupational status in daily PA and, specifically, active transportation. With regard to behavioral interventions, these probably need to be designed and evaluated specific to cultural settings according to activity lifestyle differences, for example between U.S. and German populations.

SWAmini parameter correlations to EDSS were moderate in magnitude, which is similar to previously reported coefficients between −.34 and −.70 [33, 39, 52–54]. Again, inspection of the parameter plots per EDSS score (Fig. 2) suggests reduced step count as an early feature in MS while decline in the daily amount of MVPA occurs beyond EDSS > 3, i.e. at stages with manifest decrease in walking mobility.

Corresponding IPAQ – EDSS plots revealed, that despite lower duration of MVPA in PwMS at group level, among those less severely affected, self-report of moderate activities was even higher than in HC. This paradoxical relation was even more pronounced for subjectively assessed walking duration and total EE. As discussed above, this may be interpreted as either a larger perceived exertion when physically active (despite unchanged or lower activity counts on "objective" assessment) or a systematic reporting bias in subjects aware of physical limitations, which has been reported in different populations [13]. Despite this and with only a small number of subjects remaining for IPAQ MPA and MVPA to EDSS analysis, correlations with symptom severity were similar to those observed with SWAmini. Further, IPAQ PA level assignment was related to EDSS scores. Both support the validity of IPAQ results in our PwMS cohort, although interpretations from individual absolute IPAQ results cannot be recommended.

With respect to HAQUAMS, we observed distributions of subscores similar to those reported in another German MS cohort [26] as well as expected correlations with EDSS.

However, the amount of daily moderate PA or daily step count were not related to HAQUAMS sum score, but seemed only related to the perceived impact of MS on lower limb function. This result was irrespective of the means of PA assessment (Tables 3 and 4) and adds to previous findings that PA in PwMS is only indirectly related to hrQoL, most likely mediated through physical function [55], although data on this topic are not abundant. One interventional study reported improved HAQUAMS total scores with intervention along with improvements in lower limb coordination [56]. Vice versa, decreased hrQoL as such seems unrelated to decrease in PA but related to a multitude of not directly disease-related factors [55, 57–61]. This implies, that interventions aiming to increase PA should target walking ability and physical limitations of the

lower limbs, while the quantitative assessment of lower limb function may be a potentially useful surrogate of PA for intervention monitoring.

Our findings, in line with previous reports, support the notion that both objective and subjective PA assessment may be appropriate depending on the purpose and resources of the study [39], a major limitation of both being the inherent variability in PA that requires long-term recording over several days. Further, specific limitations of different devices - questionnaires or activity monitors - have been studied in different populations [18, 42, 62, 63] and rather point to an approximation of "true" PA from different perspectives instead of one golden assessment standard. Thus, individual PA parameters may rather be interpreted as reflecting a subject's activity level than as meaningful quantitative parameters per se. Accordingly, clinically meaningful differences as determined for step count, for example, are expectedly large given the generally high standard deviations within groups of healthy subjects (here: 2397/day). It seems therefore justified to evaluate the validity of more amenable and standardized quantitative performance measures as predictors of PA in PwMS. Our data add evidence to previous findings that suggest measures related to walking and lower limb function as most promising candidates.

Conclusion

Both methods of assessment seem applicable in PwMS and able to describe reductions in daily PA at group level. Whether they can be used to track individual effects of interventions to enhance PA levels needs further exploration. The relation of PA measures with hrQoL seen with lower limb mobility suggests lower limb function not only as a major target for intervention to increase PA but also as a possible surrogate for PA changes.

Additional files

Additional file 1: Table S1. Overview of SenseWear® (SWAmini) and IPAQ (long version) parameters.

Additional file 2: Table S2. Correlations between SWAmini parameters.

Additional file 3: Figure S1. Relation of occupational status to EDSS. (DOCX 24 kb)

Additional file 4: Figure S2. Correlation of three parameters of physical activity derived from objective (SWAmini) and subjective (IPAQ) assessment after transformation into comparable units. (A) IPAQ Walking + MPA duration and SWAmini MPA duration (min/day), (B) IPAQ VPA duration and SWAmini VPA duration (min/day) and (C) IPAQ Total EE and SWAmini Active EE (MET*min/day).

Abbreviations
EDSS: Expanded Disability Status Scale; EE: Energy expenditure; HAQUAMS: Hamburg Quality of Life Questionnaire in Multiple Sclerosis;

hrQoL: Health-related quality of life; IPAQ: International Physical Activity Questionnaire; LPA: Light physical activity; MET: Metabolic equivalents; MPA: Moderate physical activity; MVPA: Moderate-to-vigorous physical activity; PA: Daily physical activity; SWAmini: SenseWear mini® Armband; VPA: Vigorous physical activity; VVPA: Very vigorous physical activity

Acknowledgments
Our technicians Susan Pikol, Cynthia Kraut and Gritt Stoffels, gave invaluable support.

Funding
This work was supported by Novartis GmbH (Roonstraße 25, 90429 Nürnberg, Germany).
There was no involvement in study design, collection, analysis, and interpretation of the data, writing of the report, and the decision to submit the article for publication.

Authors' contributions
TK was involved in study design and data analysis, collected clinical data of sample and wrote the manuscript. JRB was involved in study design, supervised clinical data acquisition and revised the manuscript. AG was involved in study design and revised the manuscript. KO, SMM and BK were involved in study design and contributed to data analysis and review of the manuscript. JBS supervised clinical data acquisition and revised the manuscript. AUB contributed to study design, data analysis and revised the manuscript. FP contributed to study design and revised the manuscript. TSH contributed to study design, data analysis, supervised and revised the manuscript. All authors read and approved the final manuscript for submission.

Competing interests
The authors declare that they have no competing interests.

Author details
[1]NeuroCure Clinical Research Center, Clinical Neuroimmunology Group, Charité – Universitätsmedizin Berlin, Charitéplatz 1, 10117 Berlin, Germany. [2]Department of Neurology, Charité – Universitätsmedizin Berlin, Charitéplatz 1, 10117 Berlin, Germany. [3]Experimental and Clinical Research Center, Charité – Universitätsmedizin Berlin and Max Delbrück Center for Molecular Medicine, Lindenberger Weg 80, 13125 Berlin, Germany. [4]Motognosis UG, Schönhauser Allee 177, 10119 Berlin, Germany.

References
1. Grilo CM. Physical activity and obesity. Biomed Pharmacother. 1994;48:127–36.
2. Bauman AE. Updating the evidence that physical activity is good for health: an epidemiological review 2000–2003. J Sci Med Sport. 2004;7:6–19.
3. Andre D, Wolf DL. Recent advances in free-living physical activity monitoring: a review. J Diabetes Sci Technol. 2007;1:760–7.
4. Learmonth YC, Motl RW. Physical activity and exercise training in multiple sclerosis: a review and content analysis of qualitative research identifying perceived determinants and consequences. Disabil Rehabil. 2016;38:1227–42.
5. Streber R, Peters S, Pfeifer K. Systematic review of correlates and determinants of physical activity in persons with multiple sclerosis. Arch Phys Med Rehabil. 2016;97:633–45.e29.
6. Gimeno-Santos E, Frei A, Steurer-Stey C, de Batlle J, Rabinovich RA, Raste Y, et al. Determinants and outcomes of physical activity in patients with COPD: a systematic review. Thorax. 2014;69:731–9.
7. Caspersen CJ, Powell KE, Christenson GM. Physical activity, exercise, and physical fitness: definitions and distinctions for health-related research. Public Health Rep. 1985;100:126–31.
8. Byrne NM, Hills AP, Hunter GR, Weinsier RL, Schutz Y. Metabolic equivalent: one size does not fit all. J Appl Physiol. 2005;99:1112–9.
9. Ainsworth BE, Haskell WL, Herrmann SD, Meckes N, Bassett DR, Tudor-Locke C, et al. 2011 compendium of physical activities: a second update of codes and MET values. Med Sci Sports Exerc. 2011;43:1575–81.
10. Hills AP, Mokhtar N, Byrne NM. Assessment of physical activity and energy expenditure: an overview of objective measures. Nutr Methodol. 2014;1:5.
11. Prince SA, Adamo KB, Hamel M, Hardt J, Connor Gorber S, Tremblay M. A comparison of direct versus self-report measures for assessing physical activity in adults: a systematic review. Int J Behav Nutr Phys Act. 2008;5:56.
12. Colbert LH, Matthews CE, Havighurst TC, Kim K, Schoeller DA. Comparative validity of physical activity measures in older adults. Med Sci Sports Exerc. 2011;43:867–76.
13. Ainsworth BE, Caspersen CJ, Matthews CE, Mâsse LC, Baranowski T, Zhu W. Recommendations to improve the accuracy of estimates of physical activity derived from self report. J Phys Act Health. 2012;9:S76–84.
14. Craig CL, Marshall AL, Sjöström M, Bauman AE, Booth ML, Ainsworth BE, et al. International physical activity questionnaire: 12-country reliability and validity. Med Sci Sports Exerc. 2003;35:1381–95.
15. Bassett DR, John D. Use of pedometers and accelerometers in clinical populations: validity and reliability issues. Phys Ther Rev. 2010;15:135–42.
16. Berntsen S. Measurement of energy expenditure by activity monitors: is it feasible to measure energy expenditure using tiny portable monitors? Phys Ther Rev. 2013;18:308–9.
17. Welk GJ, Mcclain J, Ainsworth BE. Protocols for evaluating equivalency of accelerometry-based activity monitors. Med Sci Sports Exerc. 2012;44:S39–49.
18. Coote S, O'Dwyer C. Comparative validity of accelerometer-based measures of physical activity for people with multiple sclerosis. Arch Phys Med Rehabil. 2012;93:2022–8.
19. Johannsen DL, Calabro MA, Stewart J, Franke W, Rood JC, Welk GJ. Accuracy of armband monitors for measuring daily energy expenditure in healthy adults. Med Sci Sports Exerc. 2010;42:2134–40.
20. Calabró MA, Stewart JM, Welk GJ. Validation of pattern-recognition monitors in children using doubly labeled water. Med Sci Sports Exerc. 2013;45:1313–22.
21. Calabró MA, Lee J-M, Saint-Maurice PF, Yoo H, Welk GJ. Validity of physical activity monitors for assessing lower intensity activity in adults. Int J Behav Nutr Phys Act. [Internet]. 2014 [cited 2015 Nov 8];11. Available from: http://www.ncbi.nlm.nih.gov/pmc/articles/PMC4192284/.
22. Polman CH, Reingold SC, Banwell B, Clanet M, Cohen JA, Filippi M, et al. Diagnostic criteria for multiple sclerosis: 2010 Revisions to the McDonald criteria. Ann Neurol. 2011;69:292–302.
23. Kreuz I. Das Armband Kompendium. 2006 [cited 2014 Sep 15]; Available from: http://www.body-coaches.de/wp-content/uploads/Armband_Anleitung.pdf.
24. IPAQ scoring protocol - International Physical Activity Questionnaire [Internet]. [cited 2016 Aug 5]. Available from: https://sites.google.com/site/theipaq/scoring-protocol.
25. Kurtzke JF. Disability rating scales in multiple sclerosis. Ann N Y Acad Sci. 1984;436:347–60.
26. Gold SM, Heesen C, Schulz H, Guder U, Monch A, Gbadamosi J, et al. HAQUAMS-english. Mult Scler. 2001;7:119–30.
27. Schäffler N, Schönberg P, Stephan J, Stellmann J-P, Gold SM, Heesen C. Comparison of patient-reported outcome measures in multiple sclerosis. Acta Neurol Scand. 2013;128:114–21.
28. Motl RW, McAuley E, Snook EM. Physical activity and multiple sclerosis: a meta-analysis. Mult Scler. 2005;11:459–63.
29. Currie AS, Knox KB, Glazebrook KE, Brawley LR. Physical activity levels in people with multiple sclerosis in Saskatchewan. Int J MS Care. 2009;11:114–20.
30. Cavanaugh JT, Gappmaier VO, Dibble LE, Gappmaier E. Ambulatory activity in individuals with multiple sclerosis. J Neurol Phys Ther. 2011;35:26–33.
31. Motl RW, McAuley E, Wynn D, Suh Y, Weikert M, Dlugonski D. Symptoms and physical activity among adults with relapsing-remitting multiple sclerosis. J Nerv Ment Dis. 2010;198:213–9.
32. Motl R, McAuley E. Association between change in physical activity and short-term disability progression in multiple sclerosis. J Rehabil Med. 2011;43:305–10.
33. Snook EM, Motl RW, Gliottoni RC. The effect of walking mobility on the measurement of physical activity using accelerometry in multiple sclerosis. Clin Rehabil. 2009;23:248–58.
34. Sandroff BM, Motl RW, Suh Y. Accelerometer output and its association with energy expenditure in persons with multiple sclerosis. J Rehabil Res Dev. 2012;49:467–75.
35. Klaren RE, Motl RW, Dlugonski D, Sandroff BM, Pilutti LA. Objectively quantified physical activity in persons with multiple sclerosis. Arch Phys Med Rehabil. 2013;94:2342–8.
36. Sandroff BM, Dlugonski D, Weikert M, Suh Y, Balantrapu S, Motl RW. Physical activity and multiple sclerosis: new insights regarding inactivity. Acta Neurol Scand. 2012;126:256–62.

37. Motl RW, Dlugonski D, Pilutti LA, Klaren RE. Does the effect of a physical activity behavioral intervention vary by characteristics of people with multiple sclerosis? Int J MS Care. 2015;17:65–72.

38. Dlugonski D, Pilutti LA, Sandroff BM, Suh Y, Balantrapu S, Motl RW. Steps Per Day among persons with multiple sclerosis: variation by demographic, clinical, and device characteristics. Arch Phys Med Rehabil. 2013;94:1534–9.

39. Motl RW, McAuley E, Snook EM, Scott JA. Validity of physical activity measures in ambulatory individuals with multiple sclerosis. Disabil Rehabil. 2006;28:1151–6.

40. Scheers T, Philippaerts R, Lefevre J. Objectively-determined intensity- and domain-specific physical activity and sedentary behavior in relation to percent body fat. Clin Nutr. 2013;32:999–1006.

41. Motl RW, Sandroff BM, Suh Y, Sosnoff JJ. Energy cost of walking and its association with gait parameters, daily activity, and fatigue in persons with mild multiple sclerosis. Neurorehabil Neural Repair. 2012;26:1015–21.

42. Motl RW, Snook EM, Agiovlasitis S, Suh Y. Calibration of accelerometer output for ambulatory adults with multiple sclerosis. Arch Phys Med Rehabil. 2009;90:1778–84.

43. Ezeugwu V, Klaren RE, Hubbard E A, Manns P (T), Motl RW. Mobility disability and the pattern of accelerometer-derived sedentary and physical activity behaviors in people with multiple sclerosis. Prev Med Rep. 2015;2:241–6.

44. Hubbard EA, Motl RW, Manns PJ. The descriptive epidemiology of daily sitting time as a sedentary behavior in multiple sclerosis. Disabil Health J. 2015;8:594–601.

45. Motl RW, Snook EM, McAuley E, Scott JA, Hinkle ML. Demographic correlates of physical activity in individuals with multiple sclerosis. Disabil Rehabil. 2007;29:1301–4.

46. Shook RP, Gribben NC, Hand GA, Paluch AE, Welk GJ, Jakicic JM, et al. Subjective estimation of physical activity using the international physical activity questionnaire varies by fitness level. J Phys Act Health. 2016;13:79–86.

47. Weikert M, Motl RW, Suh Y, McAuley E, Wynn D. Accelerometry in persons with multiple sclerosis: measurement of physical activity or walking mobility? J Neurol Sci. 2010;290:6–11.

48. Weikert M, Suh Y, Lane A, Sandroff B, Dlugonski D, Fernhall B, et al. Accelerometry is associated with walking mobility, not physical activity, in persons with multiple sclerosis. Med Eng Phys. 2012;34:590–7.

49. Gosney JL, Scott JA, Snook EM, Motl RW. Physical activity and multiple sclerosis: validity of self-report and objective measures. Fam Community Health. 2007;30:144–50.

50. Rice IM, Rice LA, Motl RW. Promoting physical activity through a manual wheelchair propulsion intervention in persons with multiple sclerosis. Arch Phys Med Rehabil. 2015;96:1850–8.

51. Pilutti LA, Dlugonski D, Sandroff BM, Klaren R, Motl RW. Randomized controlled trial of a behavioral intervention targeting symptoms and physical activity in multiple sclerosis. Mult Scler J. 2014;20:594–601.

52. Motl RW, Arnett PA, Smith MM, Barwick FH, Ahlstrom B, Stover EJ. Worsening of symptoms is associated with lower physical activity levels in individuals with. Mult Scler. 2008;14:140–2.

53. Fjeldstad C, Fjeldstad AS, Pardo G. Use of accelerometers to measure real-life physical activity in ambulatory individuals with multiple sclerosis. Int J MS Care. 2015;17:215–20.

54. Motl RW, Pilutti L, Sandroff BM, Dlugonski D, Sosnoff JJ, Pula JH. Accelerometry as a measure of walking behavior in multiple sclerosis. Acta Neurol Scand. 2013;127:384–90.

55. Motl RW, McAuley E, Snook EM, Gliottoni RC. Physical activity and quality of life in multiple sclerosis: Intermediary roles of disability, fatigue, mood, pain, self-efficacy and social support. Psychol Health Med. 2009;14:111–24.

56. Schulz K-H, Gold SM, Witte J, Bartsch K, Lang UE, Hellweg R, et al. Impact of aerobic training on immune-endocrine parameters, neurotrophic factors, quality of life and coordinative function in multiple sclerosis. J Neurol Sci. 2004;225:11–8.

57. Amato MP, Ponziani G, Rossi F, Liedl CL, Stefanile C, Rossi L. Quality of life in multiple sclerosis: the impact of depression, fatigue and disability. Mult Scler Houndmills Basingstoke Engl. 2001;7:340–4.

58. Beiske AG, Naess H, Aarseth JH, Andersen O, Elovaara I, Farkkila M, et al. Health-related quality of life in secondary progressive multiple sclerosis. Mult Scler. 2007;13:386–92.

59. Fernandez O, Baumstarck-Barrau K, Simeoni M-C, Auquier P, on behalf of the MusiQoL study group. Patient characteristics and determinants of quality of life in an international population with multiple sclerosis: assessment using the MusiQoL and SF-36 questionnaires. Mult Scler J. 2011;17:1238–49.

60. Benedict RHB, Wahlig E, Bakshi R, Fishman I, Munschauer F, Zivadinov R, et al. Predicting quality of life in multiple sclerosis: accounting for physical disability, fatigue, cognition, mood disorder, personality, and behavior change. J Neurol Sci. 2005;231:29–34.

61. Motl RW, McAuley E. Pathways between physical activity and quality of life in adults with multiple sclerosis. Health Psychol. 2009;28:682–9.

62. Sandroff BM, Riskin BJ, Agiovlasitis S, Motl RW. Accelerometer cut-points derived during over-ground walking in persons with mild, moderate, and severe multiple sclerosis. J Neurol Sci. 2014;340:50–7.

63. Vernillo G, Savoldelli A, Pellegrini B, Schena F. Validity of the SenseWear Armband™ to assess energy expenditure in graded walking. J Phys Act Health. 2014;12(2):178–83.

12

Self-reported physical activity correlates in Swedish adults with multiple sclerosis

Elisabeth Anens[*], Lena Zetterberg, Charlotte Urell, Margareta Emtner and Karin Hellström

Abstract

Background: The benefits of physical activity in persons with Multiple Sclerosis (MS) are considerable. Knowledge about factors that correlate to physical activity is helpful in order to develop successful strategies to increase physical activity in persons with MS. Previous studies have focused on correlates to physical activity in MS, however falls self-efficacy, social support and enjoyment of physical activity are not much studied, as well as if the correlates differ with regard to disease severity. The aim of the study was to examine associations between physical activity and age, gender, employment, having children living at home, education, disease type, disease severity, fatigue, self-efficacy for physical activity, falls self-efficacy, social support and enjoyment of physical activity in a sample of persons with MS and in subgroups with regard to disease severity.

Methods: This is a cross-sectional survey study including Swedish community living adults with MS, 287 persons, response rate 58.2%. The survey included standardized self-reported scales measuring physical activity, disease severity, fatigue, self-efficacy for physical activity, falls self-efficacy, and social support. Physical activity was measured by the Physical Activity Disability Survey – Revised.

Results: Multiple regression analyzes showed that 59% ($F_{(6,3)} = 64.9$, $p = 0.000$) of the variation in physical activity was explained by having less severe disease ($\beta = -0.30$), being employed ($\beta = 0.26$), having high falls self-efficacy ($\beta = 0.20$), having high self-efficacy for physical activity ($\beta = 0.17$), and enjoying physical activity ($\beta = 0.11$). In persons with moderate/severe MS, self-efficacy for physical activity explained physical activity.

Conclusions: Consistent with previous research in persons with MS in other countries this study shows that disease severity, employment and self-efficacy for physical activity are important for physical activity. Additional important factors were falls self-efficacy and enjoyment. More research is needed to confirm this and the subgroup differences.

Keywords: Exercise, Multiple sclerosis, Physical therapy, Rehabilitation, Self-efficacy

Background

In persons with MS (PwMS) the positive effects of physical activity (PA) are considerable. Reviews have shown positive effects on e.g. muscle strength, aerobic capacity, fatigue, quality of life and depression [1–5]. However, the benefit of exercise for populations with severe disability requires further investigation [3]. Despite the evidence of multiple health benefits in PwMS the level of PA is low [6].

Knowledge about factors that correlate to PA is helpful in order to develop successful strategies to increase PA in PwMS. Previous studies show contradictory results regarding the influence of background factors on level of PA, such as age [7, 8], gender [8, 9], and having children living at home [7, 10]. A recent systematic review showed that employment status and educational level were consistent correlates of PA [11]. This review also showed that persons with greater disability are less physically active compared to those with a milder disease, but contradictory results were found regarding the influence of fatigue on PA [11]. Self-efficacy for PA, defined as the conviction that one can successfully execute the

* Correspondence: elisabeth.anens@neuro.uu.se
Department of Neuroscience, Section for Physiotherapy, Box 593 Uppsala University, 751 24 Uppsala, Sweden

behavior required to produce a desired outcome [12] has shown to consistently facilitate PA [11]. Falls self-efficacy defined as the degree of efficacy (i.e. self-confidence) to avoid a fall [13], enjoyment of PA, and social support for PA are not extensively studied in PwMS.

A severe disease leads consistently to difficulties being physically active [6, 8, 9]. However, populations with more severe disability requires further investigation since MS participants in exercise interventions generally have a mild to moderate level of disability [3]. To get a better understanding of factors explaining PA in different subgroups and more useful results, it is of importance to investigate factors correlating to PA in PwMS with different disease severities.

The aim of this study was to examine the multivariate association between PA and age, gender, employment, having children living at home, education, type of MS, disease severity, fatigue, self-efficacy for PA, falls self-efficacy, social support and enjoyment of PA in PwMS. Subgroup analyses with regard to disease severity were also performed.

Methods

Design

This is a cross-sectional survey study.

Participants

Adults with a diagnosis of MS were recruited from the Swedish Multiple Sclerosis Registry (McDonald and/or Poser criteria). The register stratifies four types of MS; relapsing remitting, secondary progressive, primary progressive and progressive relapsing. Inclusion criteria were: having MS, age between 18 and 80 years, participants living in the county of Uppsala. All registered participants living in the county of Uppsala were invited to participate (502 subjects). Exclusion criteria were: not understanding Swedish ($n = 1$), not living independently ($n = 1$), having another neurological disease ($n = 1$), not being able to answer the survey ($n = 1$). Five participants were also excluded due to not having the required diagnosis. The final study cohort consisted of 287 subjects (response rate 58.2%). In total there were 84 men (29.3%) and 203 women (70.7%), giving a female-to-male ratio of 2.42:1. Mean age was 51.5 (SD 13.5) years. The female-to-male ratio for the 206 subjects who did not respond to the invitation was 2.38:1. Non-respondents were slightly younger, mean age 49.0 (SD 13.4) years, $p = 0.048$.

Procedure

A self-assessment questionnaire, an informatory letter, a consent form, and a stamped reply envelope were sent out by surface mail. The questionnaire was divided in two parts, with the second part sent out 2 weeks after a

reply with answers to the first part of the questionnaire was received. Two reminders were sent to participants who did not answer either of the parts within 3 weeks. All participants provided written informed consent to participate. The study was approved by the Regional Ethical Review Board, Uppsala, Sweden, D-no, 2010/278.

Outcome measures

For all measurements Swedish language versions and psychometrically sound measures were used. The amount of *PA* during the previous week was measured using the Physical Activity Disability Survey – Revised (PADS-R) [14]. The survey included six subscales; exercise, leisure time PA, general activity, therapy, employment and wheelchair use. The amount of PA during the previous week was reported for each scale. The subscale ratings were summed to give a total PADS-R. A higher score indicates more PA. *Disease severity* was measured using the Multiple Sclerosis Impact Scale (MSIS-29) [15]. The physical scale was used to classify the participants into two groups, indicating level of disease impact defined as ≤50 (minimal and mild disease), and >50 (moderate and severe disease) [16]. *Activity limitation* was measured using the ACTIV-LIM questionnaire [17]. *Fatigue* was measured with the Fatigue Severity Scale (FSS) [18]. *Self-efficacy for PA* was measured using the Exercise Self-Efficacy Scale (ESES) [19]. *Falls self-efficacy* was measured using the Falls Efficacy Scale Swedish version (FES(S)) [20]. *Social support from family for PA* was measured using Social Influences on Physical Activity (SIPA) subscale influence from family [21]. The MSIS-29, ACTIVLIM, FSS, ESES, FES(S), and SIPA are described in detail in a previous descriptive study [9]. *Enjoyment of PA* was measured using three statements (developed by our research group) about experience during, or shortly following physical activity of at least 10 min duration (e.g. walking). "I experience that it is fun to be physically active", "I experience a feeling of wellbeing when I am physically active", "I feel happy with myself when I am physically active". The answers were graded on a visual scale (from 0 to 5), and were added to a total score ranging from 0 to 15, with 15 being the highest level of enjoyment. Questions about background variables were also included in the questionnaire.

Data analysis

Data was analyzed using IBM SPSS Statistics 23. The minimum sample size was estimated as $50 + 8 k$, where k is the number of predictors, which results in a minimum sample size of 154 [22]. Missing data was handled as previously described [9]. Not all subjects answered all questions, hence the totals in the tables may differ. Forced entry multiple regression analysis was used to investigate factors that might influence PA. To evaluate the influence on PA with only the most important variables an additional regression analysis was performed, including all independent variables, with a standardized beta p- value of <0.2. No multicollinearity in the regression analysis was found by screening a correlation matrix of all included variables ($r < 0.8$) and by evaluating the variance inflation factors and tolerance statistics, except for in one case (See Discussion). There was no autocorrelation found with the Durbin-Watson test. The assumption of linearity, homoscedasticity and normally distributed residuals were met when checking the histogram and normal probability plots of the residuals. An acceptable level of outliers was found by evaluating the percentage of standardized residuals with an absolute value of greater than 2 (<5%) or 2.58 (<1%). The level of significance was set at $p < 0.05$.

Results

Background variables for the 287 participants are described in Table 1. MS subtype was relapsing remitting in 135 (47.0%) and progressive in 146 (50.9%) persons. The mean PA level was 0.18 (SD 1.47). Thirty persons (10.5%) could not walk. For 148 (51.6%) persons walking distance outdoors was more than 500 m.

Factors explaining physical activity for all participants

Including all participants and all independent factors a model including low physical disease severity, being employed, high falls self-efficacy, and high self-efficacy for PA explained 57.6% of the variation in PA. When recalculating to include only the most important factors, also enjoyment of PA remained significant, resulting in 59% of the variation in PA being explained (Table 2).

Factors explaining physical activity for persons with different disease severity

In participants with minimal and mild MS (MSIS-29 physical scale ≤50) being employed, low activity limitations, high self-efficacy for PA and high enjoyment of PA explained 39.1% of the variation in PA (Table 3). In participants with moderate and severe MS (MSIS-29 physical scale <50), 41.3% of the variation in PA was explained by high self-efficacy for PA (Table 3).

Discussion

Self-efficacy for PA consistently explained PA in the entire cohort and in all subgroups. This is consistent with previous results [11, 23]. This study confirms the importance of self-efficacy for PA also in persons with moderate and severe MS, categorized from

Table 1 Sample cohort description

Description of the cohort, n (%) or mean ± SD or median (quartiles)			
	ALL (n = 287)	Minimal/ Mild MS (n = 204)	Moderate/ Severe MS (n = 77)
Age (years)	51.5 ± 13.5	49.4 ± 13.6	57.5 ± 11.2
Gender			
Men	84 (29%)	46 (23%)	35 (46%)
Women	203 (71%)	158 (78%)	42 (55%)
Employment			
Yes	130 (45%)	116 (57%)	10 (13%)
Children at home			
Yes	71 (25%)	61 (30%)	7 (9%)
Tertiary education			
Yes	124 (43%)	96 (47%)	26 (34%)
Type of MS			
Relapsing remitting	135 (47%)	120 (59%)	12 (16%)
Secondary progressive	104 (36%)	59 (29)	43 (56%)
Primary progressive	32 (11%)	16 (7.8%)	16 (21%)
Progressive relapsing	10 (3.5%)	4 (2.0%)	5 (6.5%)
Subtype not known	6 (2.1%)	5 (2.5%)	1 (1.3%)
Progressive MS			
Yes	146 (51%)	79 (39%)	64 (83%)
Duration (years)[a]	11 (6-18)	9.5 (5-17)	13 (8-23)
MSIS-29			
Physical	28 (8-53)	18 (4-32)	66 (58-81)
Psychological	28 (11-47)	22 (8-36)	44 (31-64)
Physical activity [b]	0.18 ± 1.47	0.75 ± 1.25	- 1.23 ± 0.99

MSIS-29 Multiple Sclerosis Impact Scale. Minimal & Mild MS = MSIS-29 physical scale ≤50. Moderate & Severe MS = MSIS-29 physical scale >50
[a]Duration = time since diagnosis. [b] Physical activity was measured using the Physical Activity Disability Survey – Revised

MSIS-29. Unfortunately little research has focused on persons with moderate and severe MS. However, in a sample of 43 persons with moderate to severe MS, with an Expanded Disability Status Scale of 6.0 to 8.0, high general self-efficacy was associated with high levels of PA [24].

Falls self-efficacy, the degree of self-efficacy to avoid a fall, correlated to PA in the entire cohort. Our result is supported by a few previous studies. An exercise intervention led to increased confidence in performing activities without falling in PwMS [25]. High concerns about falling were associated with activity curtailment in PwMS [26]. The results of a review on interventions in PwMS to improve balance, indicates that programs incorporating gait, balance and functional training, especially when focusing on a

Table 2 Physical activity regression models for all persons

All persons, multiple regression, physical activity (PA) dependent variable[a]

Independent variables	All factors (n = 250)		Factors with p < 0.20 (n = 267)	
	β	P-value	β	P-value
Age	- 0.05	0.320	n.a.	n.a.
Gender	0.00	0.987	n.a.	n.a.
Employment	0.25	0.000*	0.26	0.000*
Children at home	- 0.03	0.473	n.a.	n.a.
Education	0.01	0.870	n.a.	n.a.
Progressive MS	- 0.03	0.541	n.a.	n.a.
MSIS-29 physical	- 0.30	0.002*	- 0.30	0.001*
MSIS-29 psychological	0.00	0.948	n.a.	n.a.
Fatigue	0.09	0.112	0.07	0.148
Self-efficacy for PA	0.13	0.035*	0.17	0.002*
Falls self-efficacy	0.21	0.011*	0.20	0.012*
Social support, family	0.02	0.585	n.a.	n.a.
Enjoyment of PA	0.08	0.120	0.11	0.021*
	$R^2 = 0.58$, $F_{(13,2)} = 27.0$, $p = 0.000$		$R^2 = 0.59$, $F_{(6,3)} = 64.9$, $p = 0.000$	

β = Standardized beta coefficient. * = $p < 0.05$. R^2 adjusted R square, *MSIS-29* Multiple Sclerosis Impact Scale
[a]Physical activity was measured using the Physical Activity Disability Survey – Revised

Table 3 Physical activity regression models for persons with different disease severity

Multiple regression, physical activity (PA) dependent variable[a]

Independent variables	Minimal & Mild MS Factors with p < 0.20 (n = 196)		Moderate & Severe MS Factors with p < 0.20 (n = 73)	
	β	P-value	β	P-value
Age	n.a.	n.a.	n.a.	n.a.
Gender	0.05	0.425	- 0.08	0.381
Employment	0.34	0.000*	0.15	0.132
Children at home	- 0.05	0.434	n.a.	n.a.
Education	n.a.	n.a.	n.a.	n.a.
Progressive MS	n.a.	n.a.	n.a.	n.a.
Activity limitation	0.26	0.000*	0.26	0.059
MSIS-29 psychological	n.a.	n.a.	n.a.	n.a.
Fatigue	n.a.	n.a.	0.16	0.099
Self-efficacy for PA	0.16	0.016*	0.25	0.027*
Falls self-efficacy	n.a.	n.a.	0.24	0.110
Social support, family	n.a.	n.a.	- 0.06	0.552
Enjoyment of PA	0.13	0.043*	n.a.	n.a.
	$R^2 = 0.39$, $F_{(5,2)} = 26.1$, $p = 0.000$		$R^2 = 0.41$, $F_{(5,7)} = 11.1$, $p = 0.000$	

β = Standardized beta coefficient. * = $p < 0.05$. R^2 adjusted R square, *MSIS-29* Multiple Sclerosis Impact Scale
Minimal & Mild MS = MSIS-29 physical scale ≤50. Moderate & Severe MS = MSIS-29 physical scale >50
[a]Physical activity was measured using the Physical Activity Disability Survey – Revised

high volume of challenging balance exercises, may lead to the greatest benefit in balance (and therefore potentially falls) outcomes [27].

Enjoyment of PA was associated with PA in the entire cohort, and in persons with minimal and mild MS. Experiencing enjoyment following exercise increased adherence to an exercise intervention in PwMS [28]. Most studies on correlates to PA in PwMS did not include enjoyment. However, a review showed that intrinsic motivation, or being active for the pleasure it brings, was the type of motivation that most strongly predicted longterm exercise adherence [29]. Little is known about factors that could increase enjoyment. Teixeira et al. [29] suggest e.g. emphasizing fun and skill improvement. Another review showed that experienced pleasure depends on PA intensity [30]. In addition, factors such as physical and social environment during PA might be important. The affective response during, and after PA, is probably important to consider when encouraging PA in PwMS.

In this cohort social support from family did not explain PA. Social support was inconsistently associated with PA in a previous review [11]. Possibly a more suitable questionnaire with focus on social support for PA in persons with disabilities could be of value.

Our results showed that low physical disease severity measured with MSIS-29 correlated to PA in the entire

cohort. In line with this, a consistent correlate of PA in PwMS in a recent systematic review was disability level [11]. When analyzing subgroups from MSIS-29 the physical scale, ACTIVLIM was used as a measure of disease severity, which was highly correlated to MSIS-29 in this cohort. Having low activity limitations also explained a high level of PA in persons with minimal and mild MS, and probably also in moderate to severe MS, but was not significant in this small subgroup (Table 3). Other disease related factors measured in this study were having progressive MS, level of fatigue and MSIS-29 psychological scale. None of these were found to explain PA level in this cohort. In accordance with our result, Sterber et al. [11] reported in a review that type of MS, and fatigue, were not consistent correlates to PA. Moreover, changes in PA were not associated with fatigue in the 2,5 year longitudinal study by Motl et al. [23].

We found that the second most important factor in the entire cohort was being employed, with a standardized beta of 0.26. Being employed also explained level of PA in persons with minimal and mild MS. This is in line with findings in previous studies that higher levels of PA were consistently observed in PwMS who were employed [11]. One explanation is that persons who are employed are physically active at work, and when travelling to and from work.

Educational level did not influence the level of PA in this cohort which is in contrast to a previous review in PwMS [11]. However, this was based on results from studies in the USA, and one explanation could be cultural differences. No previous study on correlates to PA in PwMS in Sweden was found. It has been shown in a large Swedish study of the general population that education ≥12 years is associated with lower PA [31]. Persons with high education often have sedentary occupations. Measures of PA may include PA at work in varying amounts, which can also explain the differing results.

We studied gender differences in this cohort and found that men were less physically active than women and more physically affected by the disease [9]. However, in the regression analysis no association was found between gender and PA. This might be explained by men having more severe disease. Similar results were found in another sample of PwMS, where a gender difference in daily step counts was found, but when considering level of disability the difference disappeared [32].

The result for persons with minimal and mild MS, is more representative to the MS population due to the larger sample and the more similar results, all independent variables except falls self-efficacy were explaining PA in both the whole sample and in persons with minimal and mild MS (Tables 2 and 3). Falls self-efficacy was not important, probably due to less limited balance in persons with minimal and mild MS. Only one factor, self-efficacy for PA explained PA in persons with moderate and severe MS, probably more factors would become significant in larger samples. Maybe other not measured factors such as accessibility to exercise facilities, and support from others to perform activities would influence the possibility to be physically active in persons with moderate and severe MS.

In this study a non-respondent bias was found, since the non-respondents were slightly younger. Despite this finding the mean age of 51.5 years in this cohort is similar to the mean age of 52.6 years in a nationwide Swedish MS study ($n = 17,485$) [33]. Our female-to-male ratio was 2.42:1, which is comparable to the female-to-male ratio of 2.35:1 in the nationwide Swedish study [33]. However, this sample had a low proportion (47%), of persons with relapsing remitting MS compared to e.g. a large Swedish sample (58.5%, $n = 16,915$) [34]. Fewer persons with relapsing remitting MS answered this survey, possible reasons for this could be that persons with less severe disease did not want to be reminded of the disease, or did not find the questions suitable (e.g. falls self-efficacy scale).

In this cross-sectional study 39-59% of the variation of PA was explained by the regression models. However, this was a cross-sectional study and high correlations are more easily obtained in cross-sectional studies compared to prospective studies. Another disadvantage with cross-sectional studies is that conclusions regarding the causal relationship between different factors cannot be drawn.

The MSIS-29 physical scale and falls self-efficacy scale correlated highly (−0.83 to −0.84), which might have influenced the regression model. However, other controls of multicollinearity were acceptable, and in addition, both factors were considered important to include. The sample size in the subgroup moderate to severe MS was quite small. However, large effects can be detected even in small sample cohorts [22].

One limitation is the use of self-reported measures. We used a subjective self-rated measure of PA, instead of an objective measure, as accelerometer. This was chosen to enable more persons to participate. We also used a self-reported measure of disease impact. However, MSIS-29 is the most widely used patient-reported outcome in MS studies, with the best psychometric properties [35]. Another limitation is that the scale to measure enjoyment of PA is new, and has not yet been psychometrically evaluated.

This study showed that persons with severe disease, those who are unemployed, and those with low self-efficacy for PA are especially prone to inactivity. The importance of self-efficacy for PA, falls self-efficacy and enjoyment is in line with Social Cognitive Theory [12]. According to Bandura [12] self-efficacy is modifiable, and e.g. positive emotions could increase self-efficacy. Strategies for behavioral changes might be applied to increase PA. A review showed that "action planning", "provide instruction" and "reinforcing effort towards behavior" were behavioral strategies that were associated with higher levels of both self-efficacy and physical activity [36]. Setting a specific detailed plan of when, where and how to perform the physical activity and providing instruction on these same categories, as well as providing positive feedback and reinforce participants efforts in attempting to become more physically active [36], are thus promising ways to promote physical activity in persons with MS. In addition, encouraging enjoyable and pleasurable physical activities, is important to enhance the PA behaviour. Gait, balance and functional training, especially when focusing on challenging balance exercises [27], and fall prevention knowledge, may increase falls self-efficacy, the degree of self-efficacy to avoid a fall.

Conclusions

This study in Swedish PwMS confirms previous research in other countries regarding the importance of disability level, employment and self-efficacy for PA for the level of PA. This study contributes to previous research in showing that the seldom studied factors falls self-efficacy and enjoyment are also important for PA, and that factors that explain physical activity differs between subgroups with different disease severity. More research preferably in prospective and intervention studies, is needed to confirm the importance of these factors, and to confirm the subgroup differences.

Abbreviations

ESES: Exercise Self-Efficacy Scale; FES(S): Falls Efficacy Scale Swedish version; FSS: Fatigue Severity Scale; MS: Multiple sclerosis; MSIS-29: Multiple Sclerosis Impact Scale; PA: Physical activity; PADS- R: Physical Activity Disability Survey – Revised; PwMS: Persons with multiple sclerosis; SIPA: Social Influences on Physical Activity

Acknowledgements

We wish to thank all of the subjects who participated. Isabell Ahlström is acknowledged for data collection. We thank the language reviewers for contributing in translating of measurements and for revising the manuscript.

Funding

This research was funded by Health Research Funds, Uppsala University, Sweden and Neuro Sweden, Sweden.

Authors` contributions

The initiative and planning of the study was a joint effort between EA, ME, and KH. EA was most responsible for the progression of the study, data analysis, interpretation of data and drafting the manuscript. LZ and CU contributed in data analysis, interpretation of data and revision of the manuscript. ME contributed also in interpretation of data and revision of the manuscript. KH contributed in data analysis, interpretation of data and revision of the manuscript. All authors read and approved the final manuscript.

Competing interests

The authors declare that they have no competing interests.

References

1. Rietberg MB, Brooks D, Uitdehaag BMJ, Kwakkel G. Exercise therapy for multiple sclerosis (review). Cochrane Database Syst Rev. 2005;25(1): CD003980.
2. Motl RW, Pilutti LA. The benefits of exercise training in multiple sclerosis. Nat Rev Neurol. 2012;8(9):487–97.
3. Latimer-Cheung AE, Pilutti LA, Hicks AL, Martin Ginis KA, Fenuta AM, MacKibbon KA, et al. Effects of exercise training on fitness, mobility, fatigue, and health-related quality of life among adults with multiple sclerosis: a systematic review to inform guideline development. Arch Phys Med Rehabil. 2013;94(9):1800–28. e1803
4. Pilutti LA, Greenlee TA, Motl RW, Nickrent MS, Petruzzello SJ. Effects of exercise training on fatigue in multiple sclerosis: a meta-analysis. Psychosom Med. 2013;75(6):575–80.
5. Ensari I, Motl RW, Pilutti LA. Exercise training improves depressive symptoms in people with multiple sclerosis: results of a meta-analysis. J Psychosom Res. 2014;76(6):465–71.
6. Klaren RE, Motl RW, Dlugonski D, Sandroff BM, Pilutti LA. Objectively quantified physical activity in persons with multiple sclerosis. Arch Phys Med Rehabil. 2013;94(12):2342–8.

7. Motl RW, Snook EM, McAuley E, Scott JA, Hinkle ML. Demographic correlates of physical activity in individuals with multiple sclerosis. Disabil Rehabil. 2007;29(16):1301–4.
8. Motl RW, Mullen S, Suh Y, McAuley E. Does physical activity change over 24 months in persons with relapsing-remitting multiple sclerosis? Health Psychol. 2014;33(4):326–31.
9. Anens E, Emtner M, Zetterberg L, Hellstrom K. Physical activity in subjects with multiple sclerosis with focus on gender differences: a survey. BMC Neurol. 2014;14(1):47.
10. Beckerman H, de Groot V, Scholten MA, Kempen JC, Lankhorst GJ. Physical activity behavior of people with multiple sclerosis: understanding how they can become more physically active. Phys Ther. 2010;90(7):1001–13.
11. Streber R, Peters S, Pfeifer K. Systematic review of correlates and determinants of physical activity in persons with multiple sclerosis. Arch Phys Med Rehabil. 2016;97(4):633–45.
12. Bandura A. Self-efficacy the exercise of control. New York: W.H. Freeman and Company; 1997.
13. Tinetti ME, Richman D, Powell L. Falls efficacy as a measure of fear of falling. J Gerontol. 1990;45(6):239–43.
14. Kayes NM, Schluter PJ, McPherson KM, Taylor D, Kolt GS. The physical activity and disability survey – revised (PADS-R): an evaluation of a measure of physical activity in people with chronic neurological conditions. Clin Rehabil. 2009;23(6):534–43.
15. Hobart J, Lamping D, Fitzpatrick R, Riazi A, Thompson A. The multiple sclerosis impact scale (MSIS-29): a new patient-based outcome measure. Brain. 2001;124(Pt 5):962–73.
16. Forbes A, While A, Mathes L, Griffiths P. Health problems and health-related quality of life in people with multiple sclerosis. Clin Rehabil. 2006;20(1):67–78.
17. Vandervelde L, Van den Bergh PY, Goemans N, Thonnard JL. ACTIVLIM: a Rasch-built measure of activity limitations in children and adults with neuromuscular disorders. Neuromuscul Disord. 2007;17(6):459–69.
18. Krupp LB, LaRocca NG, Muir-Nash J, Steinberg AD. The fatigue severity scale. Application to patients with multiple sclerosis and systemic lupus erythematosus. Arch Neurol. 1989;46(10):1121–3.
19. Kroll T, Kehn M, Ho PS, Groah S. The SCI exercise self-efficacy scale (ESES): development and psychometric properties. Int J Behav Nutr Phys Act. 2007;4:34.
20. Hellstrom K, Lindmark B. Fear of falling in patients with stroke: a reliability study. Clin Rehabil. 1999;13(6):509–17.
21. Chogahara M. A multidimensional scale for assessing positive and negative social influences on physical activity in older adults. J Gerontol B Psychol Sci Soc Sci. 1999;54(6):S356–67.
22. Field A. Discovering statistics using SPSS. 3 ed. London: SAGE; 2009.
23. Motl RW, McAuley E, Sandroff BM. Longitudinal change in physical activity and its correlates in relapsing-remitting multiple sclerosis. Phys Ther. 2013; 93(8):1037–48.
24. Vanner EA, Block P, Christodoulou CC, Horowitz BP, Krupp LB. Pilot study exploring quality of life and barriers to leisure-time physical activity in persons with moderate to severe multiple sclerosis. Disabil Health J. 2008; 1(1):58–65.
25. Cakt BD, Nacir B, Genc H, Saracoglu M, Karagoz A, Erdem HR, et al. Cycling progressive resistance training for people with multiple sclerosis: a randomized controlled study. Am J Phys Med Rehabil. 2010;89(6):446–57.
26. Peterson EW, Cho CC, Finlayson ML. Fear of falling and associated activity curtailment among middle aged and older adults with multiple sclerosis. Mult Scler. 2007;13(9):1168–75.
27. Gunn H, Markevics S, Haas B, Marsden J, Freeman J. Systematic review: the effectiveness of interventions to reduce falls and improve balance in adults with multiple sclerosis. Arch Phys Med Rehabil. 2015;96(10):1898–912.
28. McAuley E, Motl RW, Morris KS, Hu L, Doerksen SE, Elavsky S, et al. Enhancing physical activity adherence and well-being in multiple sclerosis: a randomised controlled trial. Mult Scler. 2007;13(5):652–9.
29. Teixeira PJ, Carraca EV, Markland D, Silva MN, Ryan RM. Exercise, physical activity, and self-determination theory: a systematic review. Int J Behav Nutr Phys Act. 2012;9:78.
30. Ekkekakis P, Parfitt G, Petruzzello SJ. The pleasure and displeasure people feel when they exercise at different intensities: decennial update and

progress towards a tripartite rationale for exercise intensity prescription. Sports Med. 2011;41(8):641–71.

31. Lagerros YT, Bellocco R, Adami HO, Nyren O. Measures of physical activity and their correlates: the Swedish National March Cohort. Eur J Epidemiol. 2009;24(4):161–9.

32. Dlugonski D, Pilutti LA, Sandroff BM, Suh Y, Balantrapu S, Motl RW. Steps per day among persons with multiple sclerosis: variation by demographic, clinical, and device characteristics. Arch Phys Med Rehabil. 2013;94(8):1534–9.

33. Ahlgren C, Oden A, Lycke J. High nationwide prevalence of multiple sclerosis in Sweden. Mult Scler. 2011;17(8):901–8.

34. Westerlind H, Stawiarz L, Fink K, Hillert J, Manouchehrinia A. A significant decrease in diagnosis of primary progressive multiple sclerosis: a cohort study. Mult Scler. 2016;22(8):1071–9.

35. Khurana V, Sharma H, Afroz N, Callan A, Medin J. Patient-reported outcomes in multiple sclerosis: a systematic comparison of available measures. Eur J Neurol. 2017;24(9):1099–107.

36. Williams SL, French DP. What are the most effective intervention techniques for changing physical activity self-efficacy and physical activity behaviour– and are they the same? Health Educ Res. 2011;26(2):308–22.

13

Listeria monocytogenes infection associated with alemtuzumab – a case for better preventive strategies

Trygve Holmøy[1,2]*(iD), Hedda von der Lippe[3] and Truls Michael Leegaard[2,4]

Abstract

Background: The mortality of septicaemia, meningitis and encephalitis caused by *Listeria monocytogenes* is 20–40%. Twenty-one cases of invasive listeriosis associated with alemtuzumab, including at least 16 in patients with multiple sclerosis, have been published or reported to the World Health Organization Case Safety Reports Database. Three cases were fatal, including at least one patient treated for multiple sclerosis in 2016.

Case presentation: We report a patient with multiple sclerosis who developed pyrexia, nausea and abdominal discomfort few hours after the third and last infusion of her second alemtuzumab cycle. An infusion related reaction was suspected. The patient had however eaten soft cheese and raw sausage 3 days prior to treatment, and *L. monocytogenes* septicaemia was diagnosed based on positive blood cultures.

Conclusion: Listeriosis associated with alemtuzumab is a potentially fatal condition that can mimic an infusion related reaction. As in most other previously reported cases symptoms started rapidly after the last infusion, suggesting that the patient already carried the bacteria prior to the alemtuzumab infusions. The summary of product characteristics recommends patients to avoid foods associated with listeria at least 1 month after treatment. This recommendation should include also the last weeks prior to treatment.

Keywords: Multiple sclerosis, Treatment, Alemtuzumab, Adverse events, *Listeria monocytogenes*

Background

Listeriosis is caused by the Gram positive bacteria *Listeria monocytogenes*, and is usually contracted from unpasteurized dairy products, raw fish and meat, or products made from pasteurized products contaminated with *L. monocytogenes* after production, like soft cheeses. Immunocompetent persons rarely develop severe symptoms, whereas people with defective cellular immunity may develop septicaemia, meningitis or encephalitis, with a mortality rate ranging from 20 to 40% [1, 2].

The importance of listeriosis associated with alemtuzumab in multiple sclerosis (MS) has recently been underscored by a fatal case not yet published, but that has been reported to VigiBase©, the World Health Organization international database of suspected adverse drug reactions [3] and to Sanofi Genzyme (Sanofi

Genzyme, data on file). The current case history highlights that listeriosis must be considered in patients who develop pyrexia shortly after treatment with alemtuzumab, even in the absence of meningism. It also suggests that the Summary of Product Characteristics (SPC) should be revised to minimize the risk of this potentially fatal complication.

Case presentation

The patient is a woman in her early fifties. She was diagnosed with MS after a sensory attack in the left shoulder in 2008 and a sensorimotor attack in the right leg in 2013. She was treated with interferon beta 1a from April 2013, and with fingolimod from September 2013 after a motor attack in the left leg from which she recovered partially. Treatment was changed again to natalizumab in January 2014 when macula edema was suspected. She remained clinically and radiologically stable until natalizumab was terminated in the beginning of June 2015, after she tested positive for John Cunningham virus.

---
* Correspondence: trygve.holmoy@medisin.uio.no
[1]Department of Neurology, Akershus University Hospital, Lørenskog, Norway
[2]Institute of Clinical Medicine, University of Oslo, Oslo, Norway
Full list of author information is available at the end of the article

Alemtuzumab was started at the end of July 2015. During the first cycle (12 mg for 5 days) she had transient sinus bradycardia down to 30 beats per minute but no other adverse events.

The patient remained clinically stable with an expanded disability status scale (EDSS) score at 2.5 until the second cycle (12 mg alemtuzumab preceded by 1000 mg methylprednisolone, 12 mg cetrizine and 1000 mg paracetamol for three consecutive days) in July 2016. Except for transient bradycardia there were no immediate adverse reactions, but some hours after the last infusion of alemtuzumab she became sick with nausea and fever up to 40 °C. At admission to hospital she was awake and did not have neck stiffness or other focal signs except abdominal discomfort and mild headache. She was febrile (39.5 C) and clinically dehydrated but normotensive. C-reactive protein was 180, lymphocytes were below the detection limit but the number of granulocytes was normal. As she did not have new neurological symptoms, neither detailed neurological examination, brain imaging nor lumbar puncture were performed. Four out of four blood cultures were positive for *L. monocytogenes* (confirmed by 16S RNA sequencing) which was susceptible to trimethoprim-sulphamethoxazole, ampicillin, erythromycin, meropenem and penicillin. She recovered rapidly and completely upon treatment with ampicillin and trimethoprim-sulphamethoxazole.

Discussion

To our knowledge, this is the 22nd case of listeriosis associated with alemtuzumab reported so far, either in the literature or to the WHO database VigiBase [3–6]. Including the present case, at least 16 of these have occurred in patients treated for MS (Table 1). Until January 2017 approximately 11,500 MS patients have been treated with alemtuzumab (Sanofi Genzyme, data on file), indicating that the risk of listeriosis is in the range of 0.1%. It should be noted that only one case is reported outside Europe (Australia). This could indicate that this complication of alemtuzumab might be under-reported in some areas, as the general prevalence of listeriosis in North America is comparable to that in Europe [2].

Our patient developed clinical symptoms the day after the last infusion of alemtuzumab. Notably, most previous cases of alemtuzumab-associated listeriosis in patients with MS have also presented shortly after treatment. One patient with a poor outcome (reported to VigiBase in 2014) may even have developed symptoms in the beginning of the treatment cycle.

Unlike our patient, it seems that signs of meningitis with headache have been present in most previously reported cases. Thus, headache, neck stiffness, fever, and worsening of pre-existing MS symptoms started at the day of the last infusion in a 47 year old woman [4], whereas a 43 year old man developed fever followed by headache 3 days after

the last infusion [4]. The fatal case, a 43 year old woman, was admitted to hospital with low Glasgow Coma Scale score a couple of days after the last infusion of her first alemtuzumab cycle. She developed brain edema and passed away 2 days later. Blood and CSF cultures were positive for listeria (Council for International Organizations of Medical Sciences (CIOMS) report September 16 2016, Sanofi Genzyme, data on file). One of the participants in the CAMMS-223 study, a 36 year woman, was admitted to hospital with fever, abdominal pain and headache 16 days after the last infusion (24 mg) [5], and a 33 year old woman was admitted to hospital with fever and chills 10 days after the final infusion [6].

Two other fatal cases of listeriosis associated with alemtuzumab have been reported to VigiBase. One patient who was treated for lymphoma died in 2009. Another fatal case was reported in December 2016. There are unfortunately no available information about disease characteristics or treatment details for this patient, including whether the treatment indication was MS.

In our patient listeriosis occurred in association with the second treatment cycle. Alemtuzumab-associated listeriosis has previously been reported in MS patients both after the first and the second cycle [4–6]. VigiBase does not provide direct information about treatment cycle. Eleven MS patients have however developed listeriosis in association with five infusions which are used for the first cycle, and five in association with three infusions which are used for later cycles (Table 1). This may simply reflect that not all patients have yet received the second cycle.

L. monocytogenes is occasionally present in faeces of healthy immunocompetent persons but does usually not cause disease [7]. The bacteria spread intracellularly, and CD4 and CD 8 T cells are essential for controlling the infection [1]. Alemtuzumab rapidly depletes such cells from the circulation [8], and also reduces the numbers of dendritic cells [9]. Given the long duration of T cell depletion, other factors likely contribute to the aggregation of invasive listeriosis closely after alemtuzumab infusion. Notably, alemtuzumab almost immediately and transiently impairs the release of cytokines from remaining lymphocytes as well as innate immune cells [10]. Such acute and transient effects on both innate and adaptive immunity could explain the peculiar timing of listeria infection to the period immediately after treatment [11].

The SPC for Lemtrada© recommends that patients should avoid ingestion of uncooked or undercooked meats, soft cheeses and unpasteurized dairy products for at least one month after treatment [12]. The incubation period of *L. monocytogenes* varies between 1 to 70 days [1]. Persistence of *L. monocytogenes* after food exposure can be prolonged by corticosteroids, which are now routinely administered prior to alemtuzumab infusions [13]. Our patient had eaten soft cheese and smoked sausage, both known sources of *L.*

Table 1 Characteristics of previously reported cases of listeriosis associated with alemtuzumab reported until February March 3, 2017

Source (reference)	Type of listeriosis	Gender	Indication	Number of infusions	Days from first infusion to onset	Outcome
VigiBase 2017 (3)	Meningitis	Female	Multiple sclerosis	5	Unknown	Unknown
VigiBase 2016 (3)	Meningitis	Female	Multiple sclerosis	5	8	Recovering
VigiBase 2016 (3)[a]	Listeriosis	Male	Not reported	Unknown	Unknown	Died
VigiBase 2016 (3)	Meningitis	Female	Multiple sclerosis	3	5	Recovered
VigiBase 2016 (3)	Unknown	Female	Multiple sclerosis	5	17	Unknown
VigiBase 2016 (3)	Unknown	Female	Multiple sclerosis	5	23	Unknown
Sanofi Genzyme, data on file VigiBase 2016 (3)	Meningoencephalitis	Female	Multiple sclerosis	5	7	Died
VigiBase 2016 (3)	Meningitis	Female	Multiple sclerosis	5	17	Recovered
VigiBase 2016 (3)	Unknown	Female	Multiple sclerosis	3	8	Recovered
VigiBase 2016 (3)	Unknown	Unknown	Multiple sclerosis	5	9	Unknown
VigiBase 2016 (3)	Septicaemia	Female	Multiple sclerosis	Unknown	Unknown	Unknown
VigiBase 2015 (3)	Unknown	Male	Multiple sclerosis	5	9	Recovered
VigiBase 20 14 (3)	Meningitis	Female	Multiple sclerosis	5	1	Not recovered
Rau 2015 (4)	Meningitis	Female	Multiple sclerosis	5	6	Recovered
Rau 2015 (4)	Meningitis	Female	Multiple sclerosis	5	8	Recovered
Wray 2009 (5)	Meningitis	Female	Multiple sclerosis	3	19	Recovered
Ohm 2009 (6)	Sepsis	Female	Multiple sclerosis	3	13	Not recovered
VigiBase 2010	Meningitis	Male	Unknown	NA	Unknown	Not recovered
VigiBase 2009 (3)	Unknown	Female	B cell lymphoma	NA	Unknown	Died
VigiBase 2010 (3)	Sepsis	Male	Chronic lymphocytic leukemia	NA	Unknown	Unknown
VigiBase 2011	Unknown	Unknown	Chronic lymphocytic leukemia	NA	Unknown	Unknown

[a]No information about the indication for treatment, type of listeriosis or number of infusions is provided at VigiBase for this case
Information in VigiBase comes from a variety of sources, and the likelihood that the suspected adverse reaction is drug-related is not the same in all cases. The information does not represent the opinion of the World Health Organization (3)

monocytogenes, 3 days prior to the first infusion and 6 days prior to the debut of the symptoms. She did not consume any such foods during the treatment cycle, and therefore most likely contracted the infection prior to the treatment. One of the other reported cases also consumed raw milk products a few days before the first infusion [6]. We therefore suggest that patients should avoid eating such food items the last weeks prior to alemtuzumab infusion, not only after treatment as currently recommended in the SPC. Investigators have traced outbreaks of listeria infections to a number of food products, including deli meats, hot dogs, soft cheeses (including pasteurised cheeses contaminated after production), celery, sprouts and ice cream [14]. Exposure to *L. moncytogenes* might therefore be difficult to avoid [15].

The present case history highlights that a serious infection can be difficult to distinguish from non-infectious infusion related reactions caused by cytokine release, which may occur up to 24 h after alemtuzumab infusion [16]. Such reactions are less common when infusion of alemtuzumab is preceded by corticosteroids, which are now routinely used. It should however be noted that even when preceded by 1000 mg methylprednisolone alemtuzumab may induce a rapid and transient increase in pro-inflammatory cytokines and acute phase proteins, including c-reactive protein which can rise to septic levels [10]. The differential diagnosis between infectious and non-infectious side effects shortly after alemtuzumab infusions is therefore demanding.

Conclusion

Physicians and patients should be aware of this potentially lethal side effect of alemtuzumab. The SPC should be revised and advice patients to avoid foods associated with listeria not only after, but also some weeks before treatment with alemtuzumab. The occurrence of listeriosis associated with alemtuzumab should be followed closely, and the need for antibiotic prophylaxis could be considered if prophylactic measures are insufficient.

Abbreviations
CIOMS: Council for International Organizations of Medical Sciences;
SPC: Summary of Product Characteristics; WHO: World Health Organization

Acknowledgements
The authors express their gratitude to the patient participating in the study, and to Ane Simensen for The Norwegian Medicines Agency for collecting data from Uppsala Monitoring Centre.

Funding
No funding was obtained for the preparation of this case report.

Authors' contributions
TH planned the study and wrote the manuscript. TML and HL collected data and revised the manuscript for intellectual content. All authors approved the final version of the manuscript.

Competing interests
The authors declare that they have no competing interests.

Author details
[1]Department of Neurology, Akershus University Hospital, Lørenskog, Norway. [2]Institute of Clinical Medicine, University of Oslo, Oslo, Norway. [3]Department of Infectious Diseases, Akershus University Hospital, Lørenskog, Norway. [4]Department of Microbiology, Akershus University Hospital, Lørenskog, Norway.

References
1. Hernandez-Milian A, Payeras-Cifre A. What is new in listeriosis? Biomed Res Int. 2014;2014:358051. doi:10.1155/2014/358051.
2. Maertens De NC, Devleesschauwer B, Angulo FJ, et al. The global burden of listeriosis: a systematic review and meta-analysis. Lancet Infect Dis. 14:1073–82.
3. Uppsala Monitoring Centre. VigiBase, the World Health Organization (WHO) international database of suspected adverse drug reactions. https://www.who-umc.org/vigibase/vigibase/. Accessed 3 Mar 2017.
4. Rau D, Lang M, Harth A, et al. Listeria Meningitis Complicating Alemtuzumab Treatment in Multiple Sclerosis–Report of Two Cases. Int J Mol Sci. 2015;16:14669–76.
5. Wray S. A descriptive analysis of infectious adverse reactions in alemtuzmab-treated multiple asclerosuis patients. Abstract (poster 812), 25th congress of the European Committeee for Treatment and Research, September 9–12 2009 Dusseldorf, Germany
6. Ohm S, Borchert A, Mackert BM. Alemtuzumab related Listeria infections- a growing concern? Abstract (poster 1123), 31th congress of the European Committeee for Treatment and Research, October 7–10, Barcelona 2015; Abstract
7. Grif K, Patscheider G, Dierich MP, Allerberger F. Incidence of fecal carriage of Listeria monocytogenes in three healthy volunteers: a one-year prospective stool survey. Eur J Clin Microbiol Infect Dis. 2003;22:16–20.
8. Cox AL, Thompson SA, Jones JL, et al. Lymphocyte homeostasis following therapeutic lymphocyte depletion in multiple sclerosis. Eur J Immunol. 2005; 35:3332–42.
9. Auffermann-Gretzinger S, Eger L, Schetelig J, Bornhauser M, Heidenreich F, Ehninger G. Alemtuzumab depletes dendritic cells more effectively in blood than in skin: a pilot study in patients with chronic lymphocytic leukemia. Transplantation. 2007;83:1268–72.
10. Thomas K, Eisele J, Rodriguez-Leal FA, Hainke U, Ziemssen T. Acute effects of alemtuzumab infusion in patients with active relapsing-remitting MS. Neurol Neuroimmunol Neuroinflamm. 2016;3:e228. doi:10.1212/NXI.0000000000000228.
11. Calame DG, Mueller-Ortiz SL, Wetsel RA. Innate and adaptive immunologic functions of complement in the host response to Listeria monocytogenes infection. Immunobiology. 2016;221:1407–17.
12. Genzyme. Lemtrada Summary of Products Characteristics 2016 http://www.ema.europa.eu/ema/index.jsp?curl=pages/medicines/human/medicines/003718/human_med_001678.jsp&mid=WC0b01ac058001d124. Accessed 22 Feb 2017
13. Prats N, Lopez S, Domingo M, et al. Prolonged persistence of Listeria monocytogenes after intragastric infection in corticosteroid-treated mice. Vet Microbiol. 1997;58:79–85.
14. Listeria. Center of Disease Control https://www.cdc.gov/listeria/prevention.html Accessed 20 Feb 2017.
15. Wadamori Y, Gooneratne R, Hussain MA. Outbreaks and factors influencing microbiological contamination of fresh produce. J Sci Food Agric. 2016; doi: 10.1002/jsfa.8125.
16. Moreau T, Coles A, Wing M, et al. Transient increase in symptoms associated with cytokine release in patients with multiple sclerosis. Brain. 1996;119:225–37.

14

Peginterferon beta-1a improves MRI measures and increases the proportion of patients with no evidence of disease activity in relapsing-remitting multiple sclerosis

Douglas L. Arnold[1,2], Peter A. Calabresi[3], Bernd C. Kieseier[4,5], Shifang Liu[5], Xiaojun You[5], Damian Fiore[5] and Serena Hung[5*]

Abstract

Background: Subcutaneous peginterferon beta-1a has previously been shown to reduce the number of T2-hyperintense and gadolinium-enhancing (Gd+) lesions over 2 years in patients with relapsing-remitting multiple sclerosis (RRMS), and to reduce T1-hypointense lesion formation and the proportion of patients showing evidence of disease activity, based on both clinical and radiological measures, compared with placebo over 1 year of treatment. The objectives of the current analyses were to evaluate T1 lesions and other magnetic resonance imaging (MRI) measures, including whole brain volume and magnetization transfer ratio (MTR) of normal appearing brain tissue (NABT), and the proportions of patients with no evidence of disease activity (NEDA), over 2 years.

Methods: Patients enrolled in the ADVANCE study received continuous peginterferon beta-1a every 2 or 4 weeks for 2 years, or delayed treatment (placebo in Year 1; peginterferon beta-1a every 2 or 4 weeks in Year 2). MRI scans were performed at baseline and Weeks 24, 48, and 96. Proportions of patients with NEDA were calculated based on radiological criteria (absence of Gd + and new/newly-enlarging T2 lesions) and clinical criteria (no relapse or confirmed disability progression) separately and overall.

Results: Peginterferon beta-1a every 2 weeks significantly reduced the number and volume of T1-hypointense lesions compared with delayed treatment over 2 years. Changes in whole brain volume and MTR of NABT were suggestive of pseudoatrophy during the first 6 months of peginterferon beta-1a treatment, which subsequently began to resolve. Significantly more patients in the peginterferon beta-1a every 2 weeks group compared with the delayed treatment group met MRI-NEDA criteria (41% vs 21%; odds ratio [OR] 2.56; p < 0.0001), clinical-NEDA criteria (71% vs 57%; OR 1.90; p < 0.0001) and achieved overall-NEDA (37% vs 16%; OR 3.09; p < 0.0001).

Conclusion: Peginterferon beta-1a provides significant improvements in MRI measures and offers patients a good chance of remaining free from evidence of MRI, clinical and overall disease activity over a sustained 2-year period.

Keywords: Clinical trial, Phase 3, Multiple sclerosis, Relapse-remitting multiple sclerosis, Peginterferon beta-1a, Pegylation, Interferon, Magnetic resonance imaging, NEDA, No evidence of disease activity

* Correspondence: serena.hung@biogen.com
[5]Biogen, 225 Binney St, Cambridge, MA, USA
Full list of author information is available at the end of the article

Background

Interferon beta-1a is a therapeutic protein that has been used for many years as an effective treatment for multiple sclerosis (MS). A limitation is the need for frequent administration and associated injection-site adverse events [1]. Attachment of polyethylene glycol (PEG) molecules (pegylation) has been shown to improve the pharmacokinetic and pharmacodynamic properties of protein therapeutics, including interferon beta-1a [2, 3]. The approved dosing schedule of pegylated interferon beta-1a (peginterferon beta-1a) for relapsing-remitting multiple sclerosis (RRMS) of one subcutaneous (SC) injection every 2 weeks is less frequent than other currently available injectable therapies [2–4].

The efficacy and safety of peginterferon beta-1a in patients with RRMS were demonstrated in the ADVANCE study, a 2-year, Phase 3, multicenter study with a 1-year placebo-controlled period. In Year 1, peginterferon beta-1a (125 mcg SC) administered every 2 or 4 weeks resulted in a significantly lower annualized relapse rate (ARR), risk of relapse, and 12-week confirmed disability progression than placebo, with a safety profile similar to established interferon beta-1a therapies [5]. After 96 weeks of treatment, ARR was further reduced in patients who continued on peginterferon beta-1a every 2 weeks, and was maintained in the every 4 weeks treatment group [6]. Magnetic resonance imaging (MRI) results reflected the clinical findings, showing that peginterferon beta-1a every 2 weeks significantly reduced the mean number of new or newly enlarging T2 hyperintense lesions, new T1 hypointense lesions, and gadolinium-enhancing (Gd+) lesions, and the mean volume of T2 hyperintense and T1 hypointense lesions, when compared with placebo and with the peginterferon beta-1a every 4 weeks treatment group at Week 24 and Week 48. In Year 2, there were further relative reductions in the number of new or newly enlarging T2 hyperintense lesions in both continuous peginterferon beta-1a groups compared with the delayed treatment group (patients who received placebo in Year 1, and were re-randomized to peginterferon beta-1a every 2 or 4 weeks in Year 2). The mean number of Gd + lesions at 2 years was significantly lower in the peginterferon beta-1a every 2 weeks group than in patients who crossed over from placebo to peginterferon beta-1a every 2 or 4 weeks at Week 48 (delayed treatment group) [6]. Overall, patients receiving continuous peginterferon beta-1a throughout the study displayed better efficacy than the delayed treatment group, and every 2 weeks dosing was more efficacious than every 4 weeks dosing. Peginterferon beta-1a was well tolerated across all treatment groups [6], and the safety profile was maintained over the 2 years. In total there were 9 deaths (7 had received at least 1 dose of study drug),

which an independent data safety monitoring board concluded were not likely related to study drug and did not change the risk-benefit profile of peginterferon beta-1a [6].

As treatments have improved, achievement of minimal disease activity has become a realistic goal and ARR endpoints have become a less sensitive measure with which to evaluate new therapies in RRMS [7]. No evidence of disease activity (NEDA; also known as freedom from measured disease activity [FMDA]) is a new, more stringent clinical endpoint in MS incorporating both clinical and MRI aspects of disease activity, [7, 8] and has been evaluated in several clinical trials of disease-modifying therapies (natalizumab, cladribine, combiRx [interferon beta-1a and glatiramer acetate], fingolimod, peginterferon beta-1a), although there has been variation in the definition used [9–13]. Analysis of NEDA in Year 1 of ADVANCE showed that significantly more patients receiving peginterferon beta-1a every 2 weeks achieved NEDA compared with the peginterferon beta-1a every 4 weeks and placebo groups [13]. The objectives of the present analyses were to further explore MRI results, and determine the proportion of patients who showed NEDA over the full 2 years of the Phase 3 ADVANCE study.

Methods

Study design and participants

The study design has been described previously [5, 6]. Briefly, ADVANCE was a randomized, multicenter, double-blind, placebo-controlled Phase 3 cross-over study of peginterferon beta-1a in patients with RRMS [5]. Patients who met the following key eligibility criteria were recruited between June 2009 and November 2011: diagnosis of RRMS as defined by the McDonald criteria, [14] age 18 – 65 years, Expanded Disability Status Scale [15] (EDSS) score of 0 – 5, and at least two clinically documented relapses in the previous three years (at least one within the 12 months prior to randomization). Patients with progressive forms of MS, and those who had previously received interferon treatment for MS for longer than four weeks' duration, or less than six months prior to baseline, were excluded. The protocol was approved by each site's institutional review board and was conducted according to the International Conference on Harmonization Guidelines for Good Clinical Practice and the Declaration of Helsinki. Every patient provided written informed consent prior to study entry.

Randomization and blinding

For the first year of the study, patients were randomly assigned (1:1:1) to receive SC injections of placebo, or peginterferon beta-1a 125 mcg every 2 weeks or every 4 weeks. To maintain dose blinding, all patients received an injection every 2 weeks; patients assigned to peginterferon beta-1a every 4 weeks received alternate injections of placebo and peginterferon beta-1a. During Year 2, all patients received dose-blinded peginterferon beta-1a, with patients initially randomized to active treatment continuing on the same dose regimen, and patients receiving placebo in Year 1 re-randomized to peginterferon beta-1a every 2 or 4 weeks at Week 48 [6].

All management, site personnel, investigators, and patients were blinded to treatment assignment. Each site used separate examining and treating neurologists, thereby maintaining blinding for all treatment groups.

Study procedures, definitions and endpoints

Methods for the assessment of clinical and radiologic endpoints in the ADVANCE study after 1 and 2 years [5, 6] and details of additional Year 1 MRI analyses [13] have been published in detail previously. Here we describe methods relevant to the post-hoc analyses of MRI data collected throughout the 2-year study, and assessments of NEDA.

MRI scans obtained at screening and at Weeks 24, 48, and 96 were evaluated centrally in a blinded manner at NeuroRx Research, Montreal, Canada. MRI endpoints derived from MRI scans included: number and volume of T1-hypointense, T2-hyperintense and Gd + lesions; number of new active lesions (sum of Gd+ plus non-enhancing new or newly enlarging T2 hyperintense lesions); whole brain volume; and magnetization transfer ratio (MTR) in normal-appearing brain tissue (NABT) and Gd + lesions. A summary of pulse sequences acquired and the analysis methods are provided in Additional file 1 (Document S1: MRI acquisition parameters and analysis).

Overall-NEDA, MRI-NEDA, and clinical-NEDA were all evaluated for the periods 0–96 weeks and 48–96 weeks, and were defined as follows:

- Overall-NEDA: no evidence of clinical or MRI disease activity over the stated time period. This combines MRI-NEDA and Clinical-NEDA, both defined below.
- MRI-NEDA: no Gd + lesions at any scan after the beginning of the stated time period, and no new or newly-enlarging T2 hyperintense lesions at the end compared with the beginning of the period.
- Clinical-NEDA: no relapses[1] and no onset of 12-week confirmed disability progression[2] over the stated time period.

Statistical analysis

The MRI analysis population comprised patients in the intent-to-treat (ITT) population who entered Year 2, consented to participate in MRI analysis and had any MRI data. Negative-binomial regression was used for analysis of new or newly-enlarging hyperintense lesions on T2-weighted images (adjusted for baseline number of T2 hyperintense lesions); multiple logit regression was used for the analysis of Gd + and new T1 hypointense lesions (adjusted for baseline number of respective lesions). The total number of new active lesions was determined based on Gd + and T2 lesion numbers without double counting. This was compared for each continuous peginterferon beta-1a group versus the delayed treatment group based on negative binomial regression, adjusted for baseline number of Gd + lesions. Changes from baseline in T2, T1 and Gd + lesion volumes, whole brain volume, and MTR of NABT were compared using a Wilcoxon rank-sum test. Post-hoc NEDA proportions were calculated directly, based on the definitions described above, using data from all eligible patients.

The primary analysis used last observation carried forward (LOCF) data (patients who did not have all measurements, but had no evidence of disease activity on any of the available measurements, were considered as NEDA). In a sensitivity analysis, patients who did not have all MRI measurements were excluded from the calculation of NEDA, even if they had no evidence of disease activity on available measurements. A logistic regression model was used to calculate odds ratios (ORs) and corresponding p-values for between-group comparisons. All data sets are available upon request.

Results

Patient disposition and baseline characteristics

Patient demographics and baseline characteristics in the overall study population were well balanced across the treatment groups; mean age was 36–37 years, 70–72% were women, and 81–82% were of white ethnic origin [5]. Key baseline disease characteristics relevant to the MRI and NEDA analyses are presented in Table 1. A total of 1332 patients completed Year 1 of the study and continued with active treatment in Year 2. The proportion of patients who completed Year 2 was similar across treatment groups: peginterferon beta-1a every 2 weeks, 391/438 (89%), peginterferon beta-1a every 4 weeks, 411/438 (94%), and delayed treatment 396/456 (87%) [6].

MRI Outcomes

The numbers of new/newly enlarging T2 lesions and Gd + lesions during the 2 years of this study have been reported previously and are summarized in Additional file 2: Table S1 [6]. In brief, the mean number of new/newly enlarging T2 lesions from baseline to Week 96, and mean number of Gd + lesions at Week 96, were significantly lower with peginterferon beta-1a every 2 weeks compared with both delayed treatment and continuous peginterferon beta-1a every 4 weeks [6].

Table 1 Baseline disease characteristics (Calabresi et al. [5])

Characteristic	Placebo	Peginterferon beta-1a	
		Every 4 weeks	Every 2 weeks
All patients, n	500	500	512
Relapses in the 12 months prior to enrolment, mean (SD)	1.6 (0.67)	1.5 (0.62)	1.6 (0.67)
Baseline EDSS score, mean (SD)	2.44 (1.18)	2.48 (1.24)	2.47 (1.26)
T2 lesions at baseline			
Patients with available data, n	497	499	511
Mean number of lesions (SD)	50.6 (35.7)	51.4 (36.0)	48.7 (36.8)
Patients with no T2 lesions at baseline, n (%)	0	3 (<1)	4 (<1)
Gd + lesions at baseline			
Patients with available data, n	497	498	510
Mean number of lesions (SD)	1.6 (3.8)	1.8 (5.4)	1.2 (3.4)
Patients with no Gd + lesions at baseline, n (%)	296 (59.6)	297 (59.6)	334 (65.5)

EDSS expanded disability status scale, *Gd+* gadolinium-enhancing lesions, *SD* standard deviation

In the present analysis, we evaluated new T1-hypointense lesions over 2 years, and found that, again, significantly fewer T1 lesions formed during treatment with peginterferon beta-1a every 2 weeks compared with delayed treatment or peginterferon beta-1a every 4 weeks (58% and 52% reduction, respectively; both $p < 0.0001$; Fig. 1a). Patients in the peginterferon beta-1a every 2 weeks group also had, on average, significantly fewer new active lesions from baseline to Week 96 (65% and 55% reduction vs delayed treatment and peginterferon

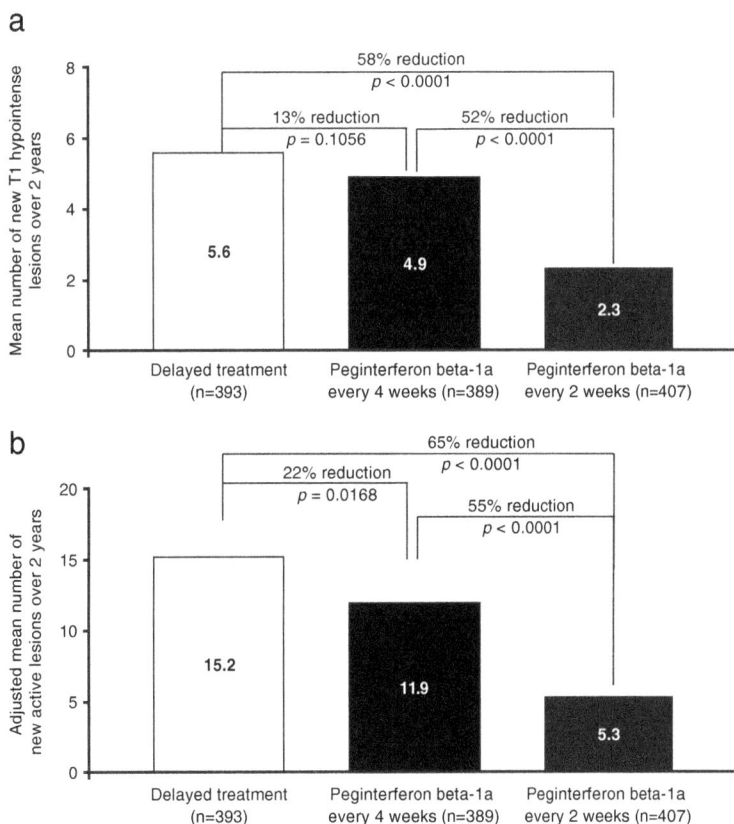

Fig. 1 MRI lesions at Week 96: **a** new T1 hypointense lesions; **b** new-active lesions Gd+, gadolinium-enhancing lesions. MRI analysis population (ITT population dosed in Year 2 with at least 1 MRI result). **a** *P* values based on multiple logit regression, adjusted for baseline number of T1 lesions. **b** *P* values based on negative binomial regression, adjusted for baseline number of Gd + lesions

beta-1a every 4 weeks, respectively; both $p < 0.0001$; Fig. 1b). Additional file 3: Figure S1 shows two illustrative examples of Gd + and T2 lesions that developed into new T1-hypointense lesions over 2 years.

Total T2 hyperintense lesion volume decreased by a mean of 0.23 cm^3 from baseline to Week 96 in the peginterferon beta-1a every 2 weeks group, while it increased in the other groups (mean increases of 0.62 cm^3 in the delayed treatment group and 0.36 cm^3 in the peginterferon beta-1a every 4 weeks; $p < 0.0001$ and $p = 0.046$, respectively, vs peginterferon beta-1a every 2 weeks; Table 2). A significantly smaller increase in T1 hypointense lesion volume was observed with continuous peginterferon beta-1a every 2 weeks compared with delayed treatment (0.48 cm^3 and 0.87 cm^3, respectively; $p < 0.0001$; Table 2). Gd + lesion volume decreased slightly in all groups, with no statistically significant difference between groups (Table 2).

During the first year of the study, whole brain volume decreased from baseline to a greater extent with peginterferon beta-1a every 2 weeks than with delayed treatment ($p < 0.01$ at Weeks 24 and 48); however, the changes were small (<1%) and by Week 96, the reduction versus baseline was numerically smallest in the peginterferon beta-1a every 2 weeks group (Fig. 2). During the period from Week 24 to 96, reduction in whole brain volume was significantly smaller with both peginterferon beta-1a every 2 weeks and peginterferon beta-1a every 4 weeks compared with delayed treatment (Fig. 2 [inset]).

MTR of NABT was reduced in all groups. At each time point, the reduction in NABT compared with baseline was smallest in the peginterferon beta-1a every 2 weeks group. At Week 48 (the end of placebo treatment for the delayed treatment group) MTR of NABT had decreased by a mean of 0.12% in the peginterferon beta-1a every 2 weeks group, compared with 0.39% in the delayed treatment group ($p = 0.05$; Fig. 3).

Analyses of no evidence of disease activity (NEDA)
Over the two years of the study, a significantly higher proportion of patients in the peginterferon beta-1a every 2 weeks group met overall-NEDA criteria compared with the delayed treatment group (36.7% vs 15.8%; OR

3.09; $p < 0.0001$). This was also significantly higher than the proportion in the peginterferon beta-1a every 4 weeks group meeting overall-NEDA criteria (23.0%; OR 1.94; $p < 0.0001$; Fig. 4a [LOCF analyses]). Both MRI and clinical components of NEDA were achieved by significantly higher proportions of patients in the peginterferon beta-1a every 2 weeks group compared with both delayed treatment and peginterferon beta-1a every 4 weeks (ORs for MRI-NEDA 2.56 and 2.08, respectively [both $p < 0.0001$]; ORs for clinical-NEDA 1.90 [$p < 0.0001$] and 1.39 [$p = 0.016$], respectively; Fig. 4a). Sensitivity analyses to exclude patients who did not have all MRI measurements for the calculation of NEDA were consistent with the primary (LOCF) NEDA analyses, with ORs the same or similar across all NEDA assessments (Fig. 4b).

The proportions of patients meeting criteria for overall-, MRI- and clinical-NEDA during Year 2 (Week 48 to Week 96) were higher in all groups than proportions achieving NEDA over the whole 2 years. Odds of achieving NEDA (overall and MRI and clinical components) remained significantly higher with continuous peginterferon beta-1a every 2 weeks compared with both delayed treatment (active treatment with peginterferon beta-1a every 2 or 4 weeks in Year 2) and continuous peginterferon beta-1a every 4 weeks (Fig. 5).

Discussion
The outcomes from this analysis of MRI data and NEDA status are consistent with those data previously reported in the ADVANCE study, supporting the efficacy of peginterferon beta-1a dosed every 2 weeks. Continuous peginterferon beta-1a every 2 weeks consistently provided significant improvements in MRI lesion-based endpoints (including reduced numbers and/or volumes of new or newly-enlarging T2 lesions, new T1 lesions, Gd + lesions, and new active lesions) versus delayed treatment. Data from the first year of the ADVANCE study showed that improvements observed in many of these endpoints was statistically significant for peginterferon beta-1a every 2 weeks versus placebo at the first brain MRI scheduled at Week 24, and sustained through to Week 48 of the ADVANCE study [13]. Alongside recently published 2-year data from the same study, [6]

Table 2 MRI lesion volumes at Week 96

Mean change from baseline (SD)	Delayed treatment	Peginterferon beta-1a	
		Every 4 weeks	Every 2 weeks
Patients with available data, n	391	389	406
T2 hyperintense lesion volume, cm^3	0.617 (2.2341)	0.362 (2.6841)[†]	-0.231 (1.6103)[a]*
T1 hypointense lesion volume, cm^3	0.869 (1.6907)	0.914 (2.4103)	0.478 (1.2417)*
Gd + lesion volume, cm^3	-0.135 (0.5478)	-0.164 (0.8676)	-0.113 (0.4460)

Gd+ gadolinium-enhancing lesions; SD standard deviation *$p < 0.0001$, [†]$p = 0.046$ versus delayed treatment by Wilcoxon rank-sum test [a]$n = 407$

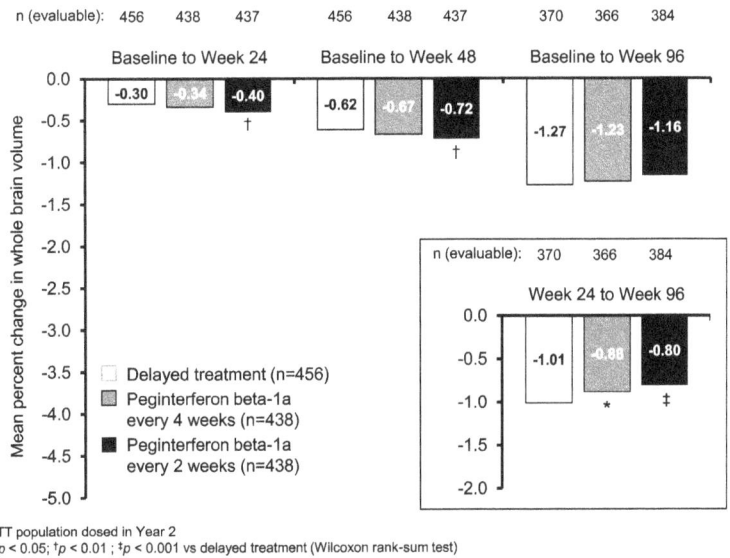

Fig. 2 Percentage reduction in whole brain volume from baseline, and from Week 24 (*inset*). ITT population dosed in Year 2. *p < 0.05; †p < 0.01; ‡p < 0.001 vs delayed treatment (Wilcoxon rank-sum test)

which shows significantly lower mean numbers of new or newly-enlarging T2 and Gd + lesions when compared to delayed treatment or peginterferon beta-1a every 4 weeks, the analyses of T1 lesions and new active lesions presented here suggest that the effect of peginterferon beta-1a every 2 weeks on reducing mean numbers of lesions is further sustained throughout the 2-year study period.

We explored additional MRI measures besides lesions. Analysis of whole brain volume at 96 weeks did not reveal statistically significant treatment effects on brain atrophy. However, this analysis could have been confounded by the occurrence of pseudoatrophy, a phenomenon whereby brain volume decreases significantly during the first 6–12 months of anti-inflammatory treatment, possibly reflecting resolution of edema and inflammation present before treatment initiation [16]. Looking at change in brain volume from Week 24 to Week 96, (to eliminate the first 6 months of treatment in the continuous peginterferon beta-1a groups, when the impact of pseudoatrophy was likely to be greatest) the trend was reversed: there was a significantly smaller

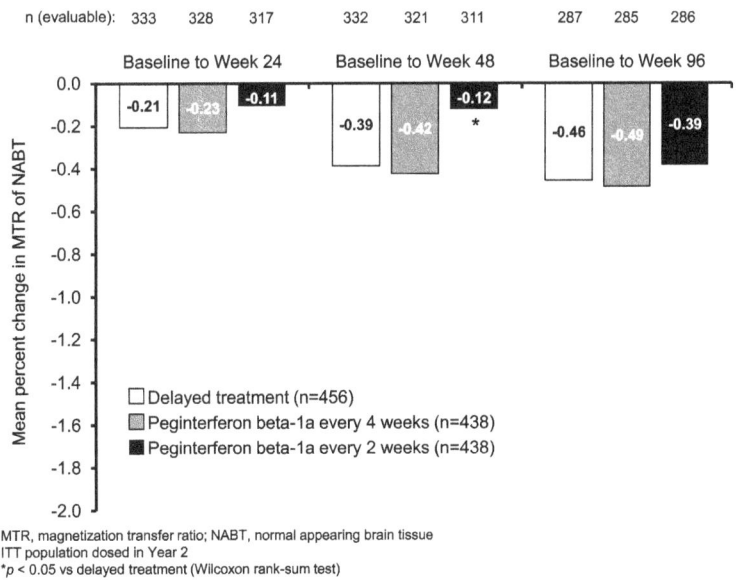

Fig. 3 Percentage reduction in MTR of NABT. MTR, magnetization transfer ratio; NABT, normal appearing brain tissue. ITT population dosed in Year 2. *p < 0.05 vs delayed treatment (Wilcoxon rank-sum test)

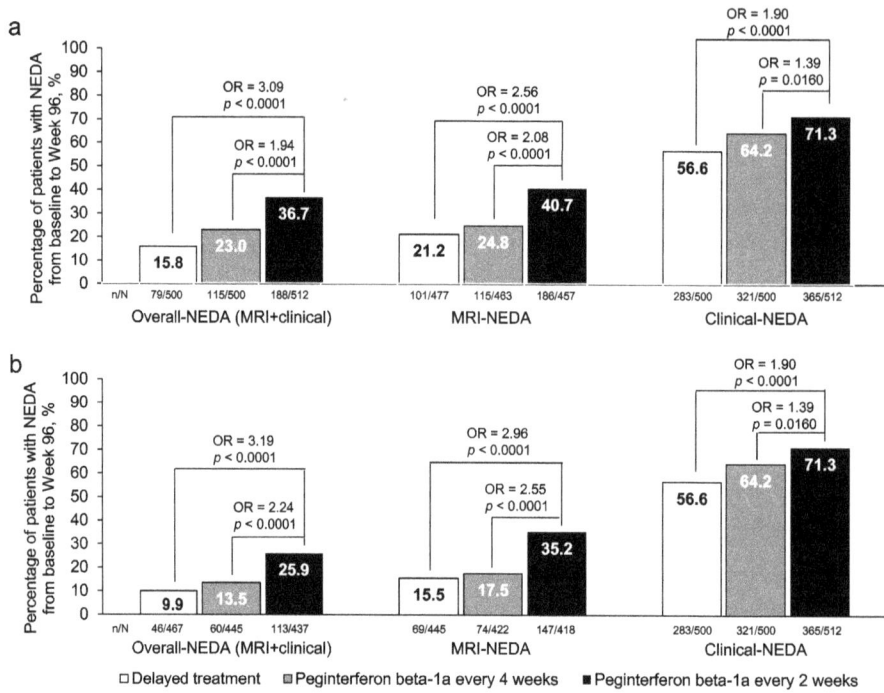

Fig. 4 Proportions of patients with NEDA over 2 years (baseline to Week 96): **a** LOCF analysis; **b** observed data[a]. MRI, magnetic resonance imaging; NEDA, no evidence of disease activity; OR, odds ratio. [a]Sensitivity analysis excluding patients with missing MRI data

reduction in whole brain volume with both peginterferon beta-1a every 2 weeks and every 4 weeks, compared with delayed treatment. This suggests that peginterferon beta-1a could slow brain atrophy in the long term, although the 2-year overall treatment duration in this study was not sufficient to overcome the effects of pseudoatrophy in the first few months, and comparisons may be further confounded by onset of pseudoatrophy on initiation of treatment in Year 2 in the delayed treatment group. Furthermore, MTR measured in NABT over 96 weeks showed a trend for improved outcomes with continuous

peginterferon every 2 weeks compared with delayed treatment. If reductions in brain volume over time were a result of true atrophy, it may be expected that this may also coincide with myelin loss (reflected by a decrease in MTR of NABT). Opposing trends for these measures during the first year of treatment with peginterferon beta-1a every 2 weeks (increased loss of brain volume coinciding with decreased reduction in MTR of NABT) support the suggestion that initial acceleration of loss of brain volume resulted from pseudoatrophy. A significant difference between peginterferon beta-1a every 2 weeks

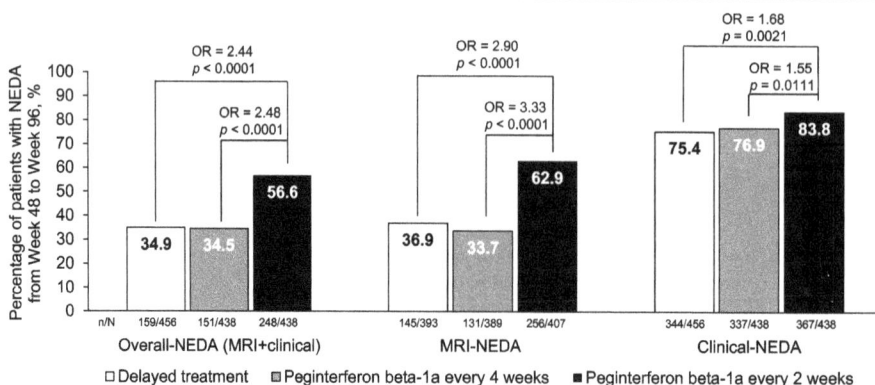

Fig. 5 Proportions of patients with NEDA in Year 2 (Week 48–96). MRI, magnetic resonance imaging; NEDA, no evidence of disease activity; OR, odds ratio. LOCF analysis (includes patients who did not have all measurements, but had no evidence of disease activity on any of the available measurements). ITT population dosed in Year 2

and delayed treatment in MTR of NABT change was apparent at Week 48, but was not sustained to Week 96; this may reflect a combination of attenuation of differences between the groups after peginterferon beta-1a treatment was commenced in the delayed treatment group and uncertainty in the point estimates given the small changes and variability in this measurement.

In addition to the MRI data, the present NEDA analyses support the efficacy of peginterferon beta-1a treatment every 2 weeks. Post-hoc analyses of efficacy data from ADVANCE showed that proportions of patients meeting criteria for overall-, MRI- and clinical-NEDA from baseline to Week 96 were significantly higher with peginterferon beta-1a every 2 weeks versus delayed treatment. MRI components of the NEDA composite appeared to be more sensitive to detecting treatment differences than clinical components; a high proportion of patients across all of the treatment groups met criteria for clinical-NEDA, supporting the value of including MRI components to support clinical-NEDA analyses. Nonetheless, NEDA criteria appear to be sufficiently robust to withstand missing MRI data, since the sensitivity analysis showed that inclusion of patients with missing MRI data in the LOCF analysis did not notably affect results. Currently, MRI-NEDA is defined as no Gd + lesions at Week 24, Week 48, or Week 96 and no new or newly-enlarging T2 hyperintense lesions compared with baseline over 96 weeks. Our analyses of MRI endpoints alongside post-hoc NEDA analyses support the use of this definition, since it reflects new active lesions detected on MRI scans. T1 lesion formation was also reduced during treatment with peginterferon beta-1a every 2 weeks, but any added value of incorporating this measure into the MRI-NEDA definition is not clear. We found limitations to potential incorporation of brain volume to the definition of NEDA: the small changes observed over periods of clinical interest, such as one or two years, and the noise in this measurement, as well as the complication of pseudoatrophy, make it unsuitable as a component of the MRI-NEDA and overall-NEDA composite endpoints.

Our results are consistent with our previous analysis of interim ADVANCE data, in which 39.8% of patients in the peginterferon beta-1a every 2 weeks group, and 17.8% in the placebo group, achieved overall NEDA in Year 1 (based on an LOCF analysis using the same NEDA definition as the current analysis) [13]. In the current analysis, overall NEDA rates over 2 years (baseline to Week 96) were 36.7% in the continuous peginterferon beta-1a group and 15.8% in the delayed treatment group. However, when we looked specifically at Year 2, these values increased to 56.6% and 34.9%, respectively. This supports the suggestion, based on our previous analysis, that it may be preferable to begin to assess NEDA status after a standard period of time (i.e., 6–12 months) following initiation of treatment, since MRI components may be affected by accrual of lesions early on before treatment efficacy becomes apparent [13].

The finding that more than half of patients on peginterferon beta-1a every 2 weeks achieved overall NEDA in Year 2 is encouraging, as recent longitudinal study in which NEDA status was monitored in a cohort of patients with MS over 7 years suggested that NEDA status at 2 years was a prognostic indicator for long term outcomes [17]. Future analyses of data from the ongoing ATTAIN study (an extension of ADVANCE) will reveal whether NEDA status is maintained for a high proportion of patients with longer-term peginterferon beta-1a treatment.

NEDA (sometimes referred to as FMDA or disease activity free [DAF]) has been assessed for many of the newer disease-modifying therapies becoming available for the treatment of MS. Rates are quite variable, with reported rates for overall-NEDA over 2 years ranging from 18% to 46% in trials of teriflunomide, dimethyl fumarate (DMF), fingolimod, natalizumab and cladribine [9, 10, 12, 18–20]. Rates should be compared with caution, as differences in study design, patient populations and MRI analysis techniques could contribute to variation, [8, 21, 22] although NEDA rates in placebo groups in these trials did not vary as widely as those in active treatment groups (7–16%). Considering differences in terms of ORs helps to account for differences in the sensitivity of the analyses, although ORs are not always provided in reporting of NEDA analyses. In a combined post-hoc analysis of data from the DEFINE and CONFIRM studies, the OR for achieving overall NEDA with DMF 240 mg twice daily versus placebo was 2.7 (23% vs 11%; $p < 0.0001$), [19] and in the CLARITY study ORs for cladribine 3.5 mg/kg and 5.25 mg/kg versus placebo were $4 \cdot 28$ and $4 \cdot 62$, respectively (44% and 46% vs 16%; both $p < 0.0001$) [10]. Peginterferon beta-1a administered continuously every 2 weeks for 2 years approximately tripled the likelihood of achieving overall-NEDA (OR 3.09) compared with delayed treatment.

Determining the relevance of this data to real-world experience will require further investigation, as patients are rarely completely lesion-free and have varying degrees of lesion activity. Interpretation is complicated by "noise" in the measurement of new lesions related to technical factors associated with the MRI acquisition and rater variability [23]. In part for these reasons, clinicians often look at a threshold for new lesions, which may be different between physicians, hospitals, and even different countries. A consensus on the use of MRI techniques and analysis may prove to be very beneficial to the study of MS, its pathophysiology, and potential treatments.

Conclusion

Analyses of MRI outcomes and NEDA outcomes, along with efficacy for clinical endpoints previously reported, [5, 6, 13] show that the efficacy of peginterferon beta-1a is extended beyond the first year of the ADVANCE study, illustrating the benefits of peginterferon beta-1a on a number of different MRI outcomes as well as clinical-NEDA status. SC peginterferon every 2 weeks is the least frequently dosed interferon therapy for the treatment of multiple sclerosis, and the present analysis further supports the use of this therapy in patients with RRMS.

Endnotes

[1]Relapses (confirmed by the independent neurologic evaluation committee) were defined as new or recurrent neurologic symptoms not associated with fever or infection, lasting for $\geq$24 h, and accompanied by new objective neurologic findings, and separated from the onset of other confirmed relapses by at least 30 days.

[2]Disability progression was defined as an increase in the EDSS score of $\geq$1.0 point in patients with a baseline score of $\geq$1.0, or an increase of $\geq$1.5 points in patients with a baseline score of 0, confirmed after 12 or 24 weeks.

Additional files

Additional file 1: Document S1. MRI acquisition parameters and analysis.

Additional file 2: Table S1. Summary of MRI endpoints over 2 years by original randomisation group [6].

Additional file 3: Gd + and T2 lesions that developed into T1 lesions: a) Gd + lesion that developed into a T1 lesion; b) new T2 lesion that developed into a T1 lesion. Figure A image 1 shows a Gd + lesion in the left prefrontal cortex at Week 48 that developed into a T1 lesion by Week 96 (image 2). Figure B image 2 shows a T2 lesion in the left prefrontal cortex at Week 48 that was not present at Week 24 (image 1). The lesion developed into a T1 lesion by Week 96 (image 3). Gd+, gadolinium-enhancing lesions.

Abbreviations

ARR: Annualized relapse rate; DAF: Disease activity free; DMF: Dimethyl fumarate; EDSS: Expanded Disability Status Scale; FMDA: Freedom from measured disease activity; Gd+: Gadolinium-enhancing; ITT: Intent-to-treat; LOCF: Last observation carried forward; MRI: Magnetic resonance imaging; MS: Multiple sclerosis; MTR: Magnetization transfer ratio; NABT: Normal appearing brain tissue; NEDA: No evidence of disease activity; OR: Odds ratio; PEG: Polyethylene glycol; RRMS: Relapsing-remitting multiple sclerosis; SC: Subcutaneous

Acknowledgements

We wish to thank the patients who volunteered for this study and the many site staff members who helped to conduct the study. Data and safety monitoring committee members: Brian Weinshenker, Willis Maddrey, Kenneth Miller, Andrew Goodman, Maria Pia Sormani, Burt Seibert. Samantha Stanbury, PhD, a professional medical writer contracted to CircleScience (Tytherington, UK), assisted with the preparation of the manuscript under the direction of the authors. Writing support was funded by the study sponsor.

Funding

This study was funding by Biogen (Cambridge, MA, USA).

Authors' contributions

All authors read and approved the final manuscript. DLA participated in the design of the study, data acquisition and interpretation, and contributed to the drafting and revision of the manuscript. PAC participated in the acquisition and interpretation of the data, conceptualization of the analyses, and contributed to the drafting and revision of the manuscript. BCK participated in the design of the study, data acquisition and interpretation, and contributed to the drafting and revision of the manuscript. SL participated in the design of the study, performed statistical analyses, and contributed to the drafting and revision of the manuscript. XY performed statistical analyses, and contributed to the drafting and revision of the manuscript. DF contributed to the drafting and revision of the manuscript. SH participated in the design of the study data interpretation and contributed to the drafting and revision of the manuscript.

Competing interests

The ADVANCE study was funded by Biogen (Cambridge, MA, USA). DA reports an equity interest in NeuroRx during the conduct of the study; personal fees from Acorda, Biogen, Genentech, Genzyme, Hoffman LaRoche, Innate Immunotherapy, MedImmune, Mitsubishi, Novartis, Receptos, Sanofi-Aventis, and Teva, outside the submitted work; as well as grants from Biogen and Novartis.

PAC has received personal consulting fees from Vertex, Abbvie and Merck. He has received grant support from Biogen, Novartis and Medimmune. BCK owns Biogen stock and is an employee of Biogen. He has received personal fees for consulting from Bayer, Biogen, Genzyme, Hoffman LaRoche, Merck Serono, Mitsubishi, Novartis, Sanofi and Teva. SL, XY, DF, SH own Biogen stock and are employees of Biogen.

Author details

[1]Montreal Neurological Institute, McGill University, Montreal, QC, Canada. [2]NeuroRx Research, Montreal, QC, Canada. [3]Department of Neurology, Johns Hopkins University, Baltimore, MD, USA. [4]Department of Neurology, Medical Faculty, Heinrich-Heine University, Düsseldorf, Germany. [5]Biogen, 225 Binney St, Cambridge, MA, USA.

References

1. Jain A, Jain SK. PEGylation: an approach for drug delivery. A review. Crit Rev Ther Drug Carrier Syst. 2008;25(5):403–47.
2. Kieseier BC, Calabresi PA. PEGylation of interferon-beta-1a: a promising strategy in multiple sclerosis. CNS Drugs. 2012;26(3):205–14.
3. Hu X, Miller L, Richman S, Hitchman S, Glick G, Liu S, et al. A novel PEGylated interferon beta-1a for multiple sclerosis: safety, pharmacology, and biology. J Clin Pharmacol. 2012;52(6):798–808.
4. Baker DP, Pepinsky RB, Brickelmaier M, Gronke RS, Hu X, Olivier K, et al. PEGylated interferon beta-1a: meeting an unmet medical need in the treatment of relapsing multiple sclerosis. J Interferon Cytokine Res. 2010;30(10):777–85.
5. Calabresi PA, Kieseier BC, Arnold DL, Balcer LJ, Boyko A, Pelletier J, et al. Pegylated interferon beta-1a for relapsing-remitting multiple sclerosis (ADVANCE): a randomised, phase 3, double-blind study. Lancet Neurol. 2014;13(7):657–65.
6. Kieseier BC, Arnold DL, Balcer LJ, Boyko AA, Pelletier J, Liu S, et al. Peginterferon beta-1a in multiple sclerosis: 2-year results from ADVANCE. Mult Scler. 2015;21(8):1025–35.
7. Lublin FD. Disease activity free status in MS. Mult Scler Relat Disord. 2012;1(1):6–7.
8. Stangel M, Penner IK, Kallmann BA, Lukas C, Kieseier BC. Towards the implementation of 'no evidence of disease activity' in multiple sclerosis treatment: the multiple sclerosis decision model. Ther Adv Neurol Disord. 2015;8(1):3–13.
9. Havrdova E, Galetta S, Hutchinson M, Stefoski D, Bates D, Polman CH, et al. Effect of natalizumab on clinical and radiological disease activity in multiple sclerosis: a retrospective analysis of the Natalizumab Safety and Efficacy in Relapsing-Remitting Multiple Sclerosis (AFFIRM) study. Lancet Neurol. 2009;8(3):254–60.

10. Giovannoni G, Cook S, Rammohan K, Rieckmann P, Sorensen PS, Vermersch P, et al. Sustained disease-activity-free status in patients with relapsing-remitting multiple sclerosis treated with cladribine tablets in the CLARITY study: a post-hoc and subgroup analysis. Lancet Neurol. 2011;10(4):329–37.

11. Lindsey JW, Scott TF, Lynch SG, Cofield SS, Nelson F, Conwit R, et al. The CombiRx trial of combined therapy with interferon and glatiramer acetate in relapsing remitting MS: Design and baseline characteristics. Mult Scler Relat Disord. 2012;1(2):81–6.

12. Kappos L, Radue EW, O'Connor P, Amato M, Zhang-Auberson LX, Tang DJ. Fingolimod treatment increases the proportion of patients who are free from disease activity in multiple sclerosis: results from a Phase 3, Placebo-Controlled Study (FREEDOMS). Neurology. 2011;76 Suppl 4:A563.

13. Arnold DL, Calabresi PA, Kieseier BC, Sheikh SI, Deykin A, Zhu Y, et al. Effect of peginterferon beta-1a on MRI measures and achieving no evidence of disease activity: results from a randomized controlled trial in relapsing-remitting multiple sclerosis. BMC Neurol. 2014;14:240.

14. Polman CH, Reingold SC, Edan G, Filippi M, Hartung HP, Kappos L, et al. Diagnostic criteria for multiple sclerosis: 2005 revisions to the "McDonald Criteria". Ann Neurol. 2005;58(6):840–6.

15. Kurtzke JF. Rating neurologic impairment in multiple sclerosis: an expanded disability status scale (EDSS). Neurology. 1983;33(11):1444–52.

16. De Stefano N, Airas L, Grigoriadis N, Mattle HP, O'Riordan J, Oreja-Guevara C, et al. Clinical relevance of brain volume measures in multiple sclerosis. CNS Drugs. 2014;28(2):147–56.

17. Rotstein DL, Healy BC, Malik MT, Chitnis T, Weiner HL. Evaluation of no evidence of disease activity in a 7-year longitudinal multiple sclerosis cohort. JAMA Neurol. 2015;72(2):152–8.

18. Freedman M OCP, Wolinsky J, et al. Teriflunomide increases the proportion of patients free from disease activity in the TEMSO phase III study. Neurology. 2012; 78 (Meeting Abstracts 1). PD5.007.

19. Havrdova EGR, Fox RJ, Kappos L, Phillips JT, Zhang A, Kurukulasuriya N, Sheikh S, Viglietta V, Dawson K, Giovannoni G. BG-12 (dimethyl fumarate) treatment for relapsing-remitting multiple sclerosis (RRMS) increases the proportion of patients free of measured clinical and neuroradiologic disease activity in the phase 3 studies. Neurology. 2013;80(Meeting Abstracts 1):07–106.

20. Nixon R, Bergvall N, Tomic D, Sfikas N, Cutter G, Giovannoni G. No evidence of disease activity: indirect comparisons of oral therapies for the treatment of relapsing-remitting multiple sclerosis. Adv Ther. 2014;31(11):1134–54.

21. Havrdova E, Galetta S, Stefoski D, Comi G. Freedom from disease activity in multiple sclerosis. Neurology. 2010;74 Suppl 3:S3–7.

22. Jacobsen C, Hagemeier J, Myhr KM, Nyland H, Lode K, Bergsland N, et al. Brain atrophy and disability progression in multiple sclerosis patients: a 10-year follow-up study. J Neurol Neurosurg Psychiatry. 2014;85(10):1109–15.

23. Elliott CMJ, Cadavid D, Richert N, Duda P, Fisher E, Narayanan S, Collins DL, Arbel T, Arnold DL. Inter-rater variability of new T2 determination in the clinic has implications for MS diagnosis and monitoring. 28th Congress of the European Committee for Treatment and Research in Multiple Sclerosis (ECTRIMS). Lyon: Mult Scler; 2012.

15

Association between multiple sclerosis, cancer risk, and immunosuppressant treatment

Paolo Ragonese*⬭, Paolo Aridon, Giulia Vazzoler, Maria Antonietta Mazzola, Vincenzina Lo Re, Marianna Lo Re, Sabrina Realmuto, Simona Alessi, Marco D'Amelio, Giovanni Savettieri and Giuseppe Salemi

Abstract

Background: The association between multiple sclerosis (MS) and cancer has long been investigated with conflicting results. Several reports suggest an increased cancer risk among MS patients treated with immunosuppressant (IS) drugs.

Methods: We performed a cohort study including MS patients recruited at the Neurological Department of the University of Palermo. Mean follow-up period was ten years for the whole cohort. We calculated cancer incidence among patients treated with IS. Incidence rates were compared in the cohort by calculating the relative risk according to length and dose of exposure to IS. Cancer incidence among MS patients was compared to cancer incidence in the general population of Sicily in similar age groups.

Results: On an overall cohort of 531 MS patients (346 women and 185 men) exposed to IS, we estimated a crude incidence rate for cancer of 2.26% (2.02% in women, 2.7% in men). Cancer risk was higher compared to rates observed among an equal number of patients not exposed to IS, and to the risk in the general population in Sicily at similar age groups (adjusted HR: 11.05; CI 1.67–73.3; $p = 0.013$).

Conclusion: The present study showed a higher cancer risk in MS patients associated only to previous IS exposure. Studies on long-term outcomes are essential to evaluate the possibility that treatment options that need to be considered for a long time-period may modify risk for life threatening diseases.

Keywords: Multiple sclerosis, Cancer, Cohort study, Immunosuppressant, Treatment

Background

The pathologic mechanisms of Multiple sclerosis (MS) are mediated by the immune system and by neurodegenerative processes causing both myelin sheath and axonal damage. MS represents one of the major causes of neurological disability, especially in young people [1]. First line treatments for MS until recently, were basically represented by immune modulating drugs like beta interferon or glatiramer acetate, while in patients with more aggressive disease courses or who did not respond to first line treatments, immune suppressors (IS) had been used [2]. For these reasons, azathioprine (AZA) was still in use, even after the introduction of disease modifying treatments (DMT). Mitoxantrone (MX) and cyclophosphamide (CP) were mostly chosen as second line treatments or as induction therapy in patients with a more aggressive disease. Their use declined significantly after the introduction of new therapies characterized by a specific mechanism of action for the treatment of MS, like monoclonal antibodies (natalizumab was approved in Italy in 2006) and fingolimod (introduced in Italy 2011) though these drugs still remain a therapeutic alternative in selected cases. The safety profile of immune treatments for MS [3–7], as well as the relationship between the disease and cancer, has been widely explored but results have been yet not conclusive [8–14]. These inconsistencies are due to methodological differences in study design, by the difficulty in selecting an appropriate reference group for comparisons, and length of follow-up,

---
* Correspondence: paolo.ragonese@unipa.it
Dipartimento di Biomedicina Sperimentale e Neuroscienze Cliniche (Department of Experimental Biomedicine and Clinical Neurosciences), Università degli Studi di Palermo, Via G. La Loggia, 1, 90129 Palermo, Italy

which is of particular relevance in clinical trials exploring the safety of drugs. Several question have not been yet well addressed. Do generally IS used for MS increase the risk for cancer or is there a particular IS which is mainly associated with increased cancer risk? Is there a difference between cancer risk among MS patients treated with IS and those who were not exposed to IS, compared to people not affected by MS (general population)? In order to contribute to assess these issues we performed a cohort study including patients affected by MS exposed to IS, and an equal number of MS patients not exposed to IS to determine cancer risk. The present study was also aimed to compare cancer incidence among people affected by MS to that in the general population in the same geographic area and in the same period.

Methods

Cohort design

During the study period (1994, to January 31st, 2011) we identified at our Neurologic Department a cohort of 531 MS patients affected by MS (346 women and 185 men) who took at least one of the three IS (AZA, MX, and CP) independently if they had been treated with interferon or glatiramer. An equal number of patients (531) with the same sex distribution but not exposed to IS was matched as reference group. To assess the above-mentioned questions in the cohort of MS patients we considered two kind of comparison groups and hence, two different approaches. A first group consisted as indicated in an equal number of individuals affected by MS consecutively selected and followed in the same time interval, among patients followed at the same Neurological Department who had never been treated with IS. We also compared cancer incidence among individuals affected by MS exposed or not to IS, with that in the Sicilian general population, considering similar age groups and calculating the standardized incidence ratio (SIR) for cancer in the two cohorts.

Treatments

MX and CP were used in our Department after other treatments had failed to reduce relapse frequency or disability worsening in patients affected by MS. Before starting MX, patients underwent a screening for cardiovascular diseases. Treatment administration was made at a monthly dose of 8 mg/m² for the first three months, and at a dose of 12 mg/m² every three months up to a cumulative dose of 140 mg/m². We used this regimen from 1994 until 2000. Afterward to limit cumulative long-term toxicity, we modified the cumulative dose limiting it to a maximum of 90 mg/m². We limited the cumulative dose of MX because of the already known possible heart toxicity. For the same reason, we used to

perform a tight monitoring of heart function by transthoracic ecocardiography. Treatment was stopped before reaching the planned final dose if signs of impaired heart function, such as confirmed left ventricular ejection fraction (LVEF) reduction to less than 50%, or a confirmed reduction of more than 10% with respect to the first examination, were observed. Reduction or termination of infusions due to adverse events was at the physician's judgment. Azathioprine was targeted to reach a maximum dose of 3 mg/Kg of body weight per day if tolerated. Decrease of IS dosages were done in the presence of severe leucopoenia, red blood cell or platelet reduction, severe infections or other clinically relevant serological markers modifications. CP was administered at a monthly dose of 500 mg/m² during the first year of treatment; it was eventually prolonged during the second year with courses repeated every two months. We included in the whole cohort MS patients who were treated with the three IS considered in the same lag-time, obtaining a cohort with a comparable follow-up. The second group of MS patients (represented as above indicated by 531 individuals) were treated with other drugs available at that time (beta interferon or glatiramer).

Statistical analyses

Calculations of outcome measures were performed considering January 31st, 2011 as the end of follow-up while the observation was started in 1994 at the time of inclusion of the first patient for MX treatment. Statistical analyses were performed by calculating univariate relative risks (RR) for cancer comparing its incidence in MS patients exposed to IS with that in those not exposed to IS. Cox proportional models were built to calculate adjusted hazard ratios (HR) considering the follow-up period as the time variable. In these models, age at MS onset, and length of the follow-up expressed in years, were calculated as continuous variables. A separate Cox model was built including also age at treatment initiation (IS or other therapies) as a covariate. We performed also a second analysis by comparing cancer incidence rates in our cohort of MS patients, with that of individuals from the Sicilian general population of the same age groups. By means of this kind of comparison, we calculated the possible difference existing in the probability to develop cancers according to the condition of being affected or not by MS itself and not only on being exposed to therapy. Since MS cohort was represented by individuals in the age classes between 18 and 54 years of age, we made comparisons by including as a reference, cancer incidence in the Sicilian population at the same age groups. These data were freely available from the Italian National tumor registry (http://www.tumori.net/). In these second analyses, we calculated SIR. All the analyses were two-sided with alpha level set at 0.05; 95% confidence intervals (CI) were also calculated.

The local ethical committee of our University Hospital approved the study and each patient gave the consent for treatment and inclusion in our clinical database.

Results

We included 531 MS patients from our database (346 women and 185 men), who had been treated with IS. 531 MS individuals who had never been exposed to IS were included for comparisons. Table 1 summarizes characteristics of the two groups of MS patients in the cohort. The two groups were not significantly different with regard to age, disease duration and cumulative length of the follow-up. Mean follow up was 9 years for patients treated with IS, and 10 years in for the others. As expected, patients treated with different kind of IS have different period of treatment exposure; AZA treatment was usually stopped after 5 years of therapy, while for CP and MX patients usually reached the planned total cumulative dose within two tears of therapy. Details about types of tumors in men and women are reported in Table 2. Gut cancers (colon or rectal cancer), female breast cancer and leukemia represented the most common type of cancer. Cancer distribution according to length of exposure and the type of IS are reported in Table 2. This variable was dichotomized according to the median time of treatment duration for each specific drug (below or above the mean). In the present cohort, we observed no cancers in those people exposed to CP alone. Table 3 reports relative risks and hazard ratios for

the association between MS and the exposure to IS. At univariate analyses, we observed a significant association between exposure to IS and cancer in MS patients. Individuals treated with AZA had a four-fold increased risk for cancer, compared to those not exposed (median time of treatment 5 years). Among MS patients who were treated with MTX (median exposure one year), cancer risk was four times higher. Cox proportional hazard models revealed an even higher risk for cancers associated to IS exposure; HR was 11.05 (95% CI 1.67–73.30; $p = 0.01$) in the most conservative model. Age at onset of MS appeared to be independently associated to cancer risk (HR 1.05; CI 1.01–1.10; $p = 0.03$). As indicated in Table 4, SIR was four times higher in MS individuals exposed to IS compared to the age matched general population. On the contrary there was no a different cancer incidence in people affected by MS who did not undergo to IS therapy, showing significant lower cancer rates (SIR 0.97; CI 0.96–0.98).

Discussion

The present study did not show an association between being affected by MS and cancer. The study revealed, a direct strong association between IS exposure among individuals affected by MS and cancer. Risk for cancer observed in individuals with MS exposed to IS seems to be related to the duration of exposure and to the cumulative dose, not to a specific IS. Our study has some limits derived from the relatively small number of cancers identified in the cohort, despite the fact that a large cohort of MS patients was included and the analyses were performed on the basis of a long follow-up period. Our aim was to investigate if the risk for cancer could be related to the disease itself or to the exposure to treatments. Therefore we chose to compare MS patients exposed to IS to MS individuals who had never been treated with IS, and to a second cohort of individuals not affected by MS. For the same reason we compared cancer incidence in MS individuals to that of the Sicilian general population. In our cohort, we did not observe any cancer among individuals who were exposed to

Table 1 Demographic and clinical characteristics of the MS cohort included in the study

Variable	Exposed to IS	Others
Sex (W/M)	531 (336/195)	531 (359/172)
Mean age at onset (years +/− SD)	29 (10)	30 (10)
Mean age at treatment start (years +/− SD)	29.4 (9.9)	40 (13.5)
Mean disease duration (SD)	19 (9)	20 (10)
Mean Follow-up (years +/− SD) for the whole cohort	9 (5)	10 (6)
Mean Follow-up (years +/− SD) for the MX group	8 (5)	–
Mean Follow-up (years +/− SD) for the CP group	5 (5)	–
Mean Follow-up (years +/− SD) for the AZA group	10 (6)	–
Mean treatment duration for the MX group (years)	1	–
Mean treatment duration for the CP group (years)	1	–
Mean treatment duration for the AZA group (years)	4	–

Table 2 Number and type of cancer by IS drug and by exposure duration

Drug	Exposure duration (years)	No. of patients	N. and site of cancer	p*
Azathioprine	< 4	169	3 (gut [a], brain, ovary)	
	≥4	177	4 (3 breast, 1 gut[a])	0,75
Mitoxantrone	<1	74	1 (pancreas)	
	≥1	188	5 (3 leukemia, 1 lung, 1 gut)	0,5

* two sided Chi square analysis comparing the frequency among MS patients exposed for the longer period, compared to those exposed for a shorter period
[a]Gut cancers include colon and rectal cancers

Table 3 Relative risks and HR calculation by investigated variables

Variable	RR (CI)^c	HR	p
Model A			
Sex (men/women)	0.78 (0.28–2.22)	1.24 (0.43–3.56)	0.69
Age at MS onset^a	1.001 (0.97–1.03)	1.05 (1.01–1.10)	0.03
Follow-up length^a	1.03 (0.98–1.08)	_	–
IS exposure (yes vs. no)^b	4.01 (1.14–14.1)	11.05 (1.67–73.3)	0.013
Model B			
Sex		1.32 (0.46–3.78)	0.6
Age at treatment^a		1.07 (1.02–1.12)	0.01
Disease duration^a		2.36 (0.71–7.84)	0.2
IS exposure (yes vs. no)^b		35.05 (3.12–403.31)	0.01

^{a}Age at onset and length of follow-up were dichotomous variables according to the median of the distribution in the whole cohort in univariate analyses, while they were calculated as continuous variables in Cox models
^{b}Model B was built including age at treatment initiation (IS or other therapies) and disease duration as covariates

cyclophosphamide only, similarly to other study [15]; it is to note however, that in our cohort, the group of patients treated with CP was the smallest and the follow-up was not as long as for the other drugs investigated. Cancer risk in the present study appears to be similar in individuals treated with MTX or AZA. These results confirm previous studies indicating a higher cancer risk related to MTX exposure, represented not only by leukemia [7, 10]. We also observed similar results for azathioprine; breast cancer was the most frequently observed in this group of patients. The results we observed need several comments. A positive association between MS and cancer has been proposed several times, suggesting that chronic inflammation could be the mechanism underneath this relationship [16]. More recent observations, anyway, do not support this association anymore, although conflicting results were reported for the association between MS and specific kind of cancers in several studies [14, 17]. A study investigating the association between autoimmunity and cancer risk [17], showed an inverse association between MS and intestinal cancers. Other studies did not confirm this association reporting on the contrary a global reduction of cancer risk and an association with other kind of tumors [8, 17, 18].

We found that MS does not appear to be associated to cancer risk by itself. Although we did not observe relevant differences between men and women for cancer risk, these results were not plotted because further stratification would have led to small numbers and very broad confidence intervals. Another limitation of this study derives from the fact that due to the study design, it was not possible to investigate the possible confounding effect of environmental risk factors for cancer like smoking habit. It would be in fact not feasible to obtain

this information for referent individuals from the general population. Another important consideration derives from the fact that all the analyses performed with the two different approaches we used, lead to the same observation in our cohort. Comparing MS patients' risk for cancer with the one in the general population with similar ages reduced also the possibility of a possible selection bias deriving from age at patients' selection. It is also important to underline that length of follow-up is crucial in this kind of studies. Carcinogenesis may occur in fact with a long latency. Studies with shorter follow-up may not be able to identify an association also because in the age groups represented by MS patients, cancer incidence depends on the anatomical and histological type of the tumor. All of the three drugs considered in this study act suppressing specific lymphocyte subpopulation but also by permanently modifying DNA expression of oncogenes; all of them activate pathways that determine an increased risk for the development of cancers [19]. For instance, suppression of natural killer cells has been associated for instance to an increased risk for leukemia and for skin cancers in several studies although not focused to MS patients [20]. This is not of course the only explanation for the association we observed. Patients with chronic diseases like MS are frequently exposed to several drugs whose interaction may contribute to alter immune function leading to increased cancer susceptibility. However, there is no information

Table 4 SIR and 95% confidence intervals calculations for MS patients exposed or not to IS drugs. Comparison were made with respect to the Sicilian general population in the correspondent age classes

Age	Exposed to IS			Not exposed to IS		
	No.	Expected	Observed	No.	Expected	Observed
15–19	1	0,00035	0	2	0,0007	0
20–24	2	0,00100	0	9	0,0050	0
25–29	17	0,01200	0	28	0,0210	0
30–34	35	0,03600	0	41	0,0420	0
35–39	71	0,10,000	1	61	0,0900	0
40–44	66	0,16,000	2	78	0,1900	0
45–49	87	0,30,000	1	78	0,2700	1
50–54	90	0,48,000	3	59	0,3160	0
55–59	62	0,47,000	1	56	0,4280	0
60–64	48	0,51,000	2	52	0,5500	0
65–69	35	0,52,000	0	34	0,5100	1
70–74	13	0,24,000	3	17	0,3100	0
75–79	4	0,08600	0	7	0,1500	0
80–84	0	0,00000	0	6	0,1400	1
85+	0	0,00000	0	3	0,0650	0
Total	531	2,91,535	13	531	3,0877	3
SIR	Tot		4,12			0,97

about how the temporal interaction between drugs may further modify the risk. We did not observe anyway in our cohort a higher risk among those patients who were exposed to more treatments. Another explanation would consider the possibility that MS patients, similarly to what has been hypothesized in other immune mediated diseases, may have a higher intrinsic susceptibility to cancer if exposed to immune modifying drugs [21]. This hypothesis is not supported by our findings showing that MS individuals who have been treated with drugs different from IS, like beta interferon or glatiramer, did not show risk of developing cancer differently from that observed in the general population [22]. Another important methodological aspect needs to be highlighted. In our cohort of patients, we observed a higher age at treatment initiation among those people who were never treated with IS therapy. This should not appear surprising considering that immune suppression was the only available therapy for more aggressive cases until the availability of natalizumab. For this reason, in patients with a less aggressive disease course, there could be a longer latency from MS onset to treatment start particularly if we consider the possible effect on this phenomenon of the diagnostic criteria used at that time and also, for a possible different disposition to treat patients with a disease course considered less aggressive. Nevertheless, as shown in Table 3, the Cox model that included also age at treatment start (IS or other drugs) as a covariate, led an even higher HR for the association between IS and cancer risk. The observation that we did not show an association between the exposures to drugs like beta interferon or glatiramer, and cancer risk, is of particular interest. The necessity to balance between the need for a high impact drug with a possible long lasting effect on MS disease curse, and the consequent acceptance of reasonable risks in terms of safety, is in fact one of the most challenging aspects for neurologists taking care of people with MS. New drugs recently introduced or those that are going to be released for MS treatment act on specific pathways of immune system. These new mechanisms of action lack of the knowledge about long term effects. This study in our opinion strengthen the need to implement surveillance programs to improve our understanding of long term side effects and safety profile of drugs already in use and of new drugs which are going to be approved to treat MS. This would be particularly helpful for not common events that may occur after a long latency from the exposure.

Conclusion

Our study showed a higher cancer risk in MS patients associated to previous IS exposure but not the disease itself. Even though not all the drugs we considered were associated to increased cancer risk, the present study indicate the need for careful selection of MS patients requiring

therapies whose efficacies are balanced by potential harmful effects, and a stringent follow-up of those patients treated with IS. Despite the increasing amount of therapeutic possibilities to cure MS, patients still exist, who do not respond to available drugs and experience an unfavorable disease course, rapidly accumulating disability, or patients who have lack of tolerance and need therefore a therapeutic alternative. In all of these patients, a strict long-term follow-up must be planned to avoid life threatening conditions.

Abbreviations
AZA: Azathioprine; CI: Confidence intervals; CP: Cyclophosphamide; DMT: Disease modifying treatments; HR: Hazard ratio; IS: Immunosuppressant drugs; LVEF: Left ventricular ejection fraction; MS: Multiple sclerosis; MX: Mitoxantrone; RR: Relative risk; SIR: Standardized incidence ratio

Acknowledgements
Not applicable.

Funding
The present study was not supported by any funding.

Authors' contributions
PR, GSal, and GSav planned the study, revised the database contributed to the analyses, discussed the results, drafted and revised the manuscript. VLR, MLR, SR, SA, contributed to selection of patients, building up of the database and retrieving all necessary information, revising the manuscript. PA, GV, MAM, and MDA contributed to revising the database, performing analyses, discussing the results, revising the manuscript. All authors read and approved the final manuscript.

Competing interests
The authors report no competing interest with respect to this study. Authors potential conflict of interest are as follows:
- Paolo Ragonese received travel expenses or honoraria for consultancy from Merck Serono, Biogen idec, Novartis, Sanophy Genzyme and Teva pharmaceuticals.
- Paolo Aridon has nothing to disclose.
- Giulia Vazzoler has nothing to disclose.
- Maria Antonietta Mazzola has nothing to disclose.
- Vincenzina Lo Re has nothing to disclose.
- Marianna Lo Re has nothing to disclose.
- Sabrina Realmuto has nothing to disclose.
- Simona Alessi has nothing to disclose.
- Marco D'Amelio received honoraria for consulting or travel expenses by Boeringher Ingheleim.
- Giovanni Savettieri received travel expenses or honoraria for consultancy from Biogen, Teva, and Merck Serono.
- Giuseppe Salemi received travel expenses or honoraria for consultancy from Biogen, Merck Serono, Novartis and Teva Pharmaceuticals.

References
1. Compston ACC, Lassmann H, McDonald I, Miller D, Noseworthy J, Smith K, et al. McAlpine's Multiple Sclerosis. fourth ed. Philadelphia: Churchill Livingstone Elsevier; 2004.
2. Wingerchuk DM, Carter JL. Multiple Sclerosis: Current and Emerging Disease-Modifying Therapies and Treatment Strategies. Mayo Clinic Procedings. 2014;89:225–40.
3. Casetta I, Iuliano G, Filippini G. Azathioprine for multiple sclerosis. Cochrane Database Syst Rev. 2007;4:CD003982.
4. Martinelli Boneschi F, Vacchi L, Rovaris M, Capra R, Comi G. Mitoxantrone for multiple sclerosis. Cochrane Database Syst Rev. 2013;4:CD002127.

5. The Canadian Cooperative Multiple Sclerosis Study Group. The Canadian cooperative trial of cyclophosphamide and plasma exchange in progressive multiple sclerosis. Lancet. 1991;337:441–6.

6. Hauser SL, Dawson DM, Lehrich JR, Lerich JL, Beal MF, Kevy SV, Propper RD, Mills JA, Weiner HL. Intensive immunosuppression in progressive multiple sclerosis: a randomized, three-arm study of high-dose intravenous cyclophosphamide, plasma exchange, and ACTH. N Engl J Med. 1983;308:173–80.

7. Marriott JJ, Miyasaki JM, Gronseth G, O'Connor PW. Evidence report: the efficacy and safety of mitoxantrone (Novantrone) in the treatment of multiple sclerosis: report of the Therapeutics and Technology Assessment Subcommittee of the American Academy of Neurology. Neurology. 2010;74: 1463–70.

8. Bahmanyar S, Montgomery SM, Hillert J, Ekbom A, Olsson T. Cancer risk among patients with multiple sclerosis and their parents. Neurology. 2009; 72:1170–7.

9. Kingwell E, Bajdik C, Phillips N, Zhu F, Oger J, Hashimoto S, Tremlett H. Cancer risk in multiple sclerosis: findings from British Columbia, Canada. Brain. 2012;135:2973–9.

10. Martinelli V, Cocco E, Capra R, Salemi G, Gallo P, Capobianco M, Pesci I, Ghezzi A, Pozzilli C, Lugaresi A, Bellantonio P, Amato MP, Grimaldi LM, Trojano M, Mancardi GL, Bergamaschi R, Gasperini C, Rodegher M, Straffi L, Ponzio M, Comi G. Italian Mitoxantrone Group. Acute myeloid leukemia in Italian patients with multiple sclerosis treated with mitoxantrone. Neurology. 2011;77:1887–95.

11. Stroet A, Hemmelmann C, Starck M, Zettl U, Dörr J, Friedemann P, Flachenecker P, Fleischer V, Zipp F, Nückel H, Kieseier BC, Ziegler A, Gold R, Chan A. Incidence of therapy-related acute leukaemia in mitoxantrone-treated multiple sclerosis patients in Germany. Ther Adv Neurol Disord. 2012;5:75–9.

12. Ragonese P, Aridon P, Salemi G, D'Amelio M, Savettieri G. Answer to: the possible risk of cancer in multiple sclerosis patients: a controversial issue. Eur J Neurol. 2011;18:e50. doi:10.1111/j.1468-1331.2010.03304.x.

13. Nielsen NM, Rostgaard K, Rasmussen S, Koch-Henriksen N, Storm HH, Melbye M, Hjalgrim H. Cancer risk among patients with multiple sclerosis: a population-based register study. Int J Cancer. 2006;118:979–84.

14. Landgren AM, Landgren O, Gridley G, Dores GM, Linet MS, Morton LM. Autoimmune disease and subsequent risk of developing alimentary tract cancers among 4.5 million US male veterans. Cancer. 2011;117:1163–71.

15. Le Bouc R, Zéphir H, Majed B, Vérier A, Marcel M, Vermersch P. No increase in cancer incidence detected after cyclophosphamide in a French cohort of patients with progressive multiple sclerosis. Mult Scler. 2012;18:55–63.

16. Erdman S, Poutahidis T. Cancer inflammation and regulatory T cells. Int J Cancer. 2010;127:768–79.

17. Achiron A, Barak Y, Gail M, Mandel M, Pee D, Ayyagari R, Rotstein Z. Cancer incidence in multiple sclerosis and effects of immunomodulatory treatments. Breast Cancer Res Treat. 2005;89:265–70.

18. Lalmohamed A, Bazelier MT, Van Staa TP, Uitdehaag BM, Leufkens HG, De Boer A, De Vries F. Causes of death in patients with multiple sclerosis and matched referent subjects: a population-based cohort study. Eur J Neurol. 2012;19:1007–14.

19. Marcus A, Gowen BG, Thompson TW, Iannello A, Ardolino M, Deng W, Wang L, Shifrin N, Raulet DH. Recognition of tumors by the innate immune system and natural killer cells. Adv Immunol. 2014;122:91–128.

20. Gale RP, Opelz G. Commentary: does immune suppression increase risk of developing acute myeloid leukemia? Leukemia. 2012;26:422–3.

21. Marrie RA, Cohen J, Stuve O, Trojano M, Sørensen PS, Reingold S, Cutter G, Reider N. A systematic review of the incidence and prevalence of comorbidity in multiple sclerosis: Overview. Mult Scler J. 2015;3:294–304.

22. Kingwell E, Evans C, Zhu F, Oger J, Hashimoto S, Tremlett H. Assessment of cancer risk with β-interferon treatment for multiple sclerosis. J Neurol Neurosurg Psychiatr. 2014;85:1096–102.

16

Anxiety, emotional processing and depression in people with multiple sclerosis

Marie-Claire Gay[1]*, Catherine Bungener[2,3], Sarah Thomas[4], Pierre Vrignaud[1], Peter W Thomas[4], Roger Baker[4], Sébastien Montel[5], Olivier Heinzlef[6], Caroline Papeix[7], Rana Assouad[7] and Michèle Montreuil[5]

Abstract

Background: Despite the high comorbidity of anxiety and depression in people with multiple sclerosis (MS), little is known about their inter-relationships. Both involve emotional perturbations and the way in which emotions are processed is likely central to both. The aim of the current study was to explore relationships between the domains of mood, emotional processing and coping and to analyse how anxiety affects coping, emotional processing, emotional balance and depression in people with MS.

Methods: A cross-sectional questionnaire study involving 189 people with MS with a confirmed diagnosis of MS recruited from three French hospitals. Study participants completed a battery of questionnaires encompassing the following domains: i. anxiety and depression (Hospital Anxiety and Depression Scale (HADS)); ii. emotional processing (Emotional Processing Scale (EPS-25)); iii. positive and negative emotions (Positive and Negative Emotionality Scale (EPN-31)); iv. alexithymia (Bermond-Vorst Alexithymia Questionnaire) and v. coping (Coping with Health Injuries and Problems-Neuro (CHIP-Neuro) questionnaire. Relationships between these domains were explored using path analysis.

Results: Anxiety was a strong predictor of depression, in both a direct and indirect way, and our model explained 48% of the variance of depression. Gender and functional status (measured by the Expanded Disability Status Scale) played a modest role. Non-depressed people with MS reported high levels of negative emotions and low levels of positive emotions. Anxiety also had an indirect impact on depression via one of the subscales of the Emotional Processing Scale ("Unregulated Emotion") and via negative emotions (EPN-31).

Conclusions: This research confirms that anxiety is a vulnerability factor for depression via both direct and indirect pathways. Anxiety symptoms should therefore be assessed systematically and treated in order to lessen the likelihood of depression symptoms.

Keywords: Multiple sclerosis, Anxiety, Depression, Emotional Processing, Coping, Mood, Predictors

Background

Multiple sclerosis (MS) is an autoimmune degenerative disease of the central nervous system associated with significant behavioural and emotional sequelae [1–3]. People with MS have to contend on a daily basis with a range of physical, cognitive and psychological symptoms, such as walking and mobility limitations, pain, fatigue, depression, memory and concentration difficulties [4]. MS impacts on all spheres of people's lives including employment, relationships and social life, leisure and activities of daily living

[5]. People with MS face considerable unpredictability and uncertainty due to the variable nature of the disease course; for example, risks of relapses, hospital admissions and of further disability developing [6]. As there is currently no cure for MS and it is typically diagnosed in the prime of life, people live with these challenging symptoms and variable disease course over many years [5].

It is, therefore, not surprising that anxiety disorders have been reported in the literature as being present in between 36 – 54% of the MS population with approximately 30% of people with MS experiencing symptoms consistent with generalised anxiety disorder [7–9]. More than half of people with MS experience depression at

* Correspondence: marieclaire.gay@gmail.com
[1]Psychology Department, University of Paris West, Nanterre, France
Full list of author information is available at the end of the article

some point during the course of their illness [10, 11]. Alexithymia, a difficulty in identifying and describing emotions, is also common; affecting up to 42% of people with MS. [12, 13] Research on coping (the way people manage their relationships with their environment to adjust to their disease) [14] suggests that symptoms are worsened by an emotion-centred approach [15, 16].

However, despite the high comorbidity of anxiety and depression in people with MS, little is known about the relationship between them. Brown et al. [17] showed that anxiety and depression predict each other with anxiety predicting later depression. Gay et al. [18] indicated that anxiety is a strong predictor of depression and that its impact on depression is heightened by the presence of alexithymia and a lack of social support.

Both anxiety and depression involve emotional disruptions or perturbations. Emotions are very rapid adaptive responses consisting of physiological, cognitive and behavioural elements [19]. These are felt by the individual in terms of positive or negative emotions.

According to Watson and Clark's model of anxiety and depression [20, 21], depression is characterised by an abnormally high level of negative emotions and an abnormally low level of positive emotions, while anxiety is linked to a high level of negative emotions but without perturbations of positive emotions. Emotional balance refers to the respective levels of positive and negative emotions experienced by an individual. There is an emotional imbalance in anxiety and depression disorders [22, 23].

Emotional perturbations can also occur as processes. Baker et al. have developed a model of emotional regulation [24, 25] that draws upon Rachman's conceptualisation of emotional processing [26]. Rachman proposes that certain behavioural signs (e.g. intrusive and repetitive emotional memories) indicate that distressing emotional events have not been properly 'emotionally processed' or 'absorbed' [26]. Difficulties can occur at different stages of emotional processing in terms of registration, appraisal, experience, awareness and expression. Five emotional dysregulation processes have been identified [25]: "suppression" referring to an excessive control of emotions; "signs of unprocessed emotion", reflecting cognitive and behavioural signs of incomplete processing; "unregulated emotion", consisting of an inability to control one's emotions; "avoidance", referring to the avoidance of negative emotions and "impoverished emotional experience" consisting of a detached experience of emotions due to poor emotional insight.

A key issue is how emotional perturbations (imbalances in positive and negative emotions and emotional processing deficits) lead to depression and whether anxiety exerts an impact directly on depression in MS or whether it influences depression via factors related to emotional processing. The aim of the current study was to explore the relationship between anxiety and depression and the relevance of emotional processing, emotional balance, and coping to depressive symptomatology.

Methods

All the required ethical authorisations were obtained from the French Ethics Committee (Comité de Protection des Personnes (CPP)) and all study participants provided written informed consent.

Participants and procedure

A cross-sectional questionnaire study was undertaken. Participants were patients recruited from the day care unit of the neurological departments in three French university hospitals (CHU Metz, CHI Poissy-Saint Germain, CHU La Pitié-Salpêtrière) with a neurologist-confirmed diagnosis of MS (revised McDonald criteria) [27]. Recruitment took place in 2013.

The research study was described to potential participants by the neurologist. If they wished to participate, a psychology Masters student, trained for the study, obtained their written informed consent and then collected socio-demographic and medical information from them. Participants completed the battery of self-reported outcome measures in the day care unit. The trainee was available to answer questions if required.

Descriptors

Socio-demographic and clinical variables

Socio-demographic variables (age, gender, education level and marital status) were obtained by the psychology student and clinical and disease-specific variables (type of MS and time since diagnosis) were obtained from medical notes.

Physical Disability

The Expanded Disability Status Scale [28] was used as a measure of physical disability. The Expanded Disability Status Scale (EDSS) was administered by an experienced neurologist and provided a measure of functional status. The EDSS is divided into eight functioning systems (pyramidal, cerebellar, brainstem, cerebral/mental, bowel and bladder, visual function, sensory, and other). Impairment in each system is graded separately by means of neurological examination. EDSS scores range as steps from 0 – 10 in 0.5 increments. Levels 1.0 – 4.5 refer to people with a high degree of ambulatory ability and the subsequent levels 5.0 – 9.5 refer to a loss of ambulatory ability. The range of main categories include (0) = normal neurologic exam; to (5) = ambulatory without aid or rest for 200 m, disability severe enough to impair full daily activities; to (10) = death due to MS.

Outcomes

All outcomes were self-reported.

Anxiety and depression

The Hospital Anxiety and Depression Scale (HADS) is a 14-item scale for use as a brief instrument for detecting the intensity of depression and anxiety in patient populations [29]. The HADS has few somatic items so is unlikely to confound depression with physical symptoms such as pain and fatigue and has been validated for use in the MS population [30]. Scores for the depression and anxiety subscales can range from 0 – 21 respectively, with a score >10 indicating probable anxiety or depression. The French adaptation of the HADS confirmed Zigmond and Snaith's [29] original two factor structure and has been shown to possess good psychometric properties [31]. Internal reliability was 0.79 for the anxiety subscale and from 0.82 for the depression subscale. The correlation between the two subscales was significant but moderate ($r = .47$), representing 22% of the common variance [31].

Emotional processing

The Emotional Processing Scale (EPS-25) is a 25-item self-report questionnaire designed to identify and measure emotional processing styles and potential deficits in healthy individuals and those with psychological or physical disorders [24, 25]. It comprises five subscales, each with five items that are rated on a 10-point (0–9) attitudinal scale: suppression (excessive control of emotional experience and expression), signs of unprocessed emotion (intrusive and persistent emotional experiences), unregulated emotion (inability to control one's emotions), avoidance (avoidance of negative emotional triggers), impoverished emotional experience (detached experience of emotions due to poor emotional insight). A higher score indicates poorer emotional processing with a possible mean score range of 0–9. In the original English language version of the EPS developed in the UK [25] these five factors explained 59.4% of the total variance and overall internal reliability (Cronbach's Alpha) was high ($\alpha = 0.92$), ranging from 0.70 – 0.80 for the five respective factors. The EPS-25 has been translated into numerous languages and norms have been produced for a wide range of clinical and non-clinical populations. A French version has been developed (Gay et al., not yet published). In the French adaptation the five factors explained 61.5% of the total variance and overall internal reliability (Cronbach's Alpha) was 0.91 and ranged from 0.68 – 0.84 for the five respective subscales. A French sample of healthy adults from the general population ($N = 75$) had a mean (SD) total EPS score of 2.5 (1.04) and mean (SD) scores for the respective subscales, as follows: Suppression = 3.0 (1.89); Signs of Unprocessed Emotion = 3.3 (1.79); Unregulated Emotion = 1.9 (1.31); Avoidance = 2.9 (1.36); Impoverished Emotional Experience = 1.4 (1.19). French data from 349 people with MS showed significant differences on every subscale compared to healthy adults with the exception of the Suppression subscale. The mean (SD) total EPS score for the MS sample was 3.2 (1.69) and means (SDs) for the respective subscales were: Suppression = 3.5 (2.39); Signs of Unprocessed Emotion = 3.7 (2.80); Unregulated Emotion = 2.6 (1.86); Avoidance = 3.5 (1.90) and Emotional Experience = 3.5 (1.89).

Emotional balance

The Positive and Negative Emotionality Scale (EPN-31) [22, 23] measures emotionality; in particular, the self-reported frequency with which 31 emotional states have been experienced in the past month. It consists of 31 items and produces three main scores: a positive emotionality score, a negative emotionality and a surprise emotionality score. The answer format is a 7-point scale, ranging from 1 "Not experienced at all" to 7 "Experienced this affect several times each day". For the French adaptation these three factors explained 58.2% of the total variance and internal reliability was good with Cronbach's Alphas between 0.80 and 0.95 for all main scores and between 0.72 and 0.90 for the six subscores (joy, tenderness, anger, fear, sadness, shame) [23]. A reference population comprising 948 French healthy adults (mean (SD) age = 41.4 (9.64) years) had a mean (SD) negative emotion score of 32.0 (14.30) and a mean positive emotion score of 70.1 (16.00) [23].

Alexithymia

The Bermond-Vorst Alexithymia Questionnaire [32, 33] (BVAQ) is a 40-item self-report measure which comprises two parallel versions, each with 20 items. We have used the B form. Five factors are assessed: difficulty in verbalising feelings, difficulty in identifying feelings, lack of emotional excitability, externally-oriented thinking, poor fantasy life. Each item is rated on a five-point Likert-type scale, ranging from 1 (strongly agree) to 5 (strongly disagree), with a maximum score of 100. A score over 52 is indicative of the presence of alexithymia. The French version of the BVAQ has demonstrated good psychometric properties with Cronbach's Alpha coefficient 0.83 for a sample of 322 Belgian students [33].

Coping

The Coping with Health Injuries and Problems-Neuro (CHIP-Neuro) Questionnaire consists of 24 items assessing the coping strategies of people with neurological conditions [34, 35]. The questionnaire includes six different coping strategies for neurological health problems: emotional regulation (seven items), seeking well-being (five items), active distraction (three items), information seeking (three items), palliative coping (three items) and cognitive avoidance (three items). Items are rated on a numerical scale ranging from 0 – "not at all" to 5 – "a lot", with a possible total score ranging from 0 – 120. A dominant coping strategy can be identified according to respondents' highest subscale score. The CHIP-Neuro has been validated with a French sample of people with multiple sclerosis and Parkinson's disease (N = 307) with 48% of the variance explained by the six factor solution. The internal reliability was good with Cronbach's Alphas ranging between 0.80 and 0.82 for the six subscales.

Statistical analysis

The variables introduced in the analysis were checked for normality by examining histograms and considering values for kurtosis and skewness. Descriptive statistics were used to summarise these data and Pearson's Product Moment Correlation Coefficients were used to explore associations between the various domains of interest.

Path analysis was used to estimate the strength of the direct and indirect relationships between the variables of interest. Chi-squared, the Root Mean Square Error of Approximation (RMSEA) and the Comparative Fit Index (CFI) statistics were used as measures of fit.

SPSS Version 21 for Windows was used to undertake the descriptive and correlational analyses and AMOS 20.0 structural equation modeling software for the path analyses. We imputed missing data using a multiple imputation method based on a Monte-Carlo Markov Chain algorithm [36]. The chosen algorithm imputes values for each case by drawing, at random, from the conditional distribution of the missing values given the observed values, with the unknown model parameters set equal to their maximum likelihood estimates.

Results

In total 189 participants completed the questionnaire battery. The mean age was 47.2 years (SD = 12.50; range = 18–78). Females (females = 121; males = 68) comprised approximately two-thirds of the sample reflecting gender prevalence ratios in the general multiple sclerosis population. Just over half the participants were married or in long term relationships and just over two-thirds had received education up to the age of 17 years. In terms of type of MS, 107 (57%) of the sample had relapsing remitting MS, 54 (29%) secondary progressive MS and 28 (15%) primary progressive MS. The Expanded Disability Status Scale (EDSS) was used as an index of functional status and the sample had a mean (SD) EDSS score of 4.7 (2.37) and a mean [(SD) range] disease duration of 15.0 [(9.29) 2–18] years.

Levels of missing total score data for the outcome measure questionnaires were very low (less than 3%) with the exception of the EPN-31 scale for which 8% of total scores were missing.

Descriptives for the self-reported outcome variables for the entire sample are presented in Table 1. Overall the sample had a self-reported level of depression in the normal range (HADS depression score M = 8.0, SD = 4.19). However, 19% of participants scored between 8 and 10 on the HADS depression subscale indicating possible depression and 28% scored over 10 indicating probable symptoms of depression. Using a cut-off score >10 on each respective subscale for probable anxiety and/or depression, 16/189 (8.5%) participants had both anxiety and depression; 8/189 (4.2%) had anxiety only; 37/189 (19.6%) had depression only and 128/189 (67.7%) had neither depression nor anxiety. There was a statistically significant difference (t(187) = 3.26, p < .001)) between HADS depression scores for females (M = 8.7, SD = 4.37) and males (M = 6.7, SD = 3.50) with females tending to score higher than males. Self-reported levels of anxiety were in the normal range (M = 5.8, SD = 3.78). However, 17% had scores between 8 and 10 suggesting possible anxiety and 13% had scores >10 indicating probable anxiety.

With the exception of the Avoidance subscale, mean EPS-25 scores were comparable to those found in the general population [26]. Thirty-six percent of the current MS sample scored more than one standard deviation above the mean on the Avoidance subscale. Females (M = 4.1; SD = 1.95) had significantly higher scores than males (M = 3.4; SD = 1.98) on the Unregulated Processing subscale, t(187) = 2.35, p = .02.

On the CHIP-Neuro questionnaire mean scores for the Emotion Regulation and Well-being subscales were twice as high as those for the other subscales suggesting these were the most common coping strategies used by respondents.

The cut-off for clinical alexithymia on the BVAQ is ≥53. The mean (SD) BVAQ total score for the current MS sample was 55.4 (14.15) with just over half (53%) the sample scoring at or above this cut-off.

The results showed a perturbation of emotional balance assessed by the EPN-31, with the sample self-reporting a much higher level of negative emotions (M = 51.0; SD = 19.64) and lower level of positive emotions (M = 47.2; SD = 11.79) compared to a healthy French adult reference population (N = 948) [30]. There was a statistically significant difference (t(187) = 2.28, p = .02) between negative emotion scores for females (M = 53.4, SD = 20.02) and males (M = 46.7, SD = 18.31) with females tending to score higher than males.

The relationships between anxiety, depression, emotions, emotional processing, and functional status

The relationships between depression and the other variables were explored using Pearson's Product Moment

Table 1 Descriptive statistics for the self-reported outcomes

Outcome measure	Descriptives Unless otherwise specified [(mean (SD) range)] Entire sample ($N = 189$)
Hospital Anxiety and Depression Scale (HADS) *(higher scores, more distress)*	
Depression subscale (HADS-D)	8.0 (4.18) 1–19
Score <8 [N (%)]	100 (52.91%)
Score 8–10 [N (%)]	36 (19.04%)
Score >10 [N (%)]	53 (28.04%)
Anxiety subscale (HADS-A)	5.8 (3.9) 0–18
Score <8 [N (%)]	133 (70.37%)
Score 8–10 [N (%)]	32 (16.93%)
Score >10 [N (%)]	24 (12.70%)
Emotional Processing Scale (EPS-25) *(higher scores, poorer emotional processing)*	
Suppression	4.0 (2.64) 0–9.0
Signs of Unprocessed Emotions	4.1 (2.35) 0–8.4
Unregulated Emotion	2.6 (1.97) 0–8.8
Avoidance	3.9 (1.99) 0–8.2
Impoverished Emotional Experience	2.6 (1.89) 0–8.2
Total EPS Score	4.3 (2.12) 0–9.0
Bermond-Vorst Alexithymia Questionnaire (BVAQ) *(higher scores, greater levels of alexithymia)*	
Difficulty in verbalising feelings	11.8 (4.09) 4–20
Poor fantasy life	11.2 (4.33) 4–20
Difficulty identifying feelings	10.9 (4.04) 4–20
Lack of emotional excitability	10.8 (4.31) 4–20
Externally-oriented thinking	10.7 (4.45) 4–20
Total BVAQ Score	55.4 (14.15) 20–95
Coping with Health Injuries and Problems – Neuro (CHIP-Neuro) *(higher scores, greater use of coping style)*	
Emotional regulation	22.0 (6.65) 7–35
Seeking Well-being	19.2 (3.18) 9–25
Active Distraction	9.1 (3.16) 3–15
Information Seeking	9.8 (4.00) 3–15
Palliative Coping	7.9 (2.99) 3–15
Cognitive Avoidance	8.3 (2.93) 3–15
Positive and Negative Emotionality (EPN-31) *(higher scores, greater emotionality)*	
Positive	47.2 (11.78) 10–70
Negative	51.0 (19.63) 18–111
Surprise	8.3 (3.98) 3–19

Correlation Coefficients (see Tables 2, 3, 4 and 5). HADS anxiety scores were moderately positively correlated with HADS depression scores ($r_p = .41$, $p < .001$). HADS anxiety scores were moderately positively correlated with total EPS scores ($r_p = .40$, $p < .001$) and moderately positively correlated with negative emotion scores on the EPN-31 ($r_p = .35$, $p < .001$). HADS anxiety scores were moderately negatively correlated with positive emotion scores ($r_p = -.64$, $p < .001$). Regarding coping, a moderate negative correlation was found with the active distraction subscale score of the CHIP-Neuro ($r_p = -.49$, $p < .001$) as well as a moderate positive association with emotional regulation-based coping ($r_p = .36$, $p < .001$).

Scores on the HADS depression subscale correlated positively and strongly with negative emotion scores on the EPN-31 ($r_p = .60$, $p < .001$) and with EPS total scores ($r_p = .57$, $p < .001$) and more specifically with the Signs of Unprocessed Emotions ($r_p = .55$, $p < .001$) and

Table 2 Correlations between HADS depression scores and EDSS, HADS anxiety, EPN-31 and EPS scores ($N = 189$)

	EDSS	HADS Anxiety	EPN-31 Negative	EPN-31 Positive	EPS Suppression	EPS Unprocessed	EPS Unregulated	EPS Avoidance	EPS Impoverished	EPS Total
HADS depression	-.19*	.42***	.62***	-.07 ns	.38***	.56***	.53***	.39***	.39**	.58***

* $p <.05$; ** $p <.01$; *** $p <.001$; ns Not significant

Unregulated Emotion subscales ($r_p = .51$, $p < .001$). HADS depression scores correlated positively and moderately with scores on the Emotional Regulation subscale of the CHIP-Neuro ($r_p = .45$, $p < .001$) and weakly and negatively with EDSS scores ($r_p = -.18$, $p < .05$).

There were no statistically significant differences between depressed and non-depressed participants in terms of alexithymia scores, $F(2,186) = 1.36$, $p = .26$, nor between anxious and non-anxious participants, $F(2,186) = 1.99$), $p = .14$.

The study of the direct and indirect effects of the variables using path analysis model

The path analysis aimed to explore the direct and indirect effects of anxiety on depression. Functional status was retained in the model to control for MS severity. A covariance relationship between functional status and anxiety was introduced into the model to take into account the existence of a link between these variables. Variables were introduced into the model if they were significantly correlated with anxiety and/or depression (see Tables 2, 3, 4). Alexithymia was therefore not included in the model. Among the variables representing emotional processing, only "Unregulated Emotion" was selected because its correlation was one of the highest with depression. Despite a high correlation with depression, "Signs of Unprocessed Emotion" was not introduced into the model because its shared variance with "Unregulated Emotion" led to a suppressing effect on this variable. As no specific hypothesis was available on the direction of a causal link between "negative emotions" and "Unregulated Emotion", their relationship was estimated as a covariance.

The path analysis model included both direct and indirect effects on the dependent variable "depression". One variable (functional status) had only direct effects. One (anxiety) had direct and indirect effects mediated by "Unregulated Emotion" and by "negative emotions". The model consists of 13 parameters. The sample size ($N = 189$) seems sufficient for a reliable estimation of these parameters at .80 power according to the R^2 value

(.46) and the direct and indirect effect sizes following results from Thoemmes et al. [37].

The non-significant Chi-squared test statistic indicated acceptable goodness-of-fit of the model (χ^2 (2) = 4.12, $p = .13$). The Root Mean Square Error of Approximation (RMSEA) was 0.075 indicating an acceptable fit (RMSEA values < 0.08 indicate an acceptable fit), the Comparative Fit Index (CFI) was 0.98 indicating an acceptable fit (values >0.90 indicate an acceptable fit) [38]. Figure 1 presents the standardised values of the regression coefficients. All the values are significant at $p = .001$.

The model explained almost half of the variance of depression ($R^2 = .46$). The direct effect of anxiety on depression is estimated at .24, the indirect effects (negative emotions, Unregulated Emotion) at .22.

Discussion

In this research our aim was to explore the relationship between anxiety and depression in a sample of people with MS and the relevance of emotional processing to depressive symptomatology. We also examined the respective contributions of several sociodemographic, clinical and psychological factors to depressive symptomatology.

In line with the literature [10, 11], the results confirmed that depression is prevalent in people with MS. HADS anxiety scores >10 were obtained by 8% of the sample which is lower than is commonly reported in the MS literature [7–9] though 17% had scores suggesting possible anxiety.

The results also indicated that people with MS had perturbations in their emotional balance, according to Watson and Clark's model [20, 21]; they reported fewer positive emotions than the general population and more negative ones. Their mean scores were similar to those observed in people with anxiety and depressive disorders [22] which is in line with previous research in MS [15].

However, in the current study people with MS with probable anxiety disorder also showed perturbation of their positive emotions. Another difference from Watson and Clark's model is that even non-depressed

Table 3 Correlations between HADS depression scores and BVAQ scores ($N = 189$)

	BVAQ Verbalisation	BVAQ Fantasy	BVAQ Identification	BVAQ Excitability	BVAQ Externality	BVAQ Total
HADS depression	.03 ns	.09 ns	-.01 ns	.09 ns	.04 ns	.07 ns

* $p <.05$; ** $p <.01$; *** $p <.001$; ns Not significant

Table 4 Correlations between HADS anxiety scores, EPN-31 and EPS scores ($N = 189$)

	EPN-31 Negative	EPN-31 Positive	EPS Suppression	EPS Unprocessed	EPS Unregulated	EPS Avoidance	EPS Impoverished	EPS Total
HADS anxiety	.36***	-.64***	.36***	.34***	.35***	.31***	.34***	.58***

* p <.05; ** p <.01; *** p <.001; ns Not significant

people with MS reported high levels of negative emotions and low levels of positive emotions. This result suggests that experiencing negative emotions is not sufficient to develop depression or to feel depressed. Negative emotions were nevertheless strongly implicated in depression, through dysfunctional emotional processing and anxiety.

Anxiety was a strong predictor of depression via both direct and indirect pathways. Indirect pathways were via one of the subscales of the Emotional Processing Scale, "Unregulated Emotion" and through negative emotions (EPN-31).

Functional status had an independent impact on depression. This impact was low, which is in line with the literature [18]. Anxiety and functional status were independent. The separation between anxiety and functional status indicated that functional status did not impact on anxiety. It may be that individuals' illness representations [39] and the anticipation of possible future consequences of MS [6] may provoke anxiety above and beyond that arising from current symptoms and functional status. In turn, this anxiety may inhibit healthy emotional processing.

Coping strategies did not appear to mediate the relationship between anxiety and emotional processing nor that between anxiety and depression. While alexithymia did not contribute to the final model we cannot exclude the possibility that this was due to the specific scale we used. Future research should also include other measures of alexithymia such as the Toronto Alexithymia Scale (TAS-20) [33].

In conclusion, our model explained 46% of the variance of depression. It is consistent with Watson and Clark's model of depression [21]; having high levels of negative emotions and few positive ones is a feature of depression. Depressed people with MS had such a configuration of emotions. The unpredictable and variable nature of MS may explain how anxiety can lead to perturbations in emotional balance.

Anxiety is a vulnerability factor for depression since it directly and indirectly induces negative emotions which can lead to depressive symptoms. A similar pattern of relationships between anxiety and depression has been demonstrated by researchers using other questionnaires specifically assessing anxiety (the State and Trait Anxiety Inventory- STAI [40]) and depression (the ZUNG Self-Rating Depression Scale [41]).

Study limitations

It could be argued that it might have been better to assess depression and anxiety using two separate scales. However, it is challenging to assess depression in people with MS since symptoms of MS overlap with depression (asthenia, fatigue, loss of energy, psychomotor impairment, appetite disorders, sleep disorders, sexual disorders, and cognitive disorders) and an advantage of the HADS depression subscale is that it contains few somatic items, has been validated in French and has been widely used with people with MS.

The study is based on self-reported measures and we know that people with depression tend to report more negatively in retrospective recall. Additionally, it would have been good to collect information on disease modifying treatments and to have included fatigue [17] and social support in the model.

There are inherent and well-recognised limitations in drawing conclusions about directionality in cross-sectional research of this kind. Prospectively designed studies would overcome such limitations.

Despite these acknowledged limitations, our research has strengths in showing how anxiety may affect depression in people with MS. The model we have proposed explained just under half the variance of depression and so clearly there are a range of other potential contributors (such as neurological dysfunction). Nevertheless, our findings suggest that anxiety plays an important role in the presence of depression.

Conclusion

This research confirmed that in the current sample of people with MS anxiety was a strong predictor of depression via both direct and indirect pathways. The model obtained suggested that anxiety may affect depression through unregulated emotion and negative emotions and highlights an important potential role for early intervention. We suggest several possible treatment approaches could be applied to target anxiety. Information provision for people with MS seems to increase disease-related knowledge, with less clear results on decision making and quality of life [42]. Cognitive Behavioural Therapy (CBT) has been shown to be effective for anxiety disorders in the general population [43] and should be considered for those with MS with signs of anxiety or anxiety disorders. Interventions should address both individual and social factors that support resilience such as promoting positive thinking and planning and engagement in meaningful activities. Positive

Table 5 Correlation matrix for potential variables for path model

	1	2	3	4	5	6	7	8	9	10	11	12	13	14	15	16	17	18	19	20	21	22
1. Depression (HADS)	-																					
2. EDSS	-.19*	-																				
3. Anxiety (HADS)	.42***	ns	-																			
4. Suppression (EPS)	.38***	ns	.36***	-																		
5. Unprocessed (EPS)	.56***	ns	.34***	.53***	-																	
6. Unregulated (EPS)	.53***	ns	.35***	.40***	.60***	-																
7. Avoidance (EPS)	.39***	ns	.31***	.52***	.53***	.48***	-															
8. Impoverished (EPS)	.39***	ns	.34**	.52**	.53**	.48***	.55***	-														
9. EPS Total	.58***	ns	.58***	.79***	.83***	.74***	.77***	.78***	-													
10. Emotional regulation (CHIP-Neuro)	.47***	ns	.37***	.36***	.32***	.47***	.31***	.45***	.45***	-												
11. Seeking well-being (CHIP-Neuro)	ns	ns	-.26**	-.17**	ns	ns	ns	ns	ns	-.21**	-											
12. Active distraction (CHIP-Neuro)	ns	ns	-.50***	-.27***	ns	ns	ns	-.17*	ns	ns	-.25**	-										
13. Information seeking (CHIP-Neuro)	.19**	ss	ns	ns	.16*	ns	ns	ns	ns	.27***	.20**	.34***	-									
14. Palliative Coping (CHIP-Neuro)	ns	ns	ns	ns	.16*	ns	.20**	.17*	ns	.26***	.26**	.16*	.16*	-								
15. Cognitive Avoidance (CHIP-Neuro)	ns	-.21**	-.22**	ns	ns	ns	ns	ns	ns	ns	.16*	.17*	.17*	ns	-							
16. BVAQ total	ns	ns	.18*	.20**	ns	ns	ns	ns	ns	ns	-.16*	ns	ns	ns	ns	-						
17. Verbalisation (BVAQ)	ns	ns	ns	ns	ns	ns	ns	ns	ns	ns	ns	ns	ns	ns	ns	.53***	-					
18. Fantasy (BVAQ)	ns	ns	ns	ns	ns	ns	ns	ns	ns	ns	ns	ns	ns	ns	.18*	.53***	ns	-				
19. Identification (BVAQ)	ns	ns	ns	.19*	ns	ns	ns	ns	ns	-.15*	-.15*	ns	ns	ns	ns	.76***	.30**	.30***	-			
20. Excitability (BVAQ)	ns	ns	ns	.20**	ns	ns	ns	.15*	.15*	ns	-.15*	ns	ns	ns	ns	.71***	.16**	ns	.44**	-		
21. Externality (BVAQ)	ns	ns	.16*	ns	ns	ns	ns	.15*	.15*	ns	-.16*	ns	ns	ns	.80***	.26**	.24**	.24**	-.61**	-.15*	-	
22. Positive Emotions (EPN-31)	ns	ns	-.64***	-.20**	ns	-.17*	-.20**	-.21**	-.21**	ns	.23**	.19*	ns	ns	-.21**	ns	ns	-.16*	-.15**	-.20**	ns	-
23. Negative Emotions (EPN-31)	.62***	ns	.36***	.30***	.42***	57***	.38***	.50***	.50***	.47***	-.15*	ns	ns	ns	ns	ns	ns	ns	ns	ns	ns	ns

* $p < .05$; ** $p < .01$; *** $p < .001$; ns Not significant

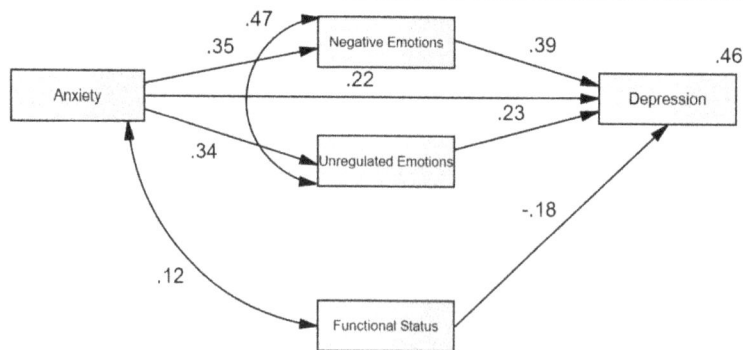

Fig. 1 Path analysis model (*N* = 189). Standardised values, all coefficients presented are significant at *p* < .001

psychological approaches that focus on eliciting positive emotions may provide a means of reducing or even neutralising the impact of aversive events on emotional experiences [44–46]. Emotion-focused or experiential therapies may be particularly helpful for people with poor awareness of their emotions and psychological functioning [47, 48]. Recognising the limits of the current research, there is a need for a more complete consideration of demographic, disease specific and psychosocial factors involved in the development of depression and of their respective contributions. National MS registers are ideally placed for the longitudinal exploration of these more complex path models [7].

Abbreviations
BVAQ: Bermond-Vorst Alexithymia Questionnaire; CHIP-Neuro: Coping with Health Injuries and Problems-Neuro; EDSS: Expanded Disability Status Scale; EPN-31: Positive and Negative Emotionality; EPS-25: Emotional Processing Scale; HADS: Hospital Anxiety and Depression Scale; MS: Multiple Sclerosis; pwMS: People with multiple sclerosis; SEM: Structural equation modelling; STAI: State and Trait Anxiety Inventory

Acknowledgements
Thanks very much to the students: Laura Caballero, Emmanuelle Pelletier, Hind Slaoui, Delphine Pluchon, Alexandra Rouette and neurologists who collected the data.
We acknowledge the Group of Scientific Interest IMSPIRE (International Multiple Sclerosis Partnership In REsearch) for providing us with inspiration.

Funding
None.

Authors' contributions
M-CG, concept and design, first author. PV, statistics. ST, methodology. PWT, statistics. RB, EPS developer. OH, MS specialist in neurology. CB, CHIP-Neuro developer. MM, concept and methodology. SM, CHIP-Neuro-developer. CP, MS Counsellor in neurology. RA, MS Counsellor in neurology.

Competing interests
None.

Author details
[1]Psychology Department, University of Paris West, Nanterre, France. [2]Laboratory of Psychopathology, University of Paris Descartes, Paris, France. [3]Health Psychology, Université Paris Sorbonne Cité, Paris, France. [4]Clinical Research Unit, Faculty of Health and Social Sciences, Bournemouth University, Bournemouth, UK. [5]Psychology Department, University of Paris 8, St Denis, France. [6]Neurology Department, Hospital of Poissy-St-Germain en Laye, Paris, France. [7]Neurology Department, GHPS Pitié Salpêtrière, Paris, France.

References
1. Compston A, Coles A. Multiple sclerosis. Lancet. 2002;359:1221–123.
2. Arnett PA. Neuropsychological presentation and treatment of demyelinating disorders. In: Halligan P, Kischna U, Marshall J, editors. Handbook of clinical neuropsychology. Oxford: Oxford University Press; 2003. p. 528–43.
3. Minden SL, Feinstein A, Kalb RC, Miller D, Mohr DC, Patten SB, et al. Evidence-based guideline: assessment and management of psychiatric disorders in individuals with multiple sclerosis. Report of the guideline development subcommittee of the american academy of neurology. Neurology. 2014;82:174–81.
4. Mitchell AJ, Benito-León J, Morales JM, González JM, Rivera-Navarro J. Quality of life and its assessment in multiple sclerosis: integrating physical and psychological components of wellbeing. Lancet Neurol. 2005;4:556–66.
5. Simmons RD. Life issues in multiple sclerosis. Nat Rev Neurol. 2010;6:603–10.
6. Mullins LL, Cote MP, Fuemmeler BF, Jean VM, Beatty WW, Paul RH. Illness intrusiveness, uncertainty, and distress in individuals with multiple sclerosis. Rehabil Psychol. 2001;46:139–53.
7. Jones KH, Ford DV, Jones PA, John A, Middleton RM, Lockhart-Jones H, et al. A large-scale study of anxiety and depression in people with multiple sclerosis: a survey via the web portal of the UK MS register. PLoS One. 2012;7:1–10.
8. Wood B, van der Mei IA, Ponsonby AL, Pittas F, Quinn S, Dwyer T, et al. Prevalence and concurrence of anxiety, depression and fatigue over time in multiple sclerosis. Mult Scler J. 2012;19:217–24.
9. Hartoonian N, Terrill AL, Beier ML, Turner AP, Day MA, Alschuler KN, et al. Predictors of anxiety in multiple sclerosis. Rehabil Psychol. 2015;60:91–8.
10. Merkelbach S, Konig J, Sittinger H. Personality traits in multiple sclerosis (MS) patients with and without fatigue experience. Acta Neurol Scand. 2003;107:195–201.
11. Viner R, Fiest KM, Bulloch AG, Williams JV, Lavorato DH, Berzins S, et al. Point prevalence and correlates of depression in a national community sample with multiple sclerosis. Gen Hosp Psychiat. 2014;36:352–4.
12. Bodini B, Mandarelli G, Tomassini V, Tarsitani L, Pestalozza I, Gasperini C, et al. Alexithymia in multiple sclerosis: relationship with fatigue and depression. Acta Neurol Scand. 2008;118:18–23.

13. Chahraoui K, Pinoit JM, Viegas N, Adnet J, Bonin B, Moreau T. Alexithymie et relation avec la dépression et l'anxiété dans la sclérose en plaques. Rev Neurol. 2008;164:242–45.

14. Lazarus RS, Folkman S. Stress, appraisal and coping. New York: Springer; 1984.

15. Bruce JM, Bruce AS, Hancock L, Lynch S. Self-reported memory problems in multiple sclerosis: influence of psychiatric status and normative dissociated experiences. Arch Clin Neuropsychol. 2010;25:39–48.

16. Kasi PM, Naqvi HA, Afghan AK, Khawar T, Khan FH, Khan UZ, et al. Coping styles in patients with anxiety and depression. ISRN Psychiatry. 2012;1–7.

17. Brown RF, Valpiani EM, Tennant CC, Dunn SM, Sharrock M, Hodgkinson S, et al. Longitudinal assessment of anxiety, depression, and fatigue in people with multiple sclerosis. Psychol Psychother. 2009;82:41–56.

18. Gay MC, Vrignaud P, Garitte C, Meunier C. Predictors of depression in multiple sclerosis. Acta Neurol Scand. 2010;121:161–70.

19. Sander D, Scherer S. Traité de psychologie des émotions. Paris: Dunod; 2009.

20. Watson D, Clark LA, Carey G. Positive and negative affectivity and their relation to anxiety and depressive disorders. J Abnorm Psychol. 1988;97:346–53.

21. Watson D, Clark LA, Harkness AR. Structures of personality and their relevance to psychopathology. J Abnorm Psychol. 1994;103:18–31.

22. Pélissolo A, Rolland JP, Perez-Diaz F, Jouvent R, Allilaire JF. Dimensional approach of emotion in psychiatry: validation of the positive and negative emotionality scale (EPN-31). Encéphale. 2007;33:256–63.

23. Diener E, Smith H, Fujita F. The personality structure of affect. J Pers Soc Psychol. 1995;69:130–41.

24. Baker R, Thomas S, Thomas PW, Owens M. Development of an emotional processing scale. J Psychosom Res. 2007;62:167–78.

25. Baker R, Thomas S, Thomas PW, Gower P, Santonastaso M, Whittlesea A. The emotional processing scale: scale refinement and abridgement (EPS-25). J Psychosom Res. 2010;68:83–8.

26. Rachman S. Emotional processing. Behav Res Ther. 1980;18:51–60.

27. Polman CH, Reingold SC, Banwell B, Clanet M, Cohen JA, Filippi M. Diagnostic criteria for multiple sclerosis: 2010 Revisions to the McDonald criteria. Ann Neurol. 2011;69:292–302.

28. Kurtzke JF. Rating neurologic impairment in multiple sclerosis: an expanded disability status scale (EDSS). Neurology. 1983;33:1422–7.

29. Zigmond AS, Snaith RP. The hospital anxiety and depressive scale. Acta Psychiatr Scand. 1983;67:361–70.

30. Honarmand K, Feinstein A. Validation of the hospital anxiety and depression scale for use with multiple sclerosis patients. Mult Scler. 2009;15:1518–24.

31. Untas A, Aguirrezabal M, Chauveau P, Leguen E, Combe C, Rascle N. Anxiété et depression en hémodialyse: validation de l'Hospital anxiety and depression scale (HADS). Nephrol Ther. 2009;5:193–200.

32. Bermond B, Vorst HC, Vingerhoets AJ, Gerritsen W. The Amsterdam alexithymia scale: its psychometric values and correlation with other personality traits. Psychother Psychosom. 1999;68:241–51.

33. Zech E, Luminet O, Rimé B, Wagner HL. Alexithymia and its measurement. Confirmatory factor analyses of the twenty-item Toronto Alexithymia Scale and the Bermond-Vorst Alexithymia Questionnaire. Eur J Pers. 1999;13:511–32.

34. Montel S, Bungener C. Coping and quality of life in 135 subjects with multiple sclerosis. Mult Scler. 2007;13:393–401.

35. Montel S, Bungener C. Validation du CHIP (questionnaire de coping) dans une population française atteinte de maladie neurologique. Rev Neurol. 2010;166:54–60.

36. Little RJA, Rubin RB. Statistical analysis with missing data. 2nd ed. Hoboken: John Wiley & Sons; 2002.

37. Thoemmes F, MacKinnon DP, Reiser MP. Power analysis for complex mediational designs using monte Carlo methods. Struct Equ Modeling. 2010;17:510–34.

38. Ullman JB. Structural equation modeling. In: Tabachnick BG, Fidell LS, editors. Using multivariate statistics (4th Ed) Needham heights. MA: Allyn & Bacon; 2001. p. 251–306.

39. Jopson NM, Moss-Morris R. The role of illness severity and illness representations in adjusting to multiple sclerosis. J Psychosom Res. 2003;54:503–11.

40. Spielberger CD. State Trait Anxiety Inventory (self-evaluation questionnaire). Palo Alto: Consulting Psychologist Press; 1983.

41. Zung WK. A self-rating depression scale. Arch Gen Psychiat. 1965;12:63–70.

42. Köpke S, Solari A, Khan F, Heesen C, Giordano A. Information provision for people with multiple sclerosis. Cochrane Rev. doi:10.1002/14651858.CD008757.pub2.

43. Hofmann SG, Smits JA. Cognitive-behavioral therapy for adult anxiety disorders: a meta-analysis of randomized placebo-controlled trials. J Clin Psychiatry. 2008;69:621–32.

44. Fredrickson BL. The role of positive emotions in positive psychology: the broaden-and-build theory of positive emotions. Am Psychol. 2001;56:218–26.

45. Silverman AM, Am V, Alschuler KN, Smith AE, Ehde DM. Bouncing back again, and again: a qualitative study of resilience in people with multiple sclerosis. Disabil Rehabil. 2016;15:1–9.

46. Csillik A. Understanding motivational interviewing effectiveness: contributions from Rogers' client-centered approach. Humanist Psychol. 2013;41:350–63.

47. Greenberg LS. Emotions, the great captains of our lives: their role in the process of change in psychotherapy. Am Psychol. 2012;67:697–707.

48. Baker R, Gale L, Abbey G, Thomas S. Emotional processing therapy for post-traumatic stress disorder. Counsell Psychol Q. 2013;26:362–85.

17

Increasing prevalence of familial recurrence of multiple sclerosis in Iran

Sharareh Eskandarieh[1,2], Narges Sistany Allahabadi[2], Malihe Sadeghi[2] and Mohammad Ali Sahraian[2,3]*

Abstract

Background: Tehran is the capital of Iran with an increasing multiple sclerosis (MS) prevalence. A retrospective population-based study was conducted to evaluate the trends of MS prevalence in Tehran.

Methods: A population-based survey was conducted for the period 1999 to 2015, based on Iranian MS Society (IMSS) registry system of Tehran, the capital city of Iran. Point regression analysis was applied on MS trend data to find annual percent change (APC).

The logistic regression analysis was used to estimate the odds ratio (OR) for individual variables in order to assess factors associating with familial recurrence of MS. P values < 0.05 were considered significant.

Results: MS prevalence has significantly increased during the study period from 1999 to 2015 (56.22 per 100,000). Total point prevalence of MS was 115.94 per 100,000 persons in 2015 compared to general population. Positive family history of MS was observed among 12.4% of patients. The strongest association amongst first-degree relatives was found in siblings, p value ≤ 0.001.

Conclusion: MS prevalence is rising in Tehran and this city is one of the regions with highest MS prevalence in Asia. In this sample, the largest proportion of relatives with MS were found among first-degree relatives, particularly siblings. Familial recurrence correlated with relative type.

Keywords: Multiple sclerosis, Prevalence, Familial recurrence, Tehran

Background

Multiple sclerosis (MS) is the second most common cause of disability in young adults, after trauma [1, 2].

It is an inflammatory autoimmune demyelinating disorder of the central nervous system resulting from a combination of genetic and environmental factors [3]. It mostly presents during 20 to 50 years of age, although there are special cases of MS presentation in pediatric and older ages [2, 4].

In 1980, Kurtzke divided the world into three regions of high ($\geq 30/100,000$), intermediate ($5-25/100,000$), and low risk for MS ($\leq 5/100,000$) [5]. According to epidemiological studies, the prevalence and incidence of MS have increased worldwide during the last decades.

MS prevalence in Iran is 51.52 /100,000 and this country is among the countries with high risk of MS in Middle East and North Africa [6]. In 2013, the areas with the highest prevalence in Iran were Isfahan (89/100,000), Tehran (88/100,000), and Fars (78/100,000) [7, 8]. The age-standardized prevalence in Tehran increased from 50.57/100,000 in 2008 to 74.28/100,000 in 2013 (113.49 for women and 37.41 for men) [6]. The female to male sex ratio of MS has increased in Canada, Australia and Japan [8]. In Iran, the average sex ratio in 2013 was 3.34:1 [7].

Familial recurrence studies in MS are useful to identify the correlated effects of genes and environment in the etiology of the disease [9]. Familial recurrence association is one of the strongest identified factors in MS, with the increased risk of MS presentation in offspring, siblings, and parents [3, 10–13].

* Correspondence: msahrai@sina.tums.ac.ir
[2]MS Research Center, Neuroscience Institute, Tehran University of Medical Sciences, Tehran, Iran
[3]MS Research Center, Sina Hospital, Hassan Abad square, Tehran, Iran
Full list of author information is available at the end of the article

In 2013, O'Gorman et al., conducted a systematic review, identifying several studies on familial factors involved in MS [14]. Although the results vary, most of them reported the highest prevalence risk in the northern countries, suggesting an association between the prevalence and country latitude [14–17]. In Canadian families with first-degree relatives affected, the risk of MS was 30–50 times greater than that for others [18]. The frequency of familial recurrence of MS is high in Canada (19.8%) [19] and it varies in Europe from 2% in Hungary [20] to 19% in the UK [10]. Its frequency in Australia varies from 10.6% to 16.2% [17]; it is 3–5% in Argentina and 10.5% in Mexico [3, 21]. In Italy, there was an increased prevalence of MS in siblings in comparison to other first-degree relatives [22].

Most of the patients who participated in projects about familial recurrence risk of MS were recruited from either clinical settings or from public solicitation, while only a few used national or regional case registries [23, 24]. This diversity in data collection methodology may decrease the validity of meta-analyses and increase the risk of sampling bias in most studies [9, 25, 26].

Some studies failed to report the familial recurrence risk because of small sample size and low statistical power [27].

In this cross-sectional population based study, a regional case registry method was used which included all MS patients in Tehran. The study aimed to evaluate the most important variables related to risk for familial recurrence of MS including pediatric onset cases, sex, age at disease onset, familial history of MS, and degree of relatives.

Methods

Study area

A population-based survey was conducted based on the Iranian MS Society (IMSS) registry system of Tehran province, the capital city of Iran. Tehran is located in the north of Iran (Latitude: 35 ° North, Longitude: 51° East) with an estimated population of 12,684,000 in 2015.

Data source

Iranian MS Society (IMSS) recorded annual incidence data from 1st April 1999 to 31st December 2015 [6, 28]. The IMSS is the single center in Tehran that registers MS patient demographic data and delivers extensive services such as medical, rehabilitation and social health facilities for the members.

All registered patients in the IMSS were residing in Tehran area. MS diagnosis was validated by neurologists using the Poser (up to 2001) [29] or McDonald criteria [30].

The McDonald criteria was used for all registered MS cases after 2001.

Neurologists are encouraged all patients to refer to the IMSS for enrollment and getting tracking code for receiving treatment. The goals of the MS registry were explained by a trained interviewer in IMSS and inform consent was taken from all patients before admitting study procedures. All patients extended their membership in IMSS every 3 years by receiving their membership card.

To design the cross-sectional population based study, the researchers tried to cover the most important epidemiological variables, which were related at the individual level to familial recurrence of MS.

All patients filled out a detailed questionnaire relating to baseline clinical and demographic data such as age, sex, birth date, age at disease onset, and familial history of MS in relatives for recognizing the familial recurrence of MS [31].

Relatives were divided into three categories: first degree relatives included mother, father, sister/brother and offspring. The second-degree relatives included grandmother, grandfather, maternal aunt/uncle and paternal aunt/uncle. The third-degree relatives included maternal cousins, paternal cousins and others [9].

We requested approval for reviewing the patients' medical records for all new cases of MS and data on which the treating neurologist completed the initial diagnosis.

Although the majority of the MS patients were registered in the IMSS, some of them might not have been registered during the years of disease onset, so the numbers may be underestimated. The Statistical Centre of Iran conducts population census regularly; however, in intervening years, the population is estimated from data obtained from various registries around the country. These population data were used to calculate the incidence and prevalence of MS on December, 2015.

Statistical analysis

Data analysis was conducted using SPSS, version 23.

The logistic regression analysis has been used to find the number of change-points in data; that is, wherever substantial changes of the annual percent change (APC) are detected [32, 33]. The prevalence was estimated by considering cases on prevalence day/total population on prevalence day.

To analyze the relationship among variables, the study made use of the Chi-squared test.

Moreover, logistic regression was used to estimate the odds ratio (OR) for individual variables in order to assess factors relating to familial recurrence of MS and age standardized in the general Iranian population in Tehran. P values < 0.05 were considered significant.

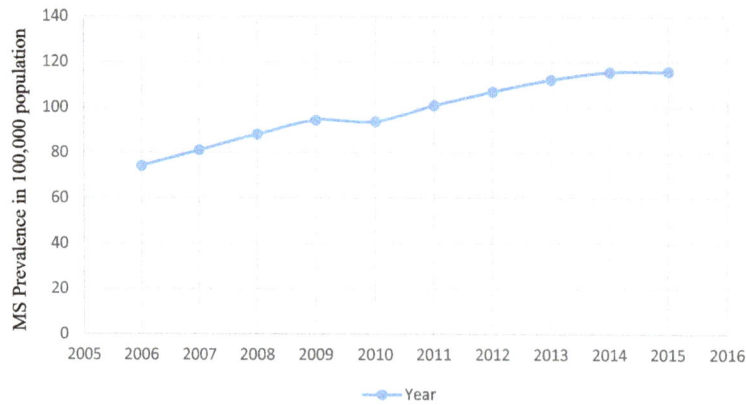

Fig. 1 Comparing prevalence trends of MS (2006–2015) in Tehran, Iran

Result

MS prevalence

A total of 16,447 registered cases of MS were included in the study. Total point prevalence of MS was 115.94 per 100,000 persons in 2015 (Fig. 1). The age standardized MS prevalence for females was 197.21 and for males was 63.23 per 100,000.

During the 2006–2015 period, a significantly increasing trend in MS prevalence was observed (Fig. 1).

Sex ratio trends

More than two-thirds of the cases (75.4%) were females.

The average female to male ratio in 2015 was 3.06:1 (Table 1).

Age at disease onset and its trends

Totally, 6316 (38.4%) patients between 18 to 27 years old at disease onset entered the study. Mean age at disease onset was 28.36 years old with a minimum and maximum of 3 and 87 years old, respectively. Mean age at disease onset for female and male patients were 28.15 and 29.01 years old, respectively (Table 1).

The logistic regression analysis revealed that age significantly associated with MS prevalence in comparing different sexes ($P < 0.00$), the association was seen in pediatric age group 18 < years old (OR = 1.24; 95% CI = 1.08–1.41); 18–27 years old (OR = 1.14; 95% CI = 1.04–1.24) and 48 ≥ (OR =0.79; 95% CI = 0.69–0.91) (Table 1).

Familial history of MS

From 1999 to 2015, a family history of MS within each sex was 1509 (12.6%) among female and 526 (13.6%) among male patients (Table 1).

The proportion of cases with familial recurrence of MS increased significantly during the study period (Fig. 2). The familial recurrence of MS was 13% for men and 12.2% for women. The 18–27 year-old group had a near-significantly greater proportion with familial recurrence compared to the 48+ age group. Amongst patients with a history of MS in their relatives, 826 (40.6%) patients had 18 to 27 years old at their disease onset (OR = 1.02; 95% CI = 0.82–1.26) (Table 2).

Crude odds ratio for familial recurrence of MS according to degree of relatives is shown in Tables 3.

Table 1 Baseline characteristics and comparing the OR of a male vs female case

Variables	Female N (%) 12,403 (75.4)	Male N (%) 4044 (24.6)	Total N (%) 16,447 (100)	P value	Crude OR (95% CI)
Familial history of MS					
No	10,507 (87.4)	3343 (86.4)	13,850 (87.2)	–	Reference
Yes	1509 (12.6)	526 (13.6)	2035 (12.8)	0.09	0.91 (0.82–1.01)
Age group (years)					
18<	**1310 (10.6)**	**362(9.0)**	**1672 (10.2)**	**0.00**	**1.24 (1.08–1.41)**
18–27	**4855 (39.2)**	**1460 (36.1)**	**6316 (38.4)**	**0.00**	**1.14 (1.04–1.24)**
28–37	3888 (31.4)	1335 (33.0)	5225 (31.8)	–	Reference
38–47	1513 (12.2)	529 (13.1)	2042 (12.4)	0.75	0.98 (0.87–1.10)
48≥	**837 (6.6)**	**358 (8.8)**	**1192 (7.2)**	**0.00**	**0.79 (0.69–0.91)**

OR = odds ratio, 95% CI= 95% confidence interval by logistic regression analysis
Bold numbers correspond to significant value

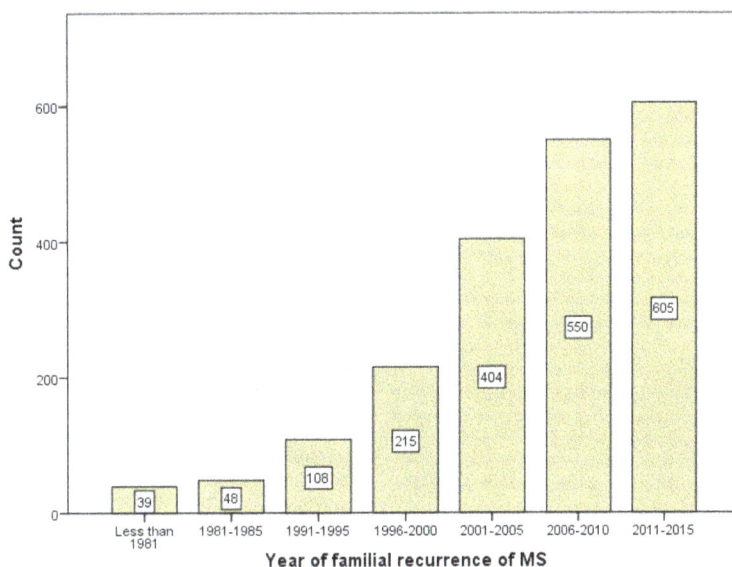

Fig. 2 Comparing familial recurrence trends of MS in Tehran, Iran

Among all patients who had familial recurrence of MS, the strongest association among first-degree relative was seen among siblings (640 (31.44%) (*P* value < 0.001) (Table 3).

With regard to second degree relatives, the strongest association was among maternal aunts/uncles.

In total, 1781 MS patients had one person in their family with MS; 153 patients had two persons, 22 patients had three persons, two patients had four persons, one patient had seven persons, and one patient had eight persons.

Discussion

The present study evaluated the changes in the prevalence of MS in Tehran with different ethnicities, during the last 16 years from 1999 to 2015. The total point prevalence of MS in Tehran shows an increase during this period; based on this data, Tehran is among the regions with the highest prevalence of MS in Asia [34].

Table 2 Comparing the OR of diffrent age groups by familial recurrence of MS

	Familial History of MS		
Age	No N (%)	Yes N (%)	OR (95% CI)
18 <	1405 (10.1)	242 (11.8)	1.15 (0.90–1.46)
18–27	5395 (39.0)	826 (40.6)	1.02 (0.82–1.26)
28–37	4524 (32.7)	618 (30.4)	Reference
38–47	1771 (12.7)	236 (11.6)	0.89 (0.70–1.13)
48 ≥	755 (5.5)	113(5.6)	0.91 (0.73–1.13)

OR odds ratio, *CI* confidence interval
P value = 0.03

MS was nearly three times more common in females than in males in 2015.

The mean age of MS onset estimated in Iran during 1999–2015 (28.3 years) is comparable to other countries in Asia such as Japan (28.3), Korea (30.4), Malaysia (28.6) and Taiwan, (30.0); it is significantly lower than China (37.4) and India (38.3) [34].

During the last two decades, the data regarding the prevalence, incidence and risk factors for the growth of MS has significantly increased [35] and familial history of MS has been introduced as one of the etiologic factors of MS by different studies [36].

Table 3 Positive familial recurrence of multiple sclerosis according to the degree of relatives

Relative	Female N (%)	Male N (%)	Total N (%)	P value
Mother	117 (72.2)	45 (27.8)	17(6.86)	0.31
Father	34 (72.3)	13 (27.7)	47 (2.20)	0.61
Sibling	**449 (70.2)**	**191 (29.8)**	**640 (30.34)**	**0.00**
Offspring	28 (77.8)	8 (22.2)	36 (1.66)	0.84
Maternal/Paternal grandmother	15 (65.2)	8 (34.8)	17 (1.13)	0.32
Maternal/Paternal grandfather	13 (76.5)	4 (23.5)	17 (0.73)	1.00
Maternal aunt/Uncle	137 (74.9)	46 (0.3)	23 (7.79)	0.86
Paternal aunt/Uncle	69 (78.4)	19 (21.6)	88 (4.32)	0.61
Maternal cousin	234 (78.3)	65 (21.7)	363 (13.54)	0.30
Paternal cousin	280 (77.1)	83 (22.9)	88 (15.43)	0.53
Others	267 (77.2)	79 (22.8)	346 (16.0)	0.52

Bold numbers correspond to significant value

Nevertheless, published data on familial recurrence forms of MS is limited [37].

Some studies have found that positive family history of MS correlated with a considerable increase in MS risk [38, 39] and positive history of MS increased from 5% in 2003 to 12.4% in 2015 in our data [40].

The results of present study specify that, in Tehran province the percentage of patients with positive family history of MS is higher than other areas of Iran (12.2%) and other countries in the Middle East like Qatar (10.4%) and Azerbaijan (8.15%) [28, 39, 41, 42].

The percentage of familial recurrence cases in this study is two times higher than that reported in Brazil (6.12%) [43], four times greater than Mexico (3%) [21] and six times higher than Hungary (2%) [20].

Among Caucasians, the highest frequency of familial recurrence of MS with one affected relative was identified in 19.8% of MS patients in Canada [44].

Despite the higher prevalence of MS amongst females, the familial recurrence was higher among males; this finding is comparable to another study conducted in Isfahan [42].

A younger age of onset is a natural feature of many inherited diseases [45]; the frequency of pediatric MS cases is diffused and varies from 3% to 5.5% [46].

According to our data, most familial recurrence of MS occurred among younger age groups compared to reference group ≥48 years old. The younger age of onset in familial recurrence of MS was seen among the MS patients in the present study which is similar to what was observed in familial recurrence among younger MS patients in Spain and Argentina [45, 47].

The amount of the familial recurrence of MS was larger among first-degree relatives, especially in siblings [43]. This finding was similar to the findings about autism among siblings [48].

This assessment confirms that MS is a multifactor disease with a considerable familial recurrence penetration.

Studying the familial recurrence risk of MS is challenging, because familial risk factors display a high degree of heterogeneity among families [49, 50].

However, it is possible that some genetic changes or additional environmental factors influence the increasing prevalence of familial recurrence of MS among Iranian population with different ethnicity.

Conclusion

The present study evaluated the trends of MS prevalence and the association of MS familial risk factors in Tehran.

Total point prevalence of MS was 115.94 per 100,000 persons in 2015. The total point prevalence increased during the study period. In fact, Tehran is among regions with the highest prevalence of MS in Asia.

The most familial recurrence of MS occurred among younger age groups. The results of the present study specify that the percentage of patients with positive family history of MS in Tehran is among the highest in the Middle East. Among all patients who had familial recurrence of MS, the strongest associations were detect among siblings.

Abbreviations
APC: Annual percent change; IMSS: Iranian MS Society; MS: Multiple sclerosis; OR: Odds ratio

Acknowledgements
We wish to acknowledge the assistance of the staff of Iranian MS Society, whose kind cooperation made this research possible. The authors would like to thank Miss Saeideh Ayobi for her helpful collaboration.

Funding
Tehran University of Medical Sciences.

Authors' contributions
We confirm that the manuscript has been read and approved by all named authors and that there are no other persons who satisfied the criteria for authorship but are not listed. MA is the corresponding author and has gathered the main data and (1) ensured that original data upon which the submission is based is preserved and retrievable for reanalysis; (2) approved data presentation as representative of the original data; and (3) foresaw and minimized obstacles to the sharing of data, materials, algorithms or reagents described in the work. SE and MA S have made substantial contributions to design, acquisition of data, analysis and interpretation of data. SE, NS and MS have worked in drafting the manuscript. SE and MA S critically revised the manuscript for important intellectual content; and all authors approved the version to be published; they all agreed to be accountable for all aspects of the work.

Competing interests
The authors declare that they have no competing interests.

Author details
[1]Brain and Spinal Cord Injury Research Center, Neuroscience Institute, Tehran University of Medical Sciences, Tehran, Iran. [2]MS Research Center, Neuroscience Institute, Tehran University of Medical Sciences, Tehran, Iran. [3]MS Research Center, Sina Hospital, Hassan Abad square, Tehran, Iran.

References
1.   Ebers GC. Environmental factors and multiple sclerosis. The Lancet Neurology. 2008;7(3):268–77.
2.   Milo R, Kahana E. Multiple sclerosis: geoepidemiology, genetics and the environment. Autoimmun Rev. 2010;9(5):A387–94.
3.   Farez MF, et al. Low familial risks for multiple sclerosis in Buenos Aires Argentina. J Neurol Sci. 2014;346(1–2):268–70.
4.   Compston, A., et al., McAlpine's multiple sclerosis (Philadelphia: Churchill Livingstone Elsevier). 2005.
5.   Kurtzke JF. Multiple sclerosis in time and space-geographic clues to cause. J Neurovirol. 2000;6(2):S134.
6.   Heydarpour P, et al. Multiple sclerosis in Tehran, Iran: a joinpoint trend analysis. Mult Scler. 2014;20(4):512.
7.   Etemadifar M, et al. Estimated prevalence and incidence of multiple sclerosis in Iran. Eur Neurol. 2014;72(5–6):370–4.
8.   Orton S-M, et al. Sex ratio of multiple sclerosis in Canada: a longitudinal study. The Lancet Neurology. 2006;5(11):932–6.
9.   Westerlind H, et al. Modest familial risks for multiple sclerosis: a registry-based study of the population of Sweden. Brain. 2014;137(Pt 3):770–8.
10. Robertson N, et al. Age–adjusted recurrence risks for relatives of patients with multiple sclerosis. Brain. 1996;119(2):449–55.

11. Dyment DA, et al. Multiple sclerosis in stepsiblings: recurrence risk and ascertainment. J Neurol Neurosurg Psychiatry. 2006;77(2):258–9.
12. Ramagopalan SV, et al. Expression of the multiple sclerosis-associated MHC class II allele HLA-DRB1* 1501 is regulated by vitamin D. PLoS Genet. 2009;5(2):e1000369.
13. Eskandarieh S, et al. Comparing epidemiology and baseline characteristic of multiple sclerosis and neuromyelitis optica: a case-control study. Mult Scler Relat Disord. 2017;12:39–43.
14. O'Gorman C, et al. Modelling genetic susceptibility to multiple sclerosis with family data. Neuroepidemiology. 2012;40(1):1–12.
15. Ebers G. A twin consensus in MS. Mult Scler. 2005;11(5):497–9.
16. Islam T, et al. Differential twin concordance for multiple sclerosis by latitude of birthplace. Ann Neurol. 2006;60(1):56–64.
17. O'Gorman C, et al. Familial recurrence risks for multiple sclerosis in Australia. J Neurol Neurosurg Psychiatry. 2011;82(12):1351–4.
18. Sadovnick AD, et al. Effect of age at onset and parental disease status on sibling risks for MS. Neurology. 1998;50(3):719–23.
19. Weinshenker BG, et al. The natural history of multiple sclerosis: a geographically based study. Brain. 1989;112(1):133–46.
20. Nagy Z, et al. Epidemiology of familial multiple sclerosis in Hungary. Mult Scler. 2007;13(2):260–1.
21. Gonzalez O, Sotelo J. Is the frequency of multiple sclerosis increasing in Mexico? J Neurol Neurosurg Psychiatry. 1995;59(5):528–30.
22. Guaschino C, et al. Familial clustering in Italian progressive-onset and bout-onset multiple sclerosis. Neurol Sci. 2014;35(5):789–91.
23. Nielsen NM, et al. Familial risk of multiple sclerosis: a nationwide cohort study. Am J Epidemiol. 2005;162(8):774–8.
24. Prokopenko I, et al. Risk for relatives of patients with multiple sclerosis in central Sardinia, Italy. Neuroepidemiology. 2003;22(5):290–6.
25. Hawkes C. Twin studies in medicine–what do they tell us? QJM: An International Journal of Medicine. 1997;90(5):311–21.
26. Hawkes C, Macgregor A. Twin studies and the heritability of MS: a conclusion. Mult Scler. 2009;15(6):661–7.
27. Johansson V, et al. Multiple sclerosis and psychiatric disorders: comorbidity and sibling risk in a nationwide Swedish cohort. Mult Scler J. 2014: 1352458514540970.
28. Sahraian MA, et al. Multiple sclerosis in Iran: a demographic study of 8,000 patients and changes over time. Eur Neurol. 2010;64(6):331–6.
29. Poser CM, et al. New diagnostic criteria for multiple sclerosis: guidelines for research protocols. Ann Neurol. 1983;13(3):227–31.
30. McDonald WI, et al. Recommended diagnostic criteria for multiple sclerosis: guidelines from the international panel on the diagnosis of multiple sclerosis. Ann Neurol. 2001;50(1):121–7.
31. Al Jumah M, et al. Familial multiple sclerosis: does consanguinity have a role? Mult Scler J. 2011;17(4):487–9.
32. Qi D, et al. Trends of prostate cancer incidence and mortality in shanghai, China from 1973 to 2009. Prostate. 2015;75(14):1662–8.
33. Rafiemanesh H, et al. Incidence trend and epidemiology of common cancers in the Center of Iran. Global journal of health science. 2015;8(3):146.
34. Eskandarieh S, et al. Multiple sclerosis epidemiology in East Asia, South East Asia and South Asia: a systematic review. Neuroepidemiology. 2016;46(3):209–21.
35. Corona T, Román GC. Multiple sclerosis in Latin America. Neuroepidemiology. 2005;26(1):1–3.
36. Moosazadeh M, et al. Prevalence of familial multiple sclerosis in Iran: a systematic review and meta-analysis. Iran J Neurol. 2017;16(2):90–5.
37. Cristiano E, Patrucco L, Rojas J. A systematic review of the epidemiology of multiple sclerosis in South America. Eur J Neurol. 2008;15(12):1273–8.
38. Maroney M, Hunter SF. Implications for multiple sclerosis in the era of the affordable care act: a clinical overview. Am J Manag Care. 2014;20(11 Suppl):s220–7.
39. Hashemilar M, et al. Multiple sclerosis in East-Azerbaijan, north west Iran. Neurology Asia. 2011;16(2):127–31.
40. Kalanie H, Gharagozli K, Kalanie AR. Multiple sclerosis: report on 200 cases from Iran. Mult Scler. 2003;9(1):36–8.
41. Deleu D, et al. Prevalence, demographics and clinical characteristics of multiple sclerosis in Qatar. Mult Scler J. 2012:1352458512459291.
42. Etemadifar M, et al. Prevalence of multiple sclerosis in Isfahan, Iran. Neuroepidemiology. 2006;27(1):39–44.
43. Papais-Alvarenga RM, et al. Familial forms of multiple sclerosis and neuromyelitis optica at an MS center in Rio de Janeiro state, Brazil. J Neurol Sci. 2015;356(1):196–201.
44. Ebers G, et al. The natural history of multiple sclerosis: a geographically based study. Brain. 2000;123(3):641–9.
45. Romero-Pinel L, et al. Anticipation of age at onset in familial multiple sclerosis. Eur J Neurol. 2010;17(4):572–5.
46. Bigi S, Banwell B. Pediatric multiple sclerosis. J Child Neurol. 2012;27(11): 1378–83.
47. Rojas J, et al. Disease onset in familial and sporadic multiple sclerosis in Argentina. Multiple Sclerosis and Related Disorders. 2016;
48. Kumar A, Juneja M, Mishra D. Prevalence of autism Spectrum disorders in siblings of Indian children with autism Spectrum disorders. J Child Neurol. 2016:0883073815624764.
49. Kerner B. Toward a deeper understanding of the genetics of bipolar disorder. Frontiers in psychiatry. 2015;6
50. Kendler KS, et al. IQ and schizophrenia in a Swedish national sample: their causal relationship and the interaction of IQ with genetic risk. Am J Psychiatr. 2015;

18

Evaluation of patients with relapsing-remitting multiple sclerosis using tract-based spatial statistics analysis: diffusion kurtosis imaging

Hai Qing Li[1†], Bo Yin[1†], Chao Quan[2†], Dao Ying Geng[1,3], Hai Yu[2], Yi Fang Bao[1], Jun Liu[4*] and Yu Xin Li[1,3*]

Abstract

Background: Diffusion kurtosis imaging (DKI) has the potential to provide microstructural insights into myelin and axonal pathology with additional kurtosis parameters. To our knowledge, few studies are available in the current literature using DKI by tract-based spatial statistics (TBSS) analysis in patients with multiple sclerosis (MS). The aim of this study is to assess the performance of commonly used parameters derived from DKI and diffusion tensor imaging (DTI) in detecting microstructural changes and associated pathology in relapsing remitting MS (RRMS).

Methods: Thirty-six patients with RRMS and 49 age and sex matched healthy controls underwent DKI. The brain tissue integrity was assessed by fractional anisotropy (FA), mean diffusivity (MD), axial diffusivity (Da), radial diffusivity (Dr), mean kurtosis (MK), axial kurtosis (Ka) and radial kurtosis (Kr) of DKI and FA, MD, Da and Dr of DTI. Group differences in these parameters were compared using TBSS ($P < 0.01$, corrected). To compare the sensitivity of these parameters in detecting white matter (WM) damage, the percentage of the abnormal voxels based on TBSS analysis, relative to the whole skeleton voxels for each parameter was calculated.

Results: The sensitivities in detecting WM abnormality in RRMS were MK (78.2%) > Kr (76.7%) > Ka (53.5%) and Dr (78.8%) > MD (76.7%) > FA (74.1%) > Da (28.3%) for DKI, and Dr (79.8%) > MD (79.5%) > FA (68.6%) > Da (40.1%) for DTI. DKI-derived diffusion parameters (FA, MD, and Dr) were sensitive for detecting abnormality in WM regions with coherent fiber arrangement; however, the kurtosis parameters (MK and Kr) were sensitive to discern abnormalities in WM regions with complex fiber arrangement.

Conclusions: The diffusion and kurtosis parameters could provide complementary information for revealing brain microstructural damage in RRMS. Dr and DKI_Kr may be regarded as useful surrogate markers for reflecting pathological changes in RRMS.

Keywords: Multiple sclerosis, relapsing–remitting, Diffusion kurtosis imaging, Diffusion tensor imaging, Tract-based spatial statistics

* Correspondence: lj7275@163.com; liyuxin@fudan.edu.cn
†Hai Qing Li, Bo Yin and Chao Quan contributed equally to this work.
⁴Department of Radiology, The Fifth People's Hospital of Shanghai, Fudan University, 128 Ruili Rd, Shanghai 200240, China
¹Department of Radiology, Huashan Hospital, Fudan University 12 Wulumuqi Rd. Middle, Shanghai 200040, China
Full list of author information is available at the end of the article

Background

Multiple sclerosis (MS) is a chronic disorder of the CNS, characterized by focal white matter (WM) plaques along with diffuse normal appearing WM (NAWM) damage and cortical demyelination [1]. Diffusion tensor imaging (DTI) is one of the most widely used methods in detecting microstructural abnormalities based on water diffusion measures with the assumption that the diffusion displacement of water molecule in an unrestricted environment has a Gaussian approximation [2].In reality, water molecules often show non-Gaussian diffusion due to the presence of barriers of cell membranes, axon sheaths, and water compartments in biological tissues [3]. So it is thought that DTI may not be capable to provide accurate values at dense intersections of fiber tracts [4]. In contrast, as a clinically feasible extension of DTI, diffusion kurtosis imaging (DKI) has been proposed to characterize the deviation of water diffusion in neural tissues from Gaussian diffusion [5, 6]. Both diffusion parameters including fractional anisotropy (FA), mean diffusivity (MD), axial diffusivity (Da), radial diffusivity (Dr) and kurtosis parameters including mean kurtosis (MK), axial kurtosis (Ka), radial kurtosis (Kr) could be obtained from DKI data. DKI can be regarded as a more sensitive indicator of diffusional heterogeneity and can be used to investigate abnormalities in tissues with isotropic structure [6, 7].

The sensitivity of DKI has been evaluated in age-related diffusion patterns in the prefrontal brain [8], reactive astrogliosis in traumatic brain injury [9], and cuprizone-induced demyelination in mice [10], which showed better demonstration of microstructural changes than with DTI. However, there were few studies to validate the merits of DKI in evaluating patients with MS [11, 12]. Tract-based spatial statistics (TBSS) provides a powerful and objective method to perform multi-subject comparisons [13].

In this study, the microstructural alterations reflected by both DKI and DTI parameters in relapsing-remitting multiple sclerosis (RRMS) were investigated using TBSS. Our aim is to assess the performances of 11 commonly used parameters derived from DKI (MK, Ka, Kr, FA, MD, Da and Dr) and DTI (FA, MD, Da and Dr) in detecting microstructural abnormalities in RRMS.

Methods

Subjects

Thirty-six (13 male and 23 female) consecutive patients with RRMS (diagnosed by McDonald criteria [14]) were prospectively enrolled in this study. All patients underwent clinical assessments, including relapse history and disability assessment using EDSS before MRI examination. Patients were excluded if they had a history of other CNS disorders, corticosteroid use or relapses within three months prior to MRI. For comparison, 49 age- and gender-matched healthy controls (17 male and 32 female), with no previous history of neurological disorders were recruited (Table 1). Approval for this study was obtained from the Ethics Committee of Huashan Hospital, Fudan University and written informed consent was obtained from all the subjects.

MRI data acquisition

All scans were acquired using Discovery MR750 3.0 T scanner (GE Healthcare, Milwaukee, WI, USA) with an eight-channel phase array head coil.

An axial FLAIR sequence (SE: repetition time/ echo time = 8800/146 ms, slice thickness = 6.0 mm, field of view = 512 × 512 mm, voxel size = 0.5 × 0.5 × 6.0 mm^3) for white matter lesion volume calculation was performed. DKI was acquired with two values of b (b = 1250 and 2500 s/mm^2) along 25 diffusion-encoding directions and b value of 0 s/ mm^2 along 25 non-diffusion-weighted images, with a spin-echo single-shot echo planar imaging (EPI) sequence (TR/TE = 4700/102 ms; matrix = 128 × 128; FOV = 240 × 240 mm; slice thickness = 4 mm without gap; 35 axial slices; acquisition time was 8 min and 42 s).

White matter lesion volume calculation

With MRIcron software (http://www.nitrc.org/projects/mricron/) we drew all the WM leisons manually on FLAIR images and calculated total WM lesion volume for each patient and summerized it in Table 1.

DKI data processing

We used the same methodology from a previously published work [15], and the differences were as following. In "calculation of diffusion and kurtosis parameters", all the data (b = 0, 1250, 2500 s/mm^2) were used for DKI fitting and only images with b = 0 and 1250 s/mm^2 were employed for DTI fitting. In "tract-based spatial statistics", group comparisons between RRMS patients and healthy controls were performed using a general linear model. The percentage of the abnormal voxels relative to the whole skeleton voxels for each parameter was calculated, so as to quantitatively compare the sensitivity of parameters from DKI and DTI in detecting brain tissue integrity impairments in RRMS.

Results

Kurtosis parameters from DKI

Compared with healthy controls, RRMS patients had significantly decreased DKI-derived kurtosis parameters in WM regions ($P < 0.01$, two-tailed, FWE corrected) with complex fiber arrangement, such as in the juxtacortical WM and corona radiata. DKI_MK, DKI_Ka and DKI_Kr could detect abnormal diffusion in 78.2%, 53.5% and 76.7% voxels of the whole WM skeleton respectively. Kurtosis parameters are shown in Fig. 1.

Table 1 Demographic and clinical characteristics of RRMS patients and healthy controls

Characteristics	RRMS patients	Healthy controls	P value
Number of subjects	36	49	
Age (years)	32.9 ± 10.6	32.3 ± 10.6	0.8*
Sex (male: female)	13:23	17:32	0.9*
EDSS	1.5 (0–5)[a]	NA	
Disease duration(month)	54.5 ± 62.8	NA	
White matter lesion volume (ml)	17.94 ± 19.00	NA	

*A Chi-square test of Pearson and *a t-test of Student were used to test the group differences in sex and age respectively. The data were shown as the mean values ± standard deviations. Abbreviations: *EDSS* expanded disability status scale, [a]median is 1.5, interquartile range is 1,1.5,2.375, minimum-maximum is 0–5. *NA* not applicable

Diffusion parameters from DKI

Compared with healthy controls, RRMS patients demonstrated reduced DKI_FA in WM regions with coherent fiber arrangement, such as the corpus callosum and anterior limb of internal capsule, and increased DKI_MD, DKI_Da and DKI_Dr ($P < 0.01$, two-tailed, FWE corrected). DKI_FA, DKI_MD, DKI_Da and DKI_Dr could detect abnormal diffusion in 74.1%, 76.7%, 28.3% and 78.8% voxels of the whole WM skeleton respectively. DKI-derived diffusion parameters are shown in Fig. 2.

Diffusion parameters from DTI

RRMS patients exhibited similar patterns with DKI-derived diffusion parameters. FA was reduced, MD, Da and Dr were increased ($P < 0.01$, two-tailed, FWE corrected). DTI_FA, DTI_MD, DTI_Da and DTI_Dr could detect abnormal diffusion in 68.6%, 79.5%, 40.1% and 79.8% voxels of the whole WM skeleton respectively. DTI-derived diffusion parameters are shown in Fig. 3.

Discussion

Although DTI has been widely used in investigating structural changes in the NAWM in MS [16, 17], it may not provide accurate parameters at dense intersections of fiber tracts [4]. In contrast, DKI can be used to quantify non-Gaussian diffusion, thus providing accurate parameters at dense intersection of fiber tracts [6]. To our knowledge, there were only a limited number of studies using DKI in MS patients [11, 12, 18, 19], Raz E et al. measured FA, MD, and MK values of the entire cross-sectional cord area, normal-appearing gray matter (NAGM) and WM in MS patients by DKI using region-of-interest (ROI) analysis, they thought that DKI could provide additional and complementary information to DTI on spinal cord pathology [11]. In another research, DKI was used to evaluate diffusional changes in NAWM regions remote from MS plaques using ROI analysis, the results indicated that DKI might be an additional sensitive indicator for detecting tissue damage in MS patients [12]. They concluded that DKI was sensitive for detecting tissue damage in MS patients and could provide information that was complementary to that of conventional DTI-derived metrics. However, most of these above-mentioned studies adopted ROI-based analysis, which had poor reproducibility of ROI positioning and only a limited number of specific regions can be

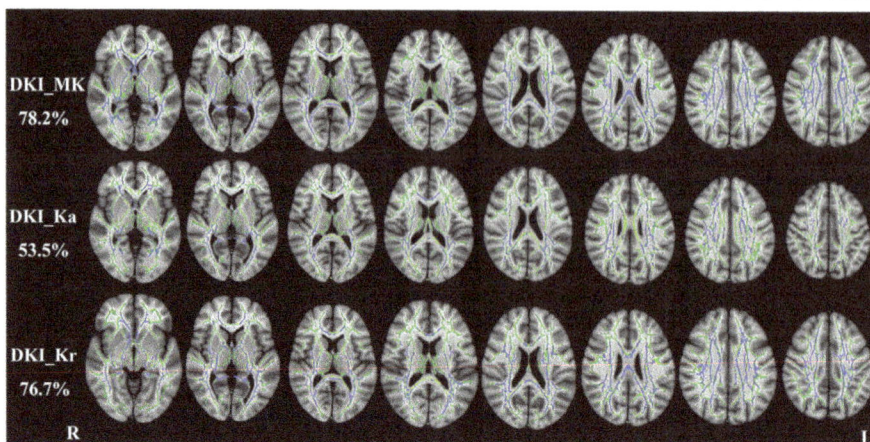

Fig. 1 TBSS shows WM regions with significant differences in the DKI_MK, DKI_Ka and DKI_Kr between RRMS patients and healthy subjects ($P < 0.01$, FWE corrected). Green represents mean FA skeleton of all participants; blue represents reduction in RRMS patients. The percentage in the left column represents the percentage of the abnormal voxels relative to the whole skeleton voxels for each parameter

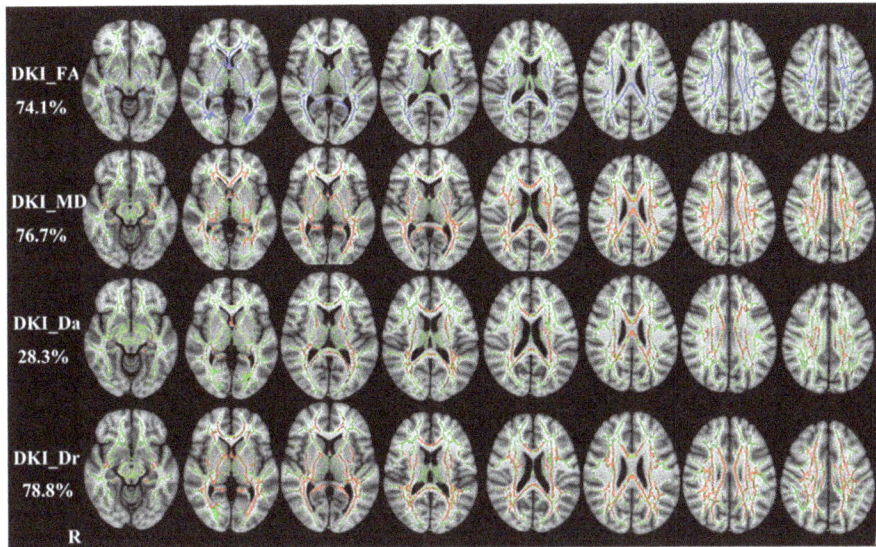

Fig. 2 TBSS shows WM regions with significant differences in the DKI_FA, DKI_MD, DKI_Da and DKI_Dr between RRMS patients and healthy subjects (*P* < 0.01, FWE corrected). Green represents mean FA skeleton of all participants; red denotes increase and blue represents reduction in RRMS patients. The percentage in the left column represents the percentage of the abnormal voxels relative to the whole skeleton voxels for each parameter

examined. In contrast, the TBSS method used in this study was relatively a novel hypothesis-free and user-independent voxel-wise analysis.

In this study, TBSS analysis of both DKI and DTI derived parameters showed widespread WM damage in RRMS patients compared with healthy controls, which was consistant with previous studies using DKI [19] or DTI [20, 21]. Similarly to a research study using DKI in schizophrenia patients, we also observed that DKI-derived kurtosis and diffusion parameters had differernt sensitivity to detect abnormality in WM areas with different fiber architecture [15]. Moreover, we found that the MK decrease in the WM of RRMS patients was predominantly caused by the Kr decrease, and the FA decrease was mainly driven by the increase of Dr.

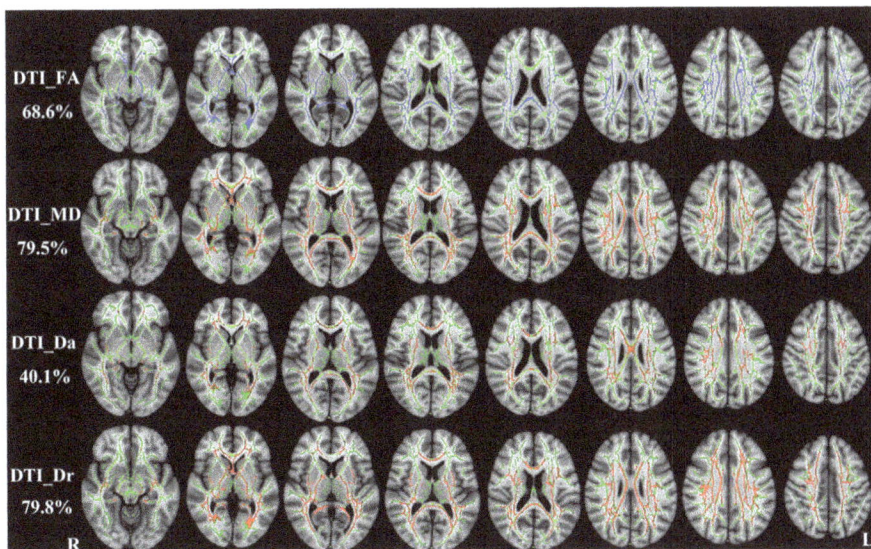

Fig. 3 TBSS shows WM regions with significant differences in the DTI_FA, DTI_MD, DTI_Da and DTI_Dr between RRMS patients and healthy subjects (*P* < 0.01, FWE corrected). Green represents mean FA skeleton of all participants; red denotes increase and blue represents reduction in RRMS patients. The percentage in the left column represents the percentage of the abnormal voxels relative to the whole skeleton voxels for each parameter

FA measures anisotropic water diffusion and is proven to be most applicable for assessing WM regions with coherent fiber arrangement. However, it is not suitable for detecting diffusion changes of complex WM architecture, such as crossing fiber regions [22, 23]. As the most characteristic parameter of DKI, MK measures the deviation of the diffusion displacement profile from a Gaussian distribution and enables to probe WM regions with complex fiber arrangement [24]. Therefore, the combination of diffusion and kurtosis parameters may provide improved sensitivity and specificity in detecting alterations in various WM structures. This theoretical prediction has been validated by a previous study in schizophrenia patients [15], and confirmed by our findings that altered diffusion parameters (especially reduced DKI_FA) were observed mainly in WM regions with coherent fiber arrangement (such as the corpus callosum and anterior limb of internal capsule). The percentage of abnormal DKI_FA voxels (74.1%) relative to the whole skeleton voxels was higher than that of DTI_FA (68.6%) in this study, which suggest that DKI_FA might have higher sensitivity than DTI_FA in detecting abnormality in WM regions, while reduced kurtosis parameters were mainly located in WM regions with complex fiber arrangement (such as the juxtacortical WM and corona radiate). The percentage of abnormal MK voxels relative to the whole skeleton voxels was 78.2%, which suggest that MK might have higher sensitivity than DTI in detecting abnormality in WM regions. Therefore, appropriate DKI derived parameters should be selected to probe altered diffusion pattern in specific WM regions in RRMS patients.

As we know, there is strong directional dependence of water distribution within myelinated WM tracts. However, once inflammation and demyelination occur, diffusivity will increase and directionality will decrease. The increase of diffusivity manifested as increase of Dr (diffusion perpendicular to the long axis) and Da (diffusion along the long axis). However, decreased Da was reported in some animal experiments [25, 26]. In our opinion, these studies may not take into account the full complexity of pathological processes occurred in RRMS. The increase of Da found in our RRMS patients was consistent with a TBSS study using DTI in RRMS patients [20]. The cause may be explained by severe decreases in axonal packing density which would lead to a whole increase in extracellular water, resulting in larger Dr increases and subsequent Da increases. Other reported reasons include fiber re-organization, increased axonal diameter and membrane permeability [27, 28]. In our study, the percentage of abnormal DKI_Dr voxels (79.8%) relative to the whole skeleton voxels is significantly higher than that of DKI_Da (28.3%), which demonstrated that the increase of MD (mean diffusivity) and

decreased FA mainly caused by the increased DKI_Dr. Similarly, this pattern of changes was also found in DTI_Da and DTI_Dr. Interestingly, when assessing the contribution of DKI_Ka and DKI_Kr in those regions showing significantly decreased DKI_MK, we found these were driven predominantly by decreases in DKI_Kr (76.5% vs DKI_Ka 53.5%). All these above-mentioned findings suggested demyelination might be regarded as a key factor among various pathological changes in RRMS. So Dr and DKI_Kr might be regarded as useful surrogate markers for reflecting pathological changes and improving clinical–radiological correlations in MS. Furthermore, Dr and DKI_Kr measured by TBSS might have great potential to be a MRI biomarker in monitoring remyelination in MS patients.

Conclusions
In conclusion, DKI-derived parameters were sensitive to detect abnormality in microstructural changes. The diffusion and kurtosis parameters could provide complementary information for revealing pathological changes in RRMS patients. Dr and DKI_Kr might be regarded as a useful surrogate marker for reflecting pathological changes and improving clinical–radiological correlations in MS patients.

Abbreviations
Da: Axial diffusivity; Dr: Radial diffusivity; GM: Gray matter; Ka: Axial kurtosis; Kr: Radial kurtosis; MK: Mean kurtosis; NAGM: Normal-appearing gray matter; NAWM: Normal-appearing white matter; WM: White matter

Acknowledgements
We would like to gratefully thank Jia Jia Zhu of Department of Radiology Affiliated Hospital, Anhui Medical University for his support and assistance. We also would like to gratefully thank Pro. Chi-Shing ZEE, Keck hospital of USC for his kindly revised the manuscript finally.

Funding
This work was supported by grants from the National Natural Science Foundation of China (81301203, 81471627 and 81200919), Science and Technology Commission of Shanghai Municipality (17411953700), Specialized Research Fund for the Doctoral Program of Higher Education of China (20130071130011) and Shanghai Health System Important Disease Joint Research Project (2013ZYJB009).

Authors' contributions
Study concept and design: YX L, J L and DY G. Acquisition of data: HQ L, B Y, C Q, H Y and YF B. Analysis and interpretation of data: HQ L, B Y, C Q, H Y and YF B. Clinical assessments: C Q and H Y. Drafting of the manuscript: HQ L, B Y and C Q. Critical revision of the manuscript for important intellectual content: YX L, J L and DY G. Statistical analysis: HQ L, B Y, C Q, H Y and YF B. Study supervision: DY G. All authors read and approved the final manuscript.

Competing interests
The authors declare that they have no competing interests.

Author details
[1]Department of Radiology, Huashan Hospital, Fudan University 12 Wulumuqi Rd. Middle, Shanghai 200040, China. [2]Department of Neurology, Huashan Hospital, Fudan University, Shanghai, China. [3]Institute of Functional and Molecular Medical Imaging, Fudan University, Shanghai, China. [4]Department of Radiology, The Fifth People's Hospital of Shanghai, Fudan University, 128 Ruili Rd, Shanghai 200240, China.

References

1. Frohman EM, Racke MK, Raine CS. Multiple sclerosis--the plaque and its pathogenesis. N Engl J Med. 2006;354(9):942–55.
2. Basser PJ, Jones DK. Diffusion-tensor MRI: theory, experimental design and data analysis - a technical review. NMR Biomed. 2002;15(7–8):456–67.
3. Tuch DS, Reese TG, Wiegell MR, Wedeen VJ. Diffusion MRI of complex neural architecture. Neuron. 2003;40(5):885–95.
4. Abdallah CG, Tang CY, Mathew SJ, Martinez J, Hof PR, Perera TD, Shungu DC, Gorman JM, Coplan JD. Diffusion tensor imaging in studying white matter complexity: a gap junction hypothesis. Neurosci Lett. 2010;475(3):161–4.
5. Hui ES, Cheung MM, Qi L, Wu EX. Towards better MR characterization of neural tissues using directional diffusion kurtosis analysis. NeuroImage. 2008; 42(1):122–34.
6. Jensen JH, Helpern JA. MRI quantification of non-Gaussian water diffusion by kurtosis analysis. NMR Biomed. 2010;23(7):698–710.
7. Jensen JH, Helpern JA, Ramani A, Lu H, Kaczynski K. Diffusional kurtosis imaging: the quantification of non-gaussian water diffusion by means of magnetic resonance imaging. Magn Reson Med. 2005;53(6):1432–40.
8. Falangola MF, Jensen JH, Babb JS, Hu C, Castellanos FX, Di Martino A, Ferris SH, Helpern JA. Age-related non-Gaussian diffusion patterns in the prefrontal brain. Journal of magnetic resonance imaging: JMRI. 2008;28(6):1345–50.
9. Zhuo J, Xu S, Proctor JL, Mullins RJ, Simon JZ, Fiskum G, Gullapalli RP. Diffusion kurtosis as an in vivo imaging marker for reactive astrogliosis in traumatic brain injury. NeuroImage. 2012;59(1):467–77.
10. Guglielmetti C, Veraart J, Roelant E, Mai Z, Daans J, Van Audekerke J, Naeyaert M, Vanhoutte G, Delgado YPR, Praet J, Fieremans E, Ponsaerts P, Sijbers J, Van der Linden A, Verhoye M. Diffusion kurtosis imaging probes cortical alterations and white matter pathology following cuprizone induced demyelination and spontaneous remyelination. NeuroImage. 2016; 125:363–77.
11. Raz E, Bester M, Sigmund EE, Tabesh A, Babb JS, Jaggi H, Helpern J, Mitnick RJ, Inglese M. A better characterization of spinal cord damage in multiple sclerosis: a diffusional kurtosis imaging study. AJNR Am J Neuroradiol. 2013; 34(9):1846–52.
12. Yoshida M, Hori M, Yokoyama K, Fukunaga I, Suzuki M, Kamagata K, Shimoji K, Nakanishi A, Hattori N, Masutani Y, et al. Diffusional kurtosis imaging of normal-appearing white matter in multiple sclerosis: preliminary clinical experience. Jpn J Radiol. 2013;31(1):50–5.
13. Smith SM, Jenkinson M, Johansen-Berg H, Rueckert D, Nichols TE, Mackay CE, Watkins KE, Ciccarelli O, Cader MZ, Matthews PM, et al. Tract-based spatial statistics: voxelwise analysis of multi-subject diffusion data. NeuroImage. 2006;31(4):1487–505.
14. Polman CH, Reingold SC, Banwell B, Clanet M, Cohen JA, Filippi M, Fujihara K, Havrdova E, Hutchinson M, Kappos L, et al. Diagnostic criteria for multiple sclerosis: 2010 revisions to the McDonald criteria. Ann Neurol. 2011;69(2): 292–302.
15. Zhu J, Zhuo C, Qin W, Wang D, Ma X, Zhou Y, Yu C. Performances of diffusion kurtosis imaging and diffusion tensor imaging in detecting white matter abnormality in schizophrenia. NeuroImage Clinical. 2015;7:170–6.
16. Vrenken H, Geurts JJ, Knol DL, van Dijk LN, Dattola V, Jasperse B, van Schijndel RA, Polman CH, Castelijns JA, Barkhof F, et al. Whole-brain T1 mapping in multiple sclerosis: global changes of normal-appearing gray and white matter. Radiology. 2006;240(3):811–20.
17. Roosendaal SD, Geurts JJ, Vrenken H, Hulst HE, Cover KS, Castelijns JA, Pouwels PJ, Barkhof F. Regional DTI differences in multiple sclerosis patients. NeuroImage. 2009;44(4):1397–403.
18. Bester M, Jensen JH, Babb JS, Tabesh A, Miles L, Herbert J, Grossman RI, Inglese M. Non-Gaussian diffusion MRI of gray matter is associated with cognitive impairment in multiple sclerosis. Mult Scler. 2015;21(7):935–44.
19. de Kouchkovsky I, Fieremans E, Fleysher L, Herbert J, Grossman RI, Inglese M. Quantification of normal-appearing white matter tract integrity in multiple sclerosis: a diffusion kurtosis imaging study. J Neurol. 2016;263(6):1146–55.
20. Liu Y, Duan Y, He Y, Yu C, Wang J, Huang J, Ye J, Parizel PM, Li K, Shu N. Whole brain white matter changes revealed by multiple diffusion metrics in multiple sclerosis: a TBSS study. Eur J Radiol. 2012;81(10):2826–32.
21. Yu HJ, Christodoulou C, Bhise V, Greenblatt D, Patel Y, Serafin D, Maletic-Savatic M, Krupp LB, Wagshul ME. Multiple white matter tract abnormalities underlie cognitive impairment in RRMS. NeuroImage. 2012;59(4):3713–22.
22. Douaud G, Jbabdi S, Behrens TE, Menke RA, Gass A, Monsch AU, Rao A, Whitcher B, Kindlmann G, Matthews PM, et al. DTI measures in crossing-fibre areas: increased diffusion anisotropy reveals early white matter alteration in MCI and mild Alzheimer's disease. NeuroImage. 2011;55(3):880–90.
23. Vos SB, Jones DK, Jeurissen B, Viergever MA, Leemans A. The influence of complex white matter architecture on the mean diffusivity in diffusion tensor MRI of the human brain. NeuroImage. 2012;59(3):2208–16.
24. Wu EX, Cheung MM. MR diffusion kurtosis imaging for neural tissue characterization. NMR Biomed. 2010;23(7):836–48.
25. Sun SW, Liang HF, Le TQ, Armstrong RC, Cross AH, Song SK. Differential sensitivity of in vivo and ex vivo diffusion tensor imaging to evolving optic nerve injury in mice with retinal ischemia. NeuroImage. 2006;32(3):1195–204.
26. Song SK, Sun SW, Ju WK, Lin SJ, Cross AH, Neufeld AH. Diffusion tensor imaging detects and differentiates axon and myelin degeneration in mouse optic nerve after retinal ischemia. NeuroImage. 2003;20(3):1714–22.
27. Lin F, Yu C, Jiang T, Li K, Chan P. Diffusion tensor tractography-based group mapping of the pyramidal tract in relapsing-remitting multiple sclerosis patients. AJNR Am J Neuroradiol. 2007;28(2):278–82.
28. Henry RG, Oh J, Nelson SJ, Pelletier D. Directional diffusion in relapsing-remitting multiple sclerosis: a possible in vivo signature of Wallerian degeneration. Journal of magnetic resonance imaging : JMRI. 2003;18(4):420–6.

19

Acquired modification of sphingosine-1-phosphate lyase activity is not related to adrenal insufficiency

Gulin Sunter[1], Ece Oge Enver[2], Azad Akbarzade[2], Serap Turan[2], Pinar Vatansever[3], Dilek Ince Gunal[1], Goncagul Haklar[3], Abdullah Bereket[2], Kadriye Agan[1] and Tulay Guran[2]*

Abstract

Background: Congenital sphingosine-1-phosphate (S1P) lyase deficiency due to biallelic mutations in *SGPL1* gene has recently been described in association with primary adrenal insufficiency and steroid-resistant nephrotic syndrome. S1P lyase, on the other hand, is therapeutically inhibited by fingolimod which is an oral drug for relapsing multiple sclerosis (MS). Effects of this treatment on adrenal function has not yet been evaluated. We aimed to test adrenal function of MS patients receiving long-term fingolimod treatment.

Methods: Nineteen patients (14 women) with MS receiving oral fingolimod (Gilenya®, Novartis) therapy were included. Median age was 34.2 years (range; 21.3–44.6 years). Median duration of fingolimod treatment was 32 months (range; 6–52 months) at a dose of 0.5 mg/day. Basal and ACTH-stimulated adrenal steroid measurements were evaluated simultaneously employing LC-MS/MS based steroid panel. Basal steroid concentrations were also compared to that of sex- and age-matched healthy subjects. Cortisol and 11-deoxycortisol, 11-deoxycorticosterone and dehydroepiandrosterone were used to assess glucocorticoid, mineralocorticoid and sex steroid producing pathways, respectively.

Results: Basal ACTH concentrations of the patients were 20.8 pg/mL (6.8–37.8 pg/mL) (normal range; 5–65 pg/mL). There was no significant difference in the basal concentrations of cortisol, 11-deoxycortisol, 11-deoxycorticosterone and dehydroepiandrosterone between patients and controls ($p = 0.11$, 0.058, 0.74, 0.15; respectively). All patients showed adequate cortisol response to 250 mcg IV ACTH stimulation (243 ng/mL, range; 197–362 ng/mL). There was no significant correlation between duration of fingolimod treatment and basal or ACTH-stimulated cortisol or change in cortisol concentrations during ACTH stimulation test ($p = 0.57$, 0.66 and 0.21, respectively).

Conclusion: Modification and inhibition of S1P lyase activity by the long-term therapeutic use of fingolimod is not associated with adrenal insufficiency in adult patients with MS. This suggests that S1P lyase has potentially a critical role on adrenal development rather than the function of a fully mature adrenal gland.

Keywords: Sphingosine-1-phosphate lyase, Fingolimod, Adrenal, Multiple sclerosis

* Correspondence: tulayguran@yahoo.com
[2]Department of Paediatric Endocrinology and Diabetes, Marmara University, Fevzi Cakmak Mh. Mimar Sinan Cd.No 41., Ustkaynarca/Pendik, 34899 Istanbul, Turkey
Full list of author information is available at the end of the article

Background

The essential role of sphingolipid metabolism has recently been emerged in adrenal disease. Three research groups almost simultaneously reported that recessive mutations in *SGPL1*, which encodes sphingosine-1-phosphate (S1P) lyase, cause a syndromic form of steroid-resistant nephrotic syndrome with adrenal insufficiency [1–3]. S1P lyase is the enzyme responsible for irreversible S1P degradation which is the final step of sphingolipid breakdown.

Sphingolipids are integral components of cell membranes in the regulation of fluidity and lipid bilayer composition, organizing the assembly of signaling molecules, and protein trafficking. Particularly, some sphingolipids like sphingosine (Sph), sphingosine-1-phosphate (S1P), and ceramide (Cer) also act as bioactive signaling molecules and are responsible for the regulation of cell growth, differentiation, senescence, or apoptosis [4].

Given a considerable role in health and disease, S1P signalling system has been extensively studied for the treatment of various inflammatory and autoimmune diseases over the last two decades. Particularly S1P lyase is still a promising target for the treatment of inflammatory and autoimmune diseases.

FTY720 (fingolimod) was designed by modification of myriocin, a naturally occurring sphingoid base analog that causes immunosuppression by interrupting sphingolipid metabolism. It was approved by the U.S. Food and Drug Administration (FDA) in 2010 for adults with relapsing forms of multiple sclerosis (MS) to reduce the frequency of clinical relapses and to delay physical disability [5].

Fingolimod has been shown to inhibit S1P lyase activity in vitro and in vivo [6, 7]. However, long-term effects of this treatment on adrenal function has not been studied so far.

Here, we have tested the adrenal function of the patients under long-term fingolimod (Gilenya®, Novartis) treatment due to relapsing-remitting MS. We aimed to explore whether therapeutic S1P receptor modulation and/or S1P lyase inhibition lead to any impairment in adrenal function on long-term.

Methods

Study was performed with the approval of the Ethics Committee of Marmara University, Faculty of Medicine, Istanbul, Turkey (09.2016.641). Patients provided written informed consent, and all studies were conducted in accordance with the principles of the Declaration of Helsinki.

We studied 19 patients (14 women, 5 men) with MS receiving oral fingolimod (Gilenya®, Novartis) therapy. Median age was 34.2 years (range; 21.3–44.6 years). Median duration of fingolimod treatment was 32 months (range; 6–52 months) at a dose of 0.5 mg/day. None of the patients was on daily steroid treatment, they had been treated with systemic steroids only during exacerbations. However, none of the patients required such treatment at least a year preceding the study.

Fifteen healthy controls (8 women, 7 men) aged from 27 to 46 years (median; 31.5 yrs) were selected randomly among the hospital staff who gave consent to contribute into the study. Baseline samples of healthy controls were collected at similar conditions as the patients' to compare normal basaline adrenal steroid secretion. Healthy controls had unremarkable past medical history and had normal blood pressure and physical examination.

We excluded patients and controls who used any anabolic medication, corticosteroids, sex steroids, or gonadotropins.

Protocol

Both patients and healthy controls provided basal blood samples between 8:00 and 10:00 AM. Then adrenocorticotrophin (ACTH) stimulation test (high dose synacthen test, HDST) was performed to the patients between 08:00 and 10:00 h. Blood samples were obtained by venipuncture before and 60 min after the application of IV 250 µg of synacthen (Novartis Pharma) [8].

All the plasma steroids were assayed simultaneously in patients and control subjects by means of liquid chromatography-mass spectrometry (LC-MS/MS).

LC-MS/MS serum steroid assays

Plasma concentrations of 17 steroid hormones (17OH-Progesterone, 21-deoxycortisol, androstenedione, dehydroepiandrosterone-sulphate (DHEA-S), dehydroepiandrosterone (DHEA), testosterone, cortisol, cortisone, corticosterone, aldosterone, 11-deoxycortisol, dihydrotestosterone, androsterone, pregnenolone, 17OH-pregnenolone, progesterone, 11-deoxycorticosterone) comprising mineralocorticoids, glucocorticoids and androgens, were determined using LC-MS/MS 8050 system (Schimadzu, Japan). Whole blood samples were collected in K2 EDTA containing tubes (Becton Dickenson, USA). Plasma samples were aliquoted and kept frozen in −20 °C degrees until the day of analysis. Internal standard mixtures which included 3 different internal standards namely the deuterated forms of aldosterone (aldo d7), cortisol (corti d4), testosterone (testo d3) for the determination of mineralocorticoids, glucocorticoids and androgens were added to each plasma sample, calibrator and control material to monitor recovery. All samples were extracted with S.r.l. Steroid Hormones kit (Eureka Lab Division, Italy). To separate substances an HPLC method was used with a RRHD Eclipse Plus C18 column (50 × 2.1 mm, 1.8 um) at a total flow rate of 0,4 mL/min at 60 °C. Total running time is 15 min and the injection volume was 20 uL. Electrospray ionization (positive mode) was used and for each hormone two multiple reaction monitoring (MRM) were recorded.

Statistical analysis

Statistical evaluation was performed using GraphPad Prism® V5.0 software (GraphPad Software Inc., San Diego, California, USA). The results for each steroid are reported as median (range) in the text. Mann-Whitney U and Spearman correlation tests were used for comparison and correlation analyses, respectively. Values were considered statistically significant when P value is less than 0.05.

Results

The ages of patient and control groups were similar ($p = 0.63$). Ages of men and women subgroups in patient and control groups were also similar ($p = 0.76$ and 0.24, respectively).

None of the patients showed proteinuria or lymphopenia (data not shown).

Basal ACTH concentrations of the patients were 20. 8 pg/mL (6.8–37.8 pg/mL) (normal range; 5–65 pg/mL). There was no significant difference in the basal concentrations of cortisol, aldosterone, dehydroepiandrosterone (DHEA), dehydroepiandrosterone sulphate (DHEAS), 11-deoxycortisol, 11-deoxycorticosterone and other key steroids in adrenal steroid pathways between patients and controls (Table 1). Despite MS patients show some variability in the measurements of 11-deoxycortisol and 11-deoxycorticosterone, median and mean values were still within the normal range of respective parameters (Fig. 1). All patients showed adequate cortisol response to ACTH stimulation (243 ng/mL, range; 197–362 ng/mL) (Fig. 2) [8].

There was no significant correlation between duration of fingolimod treatment and basal or ACTH-stimulated cortisol or change in cortisol concentrations during ACTH stimulation test ($p = 0.57$, 0.66 and 0.21, respectively).

Table 1 Comparison of basal steroid measurements of the MS patients with fingolimod treatment and healthy subjects

Parameter	Patients ($n = 19$) median (range)	Healthy controls ($n = 15$) median (range)	P value
Age (yrs)	34.2 (21.3–44.6)	31.5 (27–46)	0.63
Basal plasma cortisol (ng/ml) (N: 50–250 ng/ml)	151 (77–237)	164 (113–300)	0.11
Basal plasma aldosterone (N: < 0.24 ng/ml)	0.064 (0.023–0.20)	0.1 (0.04–0.21)	0.38
Basal plasma DHEA (ng/ml) (M: 0.61–16.3 ng/ml F: 1.02–11.85 ng/ml)	6 (2.2–11.8)	7 (2.6–14.2)	0.15
Basal plasma DHEA-S (ng/ml) (M: 480–3340 ng/ml F: 440–3220 ng/ml)	1083 (779–2825)	1427 (572–3110)	0.22
Basal plasma 11-deoxycortisol (ng/ml) (M: 0.14–1.2 ng/ml F: 0.17–1.2 ng/ml)	0.32 (0.07–1.28)	0.25 (0.07–0.54)	0.058
Basal plasma 11-deoxycorticosterone (ng/ml) (M: ≤0.15 ng/ml F: ≤0.18 ng/ml)	0.02 (0.001–0.29)	0.05 (0.01–0.11)	0.74
Basal plasma 17OH- pregnenolone (ng/ml) (M: < 1.28 ng/ml F: < 9.09 ng/ml)	1.3 (0.14–7.6)	0.52 (0.16–3.84)	0.28
Basal plasma 17OH- progesterone (M: < 2.20 ng/ml F: < 2.85 ng/ml)	0.98 (0.20–1.94)	1.25 (0.18–2.59)	0.09
Basal plasma progesterone (M: < 0.20 ng/ml F: 2.7–31 ng/ml)	0.07 (0.006–13.85)	0.08 (0.01–21.8)	0.27
Basal plasma pregnenolone (N: ≤ 3.25 ng/ml)	0.52 (0.16–2.25)	0.77 (0.42–1.12)	0.79
Basal plasma 21- deoxycortisol (N: < 0.5 ng/ml)	0.06 (0.02–0.12)	0.08 (0.03–0.31)	0.89
Basal plasma androstenedione (N: 0.20–2.50 ng/ml)	0.79 (0.32–1.50)	1.06 (0.23–2.2)	0.26

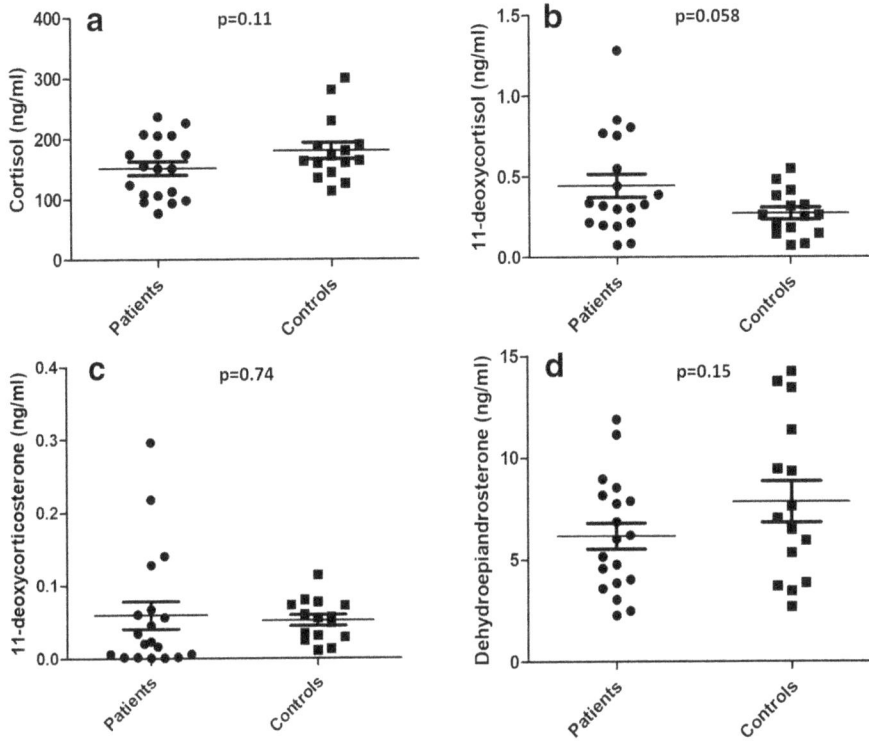

Fig. 1 LC–MS/MS based measurement of basal plasma steroids. Cortisol (**a**), 11-deoxycortisol (**b**), 11-deoxycorticosterone (**c**) and dehydroepiandrosterone (DHEA) (**d**) concentrations in patients with multiple sclerosis receiving fingolimod treatment and healthy controls are compared (p = 0.11, 0.058, 0.74, 0.15; respectively). Scatter plots represent the mean and standard errors of mean (S.E.M) of the measurements. Each symbol represents an individual case-specific measurement. Conversion to SI units: to convert nanograms per milliliter to nanomoles per liter, multiply by 2.76 for cortisol, by 2.89 for 11-deoxycortisol, by 3.03 for 11-deoxycorticosterone and by 3.467 for DHEA

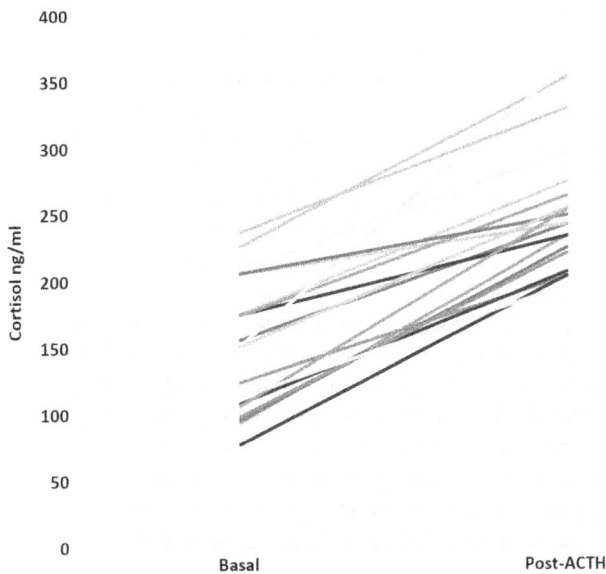

Fig. 2 LC–MS/MS based determination of basal- and ACTH-stimulated plasma concentrations of cortisol in patients with multiple sclerosis receiving fingolimod treatment. Conversion to SI units: to convert nanograms per milliliter to nanomoles per liter, multiply by 2.76 for cortisol

Discussion

Congenital sphingosine-1-phosphate (S1P) lyase deficiency due to biallelic mutations in *SGPL1*, has recently been established as a cause of primary adrenal insufficiency and steroid-resistant nephrotic syndrome [1–3]. In this study, however, we have shown that therapeutic inhibition and modification of S1P lyase activity does not impair adrenal steroid secretion in patients with multiple sclerosis.

Cortisol is a key regulator of the immune system, energy metabolism, and stress and it is well-known that psychosocial stress has frequently been associated with disease activity and acute exacerbations in MS. The hypothalamus-pituitary-adrenal (HPA) axis is generally activated in MS patients and is associated with disease progression. High cortisol levels were associated with slower disease progression, whereas patients with low cortisol levels had greater numbers of active lesions [9]. Furthermore, patients with shorter disease duration display higher cortisol stress response while MS patients with longer disease duration showed a significantly diminished HPA response. However, a recent study showed that relapsing-remitting MS patients did not differ in stress-related cortisol/catecholamine levels and glucocorticoid sensitivity than control subjects [10]. Despite these findings, very little is known about general adrenal activity and how this function is affected by current medical therapies in MS.

S1P lyase mediates the final step of the sphingolipid metabolism which is the irreversible breakdown of S1P to ethanolamine phosphate and hexadecenal [4]. Inhibition of S1P lyase activity will lead to accumulation of bioactive signaling molecules upstream of the pathway including S1P and ceramides (Cer). Cellular stress and changes in the cellular redox status can further aggravate this toxic accumulation [11, 12]. We have recently demonstrated that accumulation of S1P, Cer and potentially other upstream components of sphingolipid pathway due to congenital S1P lyase deficiency lead to a multisystemic disorder including primary adrenal insufficiency, nephrotic syndrome and ichthyosis [1].

Although the novel role of sphingolipid metabolism on adrenal function has recently been described, the anabolic, catabolic, and signaling pathways of sphingolipids have already emerged as promising targets for the treatment of diverse autoimmune disorders over the last two decades. Especially the introduction of fingolimod into market as first oral drug for the treatment of MS has boosted this effect [4, 5].

FTY720 (Fingolimod, 2-amino-2[2-(4-octylphenyl)ethyl]-1,3-propanediol) is a synthetic analogue of sphingosine. Fingolimod is phosphorylated by sphingosine kinase 2 to generate phospho-fingolimod. Phospho-fingolimod causes the internalization of S1P receptors, which sequesters lymphocytes in lymph nodes, preventing them from moving to the central nervous system and cause a relapse in MS.

Inhibition of S1P lyase is another mechanism of action of fingolimod besides modulation of S1P receptor activity. Fingolimod has been shown to inhibit S1P lyase activity in vitro and in vivo. Bandhuvula P et al. showed that the treatment with fingolimod inhibited tissue S1P lyase activity in mice and in HEK293 cells [6]. Park SM et al. further demonstrated that CD68(+) antigen presenting cells generated from human monocytes were able to internalize and irreversibly degrade S1P, and this activity was inhibited by the S1P analogue fingolimod [7]. This body of evidence warranted to explore the potential long-term effects of fingolimod treatment on adrenal function. A recent study has shown a good safety and efficacy profile of fingolimod over a 36-month treatment [13]. We have particularly confirmed that there is no impairment in adrenal steroid secretion up to 52-month of fingolimod treatment. Our patients did not also show proteinuria or lymphopenia all of which can be seen in patients with congenital S1P lyase deficiency (data not shown).

Adrenal glands of *Sgpl1−/−* mice show compromised zonation between zona glomerulosa (ZG) and zona fasciculate (ZF), and between ZF and X-zone. They also have lower expression of cytochrome P450 side-chain cleavage (CYP11A1), which facilitates the first and rate-limiting step of steroidogenesis [1]. Congenital S1P lyase deficiency causes adrenal insufficiency in early life in humans. Patients present with glucocorticoid, mineralocorticoid and sex steroid deficiency. These data suggest that *SGPL1* may have a developmental role in human adrenal. In our study, however, we tested adult human adrenal function under acquired modification and inhibition of S1P lyase activity. The use of LC-MS/MS based steroid panel enabled us to evaluate the glucocorticoid, mineralocorticoid and sex steroid producing pathways simultaneously. Concentrations of cortisol and 11-deoxycortisol, 11-deoxycorticosterone and dehydroepiandrosterone representing the secretion of zona fasciculata, zona glomerulosa and reticularis, respectively, were similar with healthy controls. Furthermore, all of the patients on fingolimod treatment showed sufficient cortisol response to ACTH stimulation regardless of treatment duration. Our data may suggest that the effect of genetic deficiency of SGPL1 must be related to developmental effects on the adrenal gland. While this may be true, especially in view of the disordered zonation observed in the SGPL1-deficient mice, it seems possible that additional effects of fingolimod, e.g., its agonist activity towards S1P receptors once it is phosphorylated, could also compensate for any ability of fingolimod to suppress adrenal steroid production through its inhibition of SGPL1.

Conclusion

In conclusion, modification and inhibition of S1P lyase activity by the long-term therapeutic use of fingolimod is safe for the adrenal function in adult patients with MS. These findings support that S1P lyase may have a critical role on adrenal development rather than the function of a fully mature adrenal gland.

Abbreviations
ACTH: Adrenocorticotrophin; Cer: Ceramide; DHEA: Dehydroepiandrosterone; DHEA-S: Dehydroepiandrosterone-sulphate; LC-MS/MS: Liquid chromatography-mass spectrometry; S1P: Sphingosine-1-phosphate; Sph: Sphingosine

Acknowledgements
We would like to acknowledge the technical assistance of Mrs. Makbule Ors from the department of biochemistry, Marmara University. We are deeply grateful to the patients and healthy controls without whom this study could not have been performed.

Funding
Our research did not receive any specific grant from any funding agency in the public, commercial or not-for-profit sector.

Authors' contributions
TG and AB designed the study. GS, KA, DIG, AA, ST recruited and clinically characterized patients. EOE performed ACTH stimulation tests. PV and GH performed biochemical studies. TG prepared the draft manuscript. All authors contributed to the discussion of results, edited and approved the final manuscript.

Competing interests
The authors declare that they have no competing interests.

Author details
[1]Department of Neurology, Marmara University, Istanbul, Turkey.
[2]Department of Paediatric Endocrinology and Diabetes, Marmara University, Fevzi Cakmak Mh. Mimar Sinan Cd.No 41., Ustkaynarca/Pendik, 34899 Istanbul, Turkey. [3]Department of Biochemistry, Marmara University, Istanbul, Turkey.

References
1. Prasad R, Hadjidemetriou I, Maharaj A, Meimaridou E, Buonocore F, Saleem M, Hurcombe J, Bierzynska A, Barbagelata E, Bergadá I, Cassinelli H, Das U, Krone R, Hacihamdioglu B, Sari E, Yesilkaya E, Storr HL, Clemente M, Fernandez-Cancio M, Camats N, Ram N, Achermann JC, Van Veldhoven PP, Guasti L, Braslavsky D, Guran T, Metherell LA. Sphingosine-1-phosphate lyase mutations cause primary adrenal insufficiency and steroid-resistant nephrotic syndrome. J Clin Invest. 2017;127(3):942–53.
2. Lovric S, Goncalves S, Gee HY, Oskouian B, Srinivas H, Choi WI, Shril S, Ashraf S, Tan W, Rao J, Airik M, Schapiro D, Braun DA, Sadowski CE, Widmeier E, Jobst-Schwan T, Schmidt JM, Girik V, Capitani G, Suh JH, Lachaussée N, Arrondel C, Patat J, Gribouval O, Furlano M, Boyer O, Schmitt A, Vuiblet V, Hashmi S, Wilcken R, Bernier FP, Innes AM, Parboosingh JS, Lamont RE, Midgley JP, Wright N, Majewski J, Zenker M, Schaefer F, Kuss N, Greil J, Giese T, Schwarz K, Catheline V, Schanze D, Franke I, Sznajer Y, Truant AS, Adams B, Désir J, Biemann R, Pei Y, Ars E, Lloberas N, Madrid A, Dharnidharka VR, Connolly AM, Willing MC, Cooper MA, Lifton RP, Simons M, Riezman H, Antignac C, Saba JD, Hildebrandt F. Mutations in sphingosine-1-phosphate lyase cause nephrosis with ichthyosis and adrenal insufficiency. J Clin Invest. 2017;127(3):912–28.
3. Janecke AR, Xu R, Steichen-Gersdorf E, Waldegger S, Entenmann A, Giner T, Krainer I, Huber LA, Hess MW, Frishberg Y, Barash H, Tzur S, Schreyer-Shafir N, Sukenik-Halevy R, Zehavi T, Raas-Rothschild A, Mao C, Müller T. Deficiency of the sphingosine-1-phosphate lyase SGPL1 is associated with congenital nephrotic syndrome and congenital adrenal calcifications. Hum Mutat. 2017; 38(4):365 72.
4. Vogt D, Stark H. Therapeutic strategies and pharmacological tools influencing S1P signaling and metabolism. Med Res Rev. 2017;37(1):3–51.
5. Brinkmann V, Billich A, Baumruker T, Heining P, Schmouder R, Francis G, Aradhye S, Burtin P. Fingolimod (FTY720): discovery and development of an oral drug to treat multiple sclerosis. Nat Rev Drug Discov. 2010;9(11):883–97.
6. Bandhuvula P, Tam YY, Oskouian B, Saba JD. The immune modulator FTY720 inhibits sphingosine-1-phosphate lyase activity. J Biol Chem. 2005; 280(40):33697–700.
7. Park SM, Angel CE, McIntosh JD, Brooks AE, Middleditch M, Chen CJ, Ruggiero K, Cebon J, Rod Dunbar P. Sphingosine-1-phosphate lyase is expressed by CD68+ cells on the parenchymal side of marginal reticular cells in human lymph nodes. Eur J Immunol. 2014;44(8):2425–36.
8. Stewart PM, Krone N. The adrenal cortex. In: Melmed S, Polonsky KS, Larsen PR, Kronenberg HM, editors. Williams textbook of endocrinology, vol. 1. 12th ed. Philadelphia: Saunders Elsevier; 2011. p. 479–544.
9. Melief J, de Wit SJ, van Eden CG, Teunissen C, Hamann J, Uitdehaag BM, Swaab D, Huitinga I. HPA axis activity in multiple sclerosis correlates with disease severity, lesion type and gene expression in normal-appearing white matter. Acta Neuropathol. 2013;126(2):237–49.
10. Kern S, Rohleder N, Eisenhofer G, Lange J, Ziemssen T. Time matters - acute stress response and glucocorticoid sensitivity in early multiple sclerosis. Brain Behav Immun. 2014;41:82–9.
11. Goldkorn T, Balaban N, Shannon M, Chea V, Matsukuma K, Gilchrist D, et al. H2O2 acts on cellular membranes to generate ceramide signaling and initiate apoptosis in tracheobronchial epithelial cells. J Cell Sci. 1998;111(Pt 21):3209–20.
12. Liu B, Andrieu-Abadie N, Levade T, Zhang P, Obeid LM, Hannun YA. Glutathione regulation of neutral sphingomyelinase in tumor necrosis factor-alpha-induced cell death. J Biol Chem. 1998;273(18):11313–20.
13. Saida T, Itoyama Y, Kikuchi S, Hao Q, Kurosawa T, Ueda K, Auberson LZ, Tsumiyama I, Nagato K, Kira JI. Long-term efficacy and safety of fingolimod in Japanese patients with relapsing multiple sclerosis: 3-year results of the phase 2 extension study. BMC Neurol. 2017;17(1):17.

20

Predictive value of early magnetic resonance imaging measures is differentially affected by the dose of interferon beta-1a given subcutaneously three times a week: an exploratory analysis of the PRISMS study

Anthony Traboulsee[1*], David K. B. Li[1], Mark Cascione[2], Juanzhi Fang[3], Fernando Dangond[4] and Aaron Miller[5]

Abstract

Background: On-treatment magnetic resonance imaging lesions may predict long-term clinical outcomes in patients receiving interferon β-1a. This study aimed to assess the effect of active T2 and T1 gadolinium-enhancing (Gd+) lesions on relapses and 3-month confirmed Expanded Disability Status Scale (EDSS) progression in the PRISMS clinical trial.

Methods: Exploratory analyses assessed whether active T2 and T1 Gd + lesions at Month 6, or active T2 lesions at Month 12, predicted clinical outcomes over 4 years in PRISMS.

Results: Mean active T2 lesion number at Month 6 was significantly lower with interferon beta-1a given subcutaneously (IFN β-1a SC) 44 μg and 22 μg 3×/week (tiw) than with placebo ($p < 0.0001$). The presence of ≥4 versus 0 active T2 lesions predicted disability progression at Years 3–4 in the IFN β-1a SC 22 μg group only ($p < 0.05$), whereas the presence of ≥2 versus 0–1 active T2 lesions predicted disability progression in the placebo/delayed treatment (DTx) (Years 2–4; $p < 0.05$) and IFN β-1a SC 22 μg groups (Years 3–4; $p < 0.05$). Greater active T2 lesion number at 6 months predicted relapses in the placebo/DTx group only (≥4 vs. 0, Years 1–4; ≥2 vs. 0–1, Years 2–4; $p < 0.05$), and the presence of T1 Gd + lesions at 6 months predicted disability progression in the IFN β-1a SC 44 μg group only (Year 1; $p < 0.05$). The presence of ≥2 versus 0–1 active T2 lesions at 12 months predicted disability progression over 3 and 4 years in the IFN β-1a SC 44 μg group.

Conclusion: Active T2 lesions at 6 months predicted clinical outcomes in patients receiving placebo or IFN β-1a SC 22 μg, but not in those receiving IFN β-1a SC 44 μg. Active T2 lesions at 12 months may predict outcomes in those receiving IFN β-1a SC 44 μg and are possibly more suggestive of poor response to therapy than T2 results at 6 months.

Keywords: MRI, Multiple sclerosis, T2 lesions, Gadolinium-enhancing lesions, Treatment response, Beta-interferon

* Correspondence: t.traboulsee@ubc.ca
[1]University of British Columbia, S113-2211 Wesbrook Mall, Vancouver, BC V6T 1Z7, Canada
Full list of author information is available at the end of the article

Background

Considerable evidence indicates that early treatment of relapsing forms of multiple sclerosis (RMS) is critical in order to delay disease progression and accumulation of irreversible disability. Therefore, as the repertoire of disease-modifying drugs (DMDs) for RMS has grown, it is increasingly important for physicians who treat patients with RMS to know when to consider treatment changes in order to derive maximum benefit from the available treatment options within the available window of opportunity. There is currently no single evidence-based algorithm to guide these decisions due to the inherent heterogeneity of RMS. In its absence, clinical and subclinical indicators of continued disease activity are being evaluated for their ability to define breakthrough disease and potential to predict long-term outcomes.

Randomized clinical trials assessing DMDs for RMS rely on clinical disease endpoints: the occurrence of relapses and confirmed disability progression [1–3]. However, modern MS clinical trial populations show lower levels of clinical disease activity compared with previously reported cohorts [3–6]. The reduced level of disease activity has led to a greater focus on alternative outcomes capable of acting as sensitive surrogates for relapses or disability progression [7–10].

MRI lesions, including T2-weighted hyperintense or T1 gadolinium-enhancing (Gd+) lesions, indicate focal inflammatory activity in RMS and may be present in patients who are clinically stable. These lesions have been proposed as a surrogate marker capable of predicting long-term treatment outcomes in patients with RMS. Although the pathophysiological relationship between MRI lesions and disease progression in MS is complex, MRI is an important component of MS diagnosis, and MRI lesion loads may allow treatment success to be predicted at early time points [9, 11]. Multiple studies of patients treated with interferon (IFN) β-1a therapies have suggested an association between the presence of early on-treatment T2 or T1 Gd + MRI lesions and an increased risk of relapse or disease progression at subsequent time points [7, 9, 10, 12, 13]. MRI results at early time points may, therefore, prove to be a useful tool for assessing the overall efficacy of DMDs, identifying breakthrough disease, and predicting long-term responses of individual patients to therapy.

PRISMS-2 was a 2-year randomized clinical trial designed to evaluate the use of IFN β-1a injected subcutaneously (SC) three times weekly (tiw) in patients with relapsing–remitting MS (RRMS) [3]. Both the 44- and 22-μg doses of IFN β-1a SC tiw demonstrated significant improvements on clinical and MRI measures of disease, compared with placebo [3]. A long-term follow-up study (PRISMS-4), in which patients treated with placebo in the original PRISMS study were reassigned to either IFN β-1a 44 or 22 μg SC tiw, assessed the efficacy of IFN β-1a SC tiw over a 4-year period [14]. Therapy with IFN β-1a SC tiw maintained a treatment benefit after 4 years of treatment, and outcomes were superior in patients who were treated with IFN β-1a SC tiw for all 4 years of the study, compared with those who began IFN β-1a SC tiw treatment after 2 years [14].

This study investigated whether early T2 and T1 Gd + MRI lesions predicted subsequent clinical outcomes in patients treated with IFN β-1a 44 μg SC tiw, IFN β-1a 22 μg SC tiw, or placebo/delayed treatment over a 4-year period in the PRISMS clinical trial.

Methods

Study design and treatment

The details of the PRISMS-2 study design have been published previously [3]. Briefly, patients with RRMS, an Expanded Disability Status Scale (EDSS) score of ≤5, and no prior treatment with IFN β were randomized 1:1:1 to IFN β-1a 44 μg SC tiw, IFN β-1a 22 μg SC tiw, or placebo. All patients had proton density (PD)/T2-weighted MRI scans twice a year. A subgroup also had monthly T2 and T1 Gd + scans before and during the first 9 months of treatment (frequent-MRI cohort).

Exploratory analyses

Exploratory analyses assessed the number of T2 lesions per patient at Month 6 and Month 12. The number of active T2 lesions was calculated as the sum of new, newly enlarging, and recurring T2 lesions on the 6-month MRI scan with reference to the baseline MRI scan. Further exploratory analyses investigated the predictive value of active T2 and T1 Gd + lesions at 6 months on EDSS progression (increase of ≥0.5 points if baseline EDSS was ≥6.0 or increase of ≥1 point if baseline EDSS was < 6.0, confirmed 3 months later) and relapses over Years 1 and 2 (PRISMS-2) and Years 3 and 4 (PRISMS-4). The effect of active T2 lesions at 6 months on time to EDSS progression was calculated over a 4-year period. Additional exploratory analyses evaluated the predictive effect of active T2 lesions at 12 months on EDSS progression and relapses over Years 1, 2, 3, and 4, as well as time to EDSS progression over 4 years.

Statistical analyses

Between-treatment comparisons of mean active T2 lesion number per patient used a negative binomial regression model with baseline burden of disease and treatment as independent factors. The effect of T2 lesions (≥4 vs. 0 and ≥ 2 vs. 0–1) on relapse and EDSS progression was assessed in the entire cohort using a logistic regression model. The logistic regression models examining the predictive value of T1 Gd + lesions analyzed data from the frequent-MRI cohort. Hazard ratios

(HRs) and *p*-values for between-group differences in time to first EDSS progression were calculated using a Cox-proportional hazards model.

Results

In total, 560 patients were randomized: 187 to the placebo group, 184 to the IFN β-1a 44 μg SC tiw group, and 189 to the IFN β-1a 22 μg SC tiw group. Baseline characteristics were similar among all three treatment groups, as has been previously reported (Table 1) [3]. The proportions of patients who experienced relapses and sustained disability progression by Years 2 and 4 are shown in Table 2.

Early T2 MRI scan results in PRISMS-2

In total, among subjects with data, 147 of 186 patients (79.0%) in the placebo/delayed treatment group had one or more active T2 lesions at 6 months, compared with 100 of 185 (54.1%) and 87 of 182 (47.8%) patients in the IFN β-1a 22 and 44 μg SC tiw groups, respectively. The mean (standard deviation [SD]) number of active T2 lesions per patient at 6 months was 4.1 (5.72) in the placebo group, compared with 2.1 (4.28) in the IFN β-1a 22 μg SC tiw group and 1.3 (2.34) in the IFN β-1a 44 μg SC tiw group (*p* < 0.0001 for each IFN β-1a group vs. placebo).

Relationship between active T2 lesions at 6 months and EDSS progression

No statistically significant differences in the proportions of patients with EDSS progression at Years 1, 2, 3, and 4 were seen between patients with ≥4 versus 0 active T2 lesions at Month 6 in the IFN β-1a 44 μg SC tiw or placebo/delayed treatment groups (Fig. 1a and c). However, the presence of ≥4 versus 0 active T2 lesions at Month 6 predicted EDSS progression at Years 3 and 4 in the IFN β-1a 22 μg SC tiw group (Fig. 1b). The presence of ≥2 versus 0–1 active T2 lesions at 6 months predicted EDSS

progression in the placebo/delayed treatment (Years 2, 3, and 4) and IFN β-1a 22 μg SC tiw (Years 3 and 4) groups, but not in the IFN β-1a 44 μg SC tiw group (Figure S1a–c shows this in more detail [see Additional file 1]). Notably, EDSS progression in patients treated with IFN β-1a 44 μg SC tiw who had ≥4 or 0 active T2 lesions at Month 6 occurred at a rate similar to that in patients treated with placebo who had no active T2 lesions at Month 6 (Figure S2 shows this in more detail [see Additional file 2]). The predictive performance of active T2 lesions on EDSS progression is shown in Table S1(a) (see Additional file 3). Positive and negative predictive values for EDSS progression according to active T2 lesions at Month 6 (≥4 vs. 0) were consistently higher in the placebo/delayed treatment group than in the IFN β-1a 44 μg SC tiw group.

Time to first EDSS progression over 4 years was significantly reduced for patients with ≥4 versus 0 active T2 lesions at Month 6 in the IFN β-1a 22 μg SC tiw group, but not in the IFN β-1a 44 μg SC tiw or the placebo/delayed treatment group (Fig. 2a–c). For patients with ≥2 versus 0–1 active T2 lesions, significant reductions in time to EDSS progression were seen in the placebo/delayed treatment group (*p* = 0.0132), but not in either IFN β-1a SC tiw group (Figure S3 shows this in more detail [see Additional file 4]).

Relationship between active T2 lesions at 6 months and relapses

The presence of ≥4 versus 0 active T2 lesions at Month 6 predicted relapses in the placebo/delayed treatment group (Years 1–4; Fig. 3a), but not in either IFN β-1a SC tiw group (Fig. 3b and c). Similar results were seen when patients with ≥2 versus 0–1 active T2 lesions at Month 6 were compared (Figure S4 shows this in more detail [see Additional file 5]). The predictive performance of active T2 lesions at 6 months on relapse at Year 2 and Year 4 is shown in Table S1(b) (see Additional file 3).

Table 1 Demographic characteristics at baseline

	Placebo			IFN β-1a 22 μg SC tiw			IFN β-1a 44 μg SC tiw		
	Number of active T2 lesions at 6 months		All (*n* = 187)	Number of active T2 lesions at 6 months		All (*n* = 189)	Number of active T2 lesions at 6 months		All (*n* = 184)
	0 (*n* = 39)	≥4 (*n* = 64)		0 (*n* = 85)	≥4 (*n* = 28)		0 (*n* = 95)	≥4 (*n* = 24)	
Age, years, mean (SD)	36.4 (7.3)	33.4 (7.8)	34.7 (7.5)	35.6 (6.5)	30.2 (7.3)	34.8 (7.0)	35.5 (8.0)	33.0 (6.7)	35.2 (7.9)
Sex, female, *n* (%)	31 (79)	47 (73)	141 (75)	53 (62)	21 (75)	126 (67)	63 (66)	14 (58)	122 (66)
Race, white, *n* (%)	38 (97)	63 (98)	184 (98)	84 (99)	28 (100)	188 (99)	94 (99)	24 (100)	182 (99)
Time since MS onset, years, mean (SD)	6.6 (5.4)	5.3 (4.3)	6.1 (4.8)	7.9 (6.45)	5.4 (4.3)	7.7 (6.1)	7.1 (5.6)	7.4 (6.9)	7.8 (6.3)
Number of relapses in past 2 years, mean (SD)	2.7 (0.8)	3.3 (1.4)	3.0 (1.3)	2.9 (1.0)	3.2 (1.2)	3.0 (1.1)	2.9 (1.0)	3.5 (1.6)	3.0 (1.1)
EDSS score, median	2.0	2.5	2.5	2.5	2.0	2.5	2.5	3.0	2.5

EDSS Expanded Disability Status Scale, *IFN β-1a* interferon beta-1a, *SC* subcutaneously, *SD* standard deviation, *tiw* three times weekly

Table 2 Proportion of patients with relapses or confirmed disability progression, Year 2 (PRISMS-2) and 4 (PRISMS-4)

	Placebo/delayed treatment (n = 187)	IFN β-1a 22 μg SC tiw (n = 189)	IFN β-1a 44 μg SC tiw (n = 184)
Relapse by Year 2 (%)	84.5	73.0	67.9
Relapse by Year 4 (%)	90.4	82.0	78.8
Confirmed EDSS progression by Year 2 (%)	39.0	31.2	27.7
Confirmed EDSS progression by Year 4 (%)	48.1	45.0	39.7

EDSS progression was defined as an increase of ≥0.5 points if baseline EDSS was ≥6 or increase of ≥1 point if baseline EDSS was < 6, confirmed 3 months later
EDSS Expanded Disability Status Scale, *IFN β-1a* interferon beta-1a, *SC* subcutaneously, *tiw* three times weekly

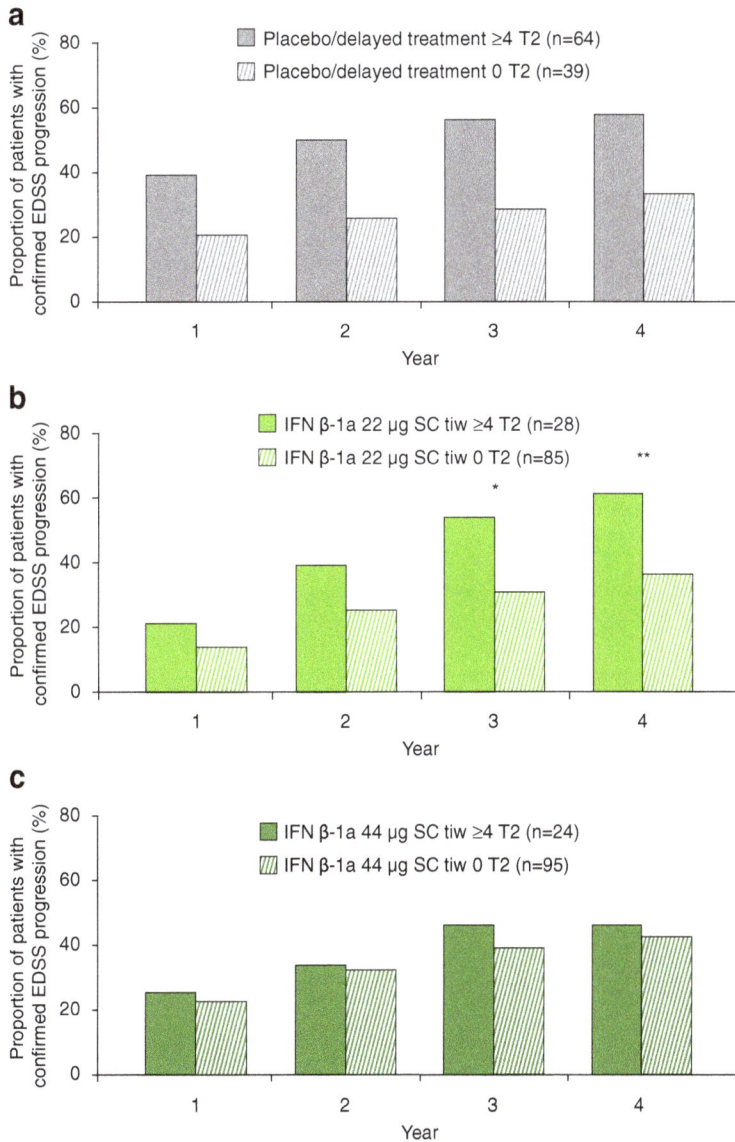

Fig. 1 Proportion progressed at each year by ≥4 versus 0 active T2 lesions at 6 months. **a** Placebo/delayed treatment, ≥4 versus 0 T2 lesions at 6 months; **b** IFN β-1a 22 μg SC tiw, ≥4 versus 0 T2 lesions at 6 months; **c** IFN β-1a 44 μg SC tiw, ≥4 versus 0 T2 lesions at 6 months. *p* values indicate differences between patients with differing lesion loads at 6 months within the treatment group. No statistically significant differences were seen in the placebo/delayed treatment or IFN β-1a 44 μg SC tiw group. Values were calculated with a logistic regression model with predictor (≥4 vs. 0 T2 lesions) as a fixed effect; number of relapses within the previous 2 years, age, baseline EDSS score, and baseline burden of disease were independent variables, and *p* values were calculated for the predictive effect of T2 lesion subgroups. *p < 0.05; **p < 0.01. EDSS: Expanded Disability Status Scale; IFN β-1a: interferon beta-1a; SC: subcutaneously; tiw: three times weekly

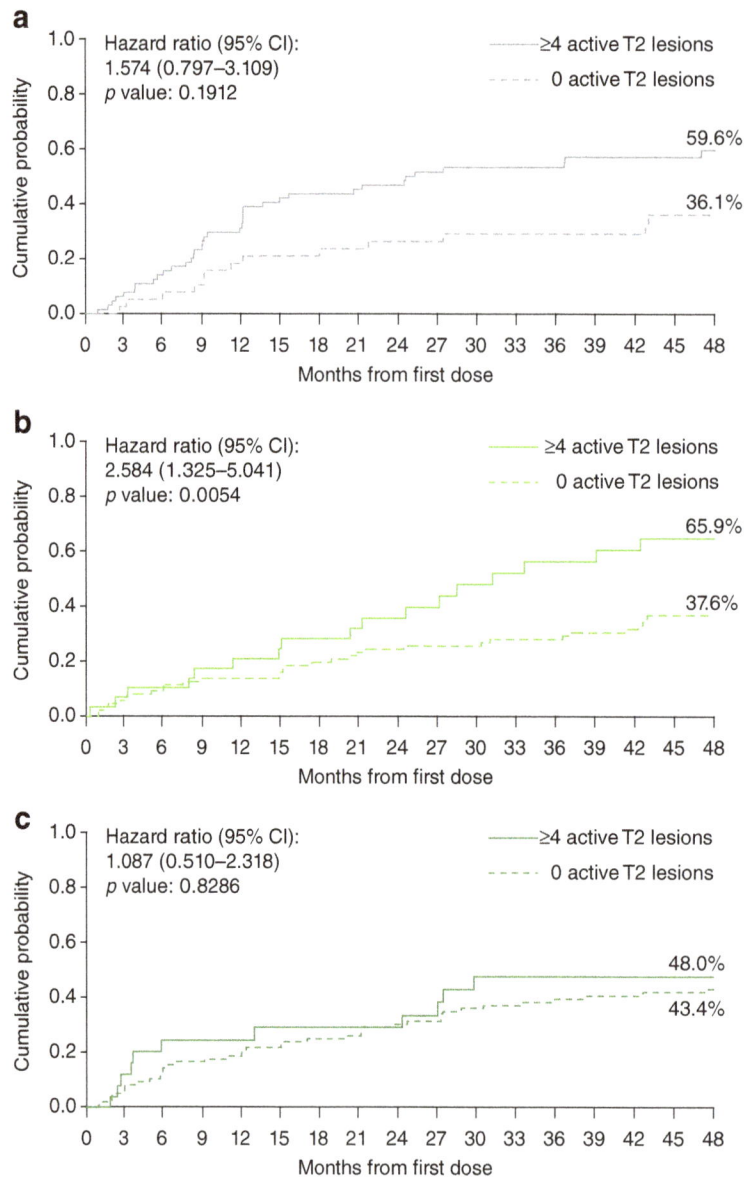

Fig. 2 Time to sustained EDSS progression by ≥4 versus 0 active T2 lesions at 6 months. **a** Placebo/delayed treatment group; **b** IFN β-1a 22 μg SC tiw group; **c** IFN β-1a 44 μg SC tiw group. A Cox proportional hazards model, adjusted for number of relapses in the previous 2 years, age, baseline EDSS score, and baseline burden of disease, was used to estimate hazard ratios and p values. p values are for time to first progression over 4 years. CI: confidence interval; EDSS: Expanded Disability Status Scale; IFN β-1a: interferon beta-1a; SC: subcutaneously; tiw: three times weekly

Relationship between T1 Gd + lesions at 6 months and clinical outcomes (relapses and EDSS progression)

The presence of T1 Gd + lesions at 6 months did not predict EDSS progression in the placebo/delayed treatment group or the IFN β-1a 22 μg SC tiw group in Years 1–4 (Fig. 4a and b). A significantly higher proportion of patients in the IFN β-1a 44 μg SC tiw group who had T1 Gd + lesions at 6 months experienced EDSS progression at Year 4 versus those

without T1 Gd + lesions ($p < 0.05$; Fig. 4c). Presumably due to the effectiveness of treatment, the number of patients in the IFN β-1a 44 μg SC tiw group with T1 Gd + lesions at 6 months was small ($n = 9$). However, when comparing patients with ≥2 T1 Gd + lesions versus those with 0–1 T1 Gd + lesions at Month 6, there was a statistically significant difference in the proportion of patients who experienced EDSS progression at Year 2 in the IFN β-1a 44 μg SC tiw

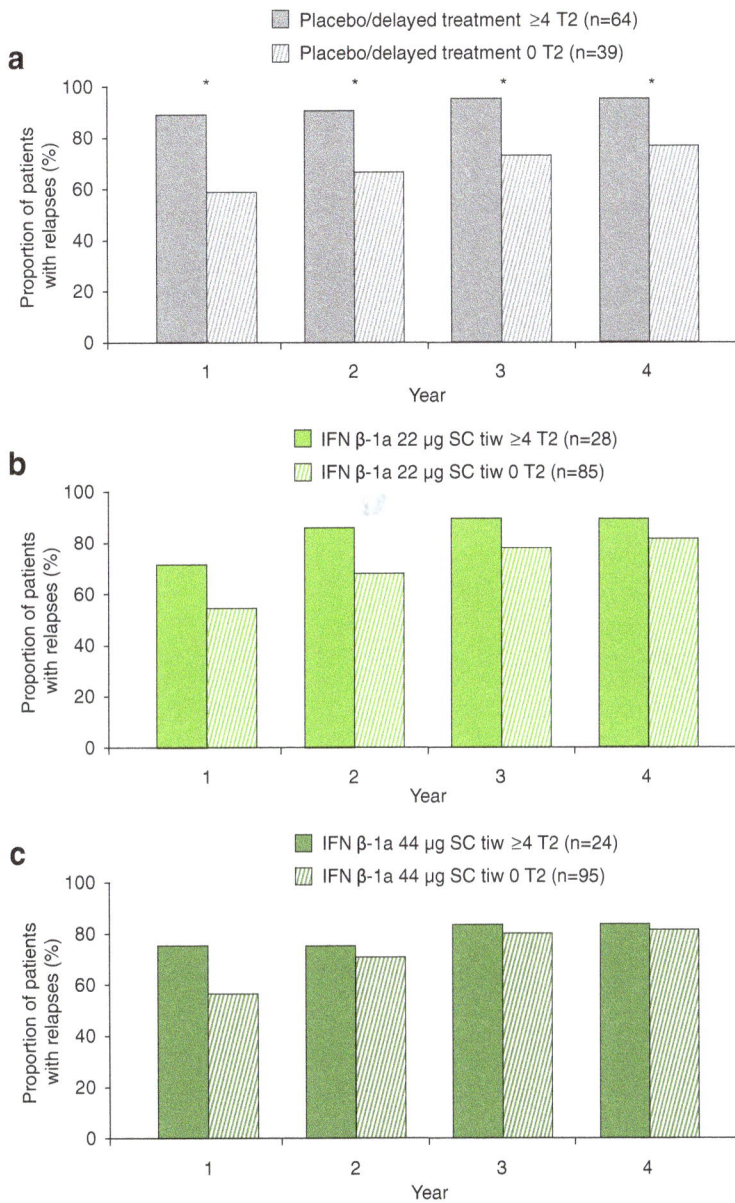

Fig. 3 Proportion relapsed at each year: ≥4 versus 0 active T2 lesions at 6 months **a** Placebo/delayed treatment group; **b** IFN β-1a 22 μg SC tiw group; **c** IFN β-1a 44 μg SC tiw group. *p* values indicate differences between patients with differing lesion loads at 6 months within the treatment group. No statistically significant differences were seen in the placebo/delayed treatment or IFN β-1a 44 μg SC tiw group. Values were calculated with a logistic regression model; number of relapses within previous 2 years, age, baseline EDSS score, and baseline burden of disease were independent variables, and *p* values were calculated for the predictive effect of T2 lesion subgroups. *$p < 0.05$. EDSS: Expanded Disability Status Scale; IFN β-1a: interferon beta-1a; SC: subcutaneously; tiw: three times weekly

group ($p = 0.0375$). Notably, the number of patients in the IFN β-1a 44 μg SC tiw group with ≥2 T1 Gd + lesions at 6 months was very small ($n = 3$).

The presence of T1 Gd + lesions at 6 months did not predict relapses in any of the treatment groups (Fig. 5a–c). Similar results were seen when comparing patients with ≥2 T1 Gd + lesions versus those with 0–1 T1 Gd + lesions at Month 6 (data not shown).

Relationship between active T2 lesions at 12 months and EDSS progression

No statistically significant differences in the proportions of patients with EDSS progression at Years 1, 2, 3, and 4 were seen between patients with ≥4 versus 0 active T2 lesions at Month 12 in any of the treatment groups. However, numerically greater proportions of patients with ≥4 versus 0 lesions exhibited EDSS progression

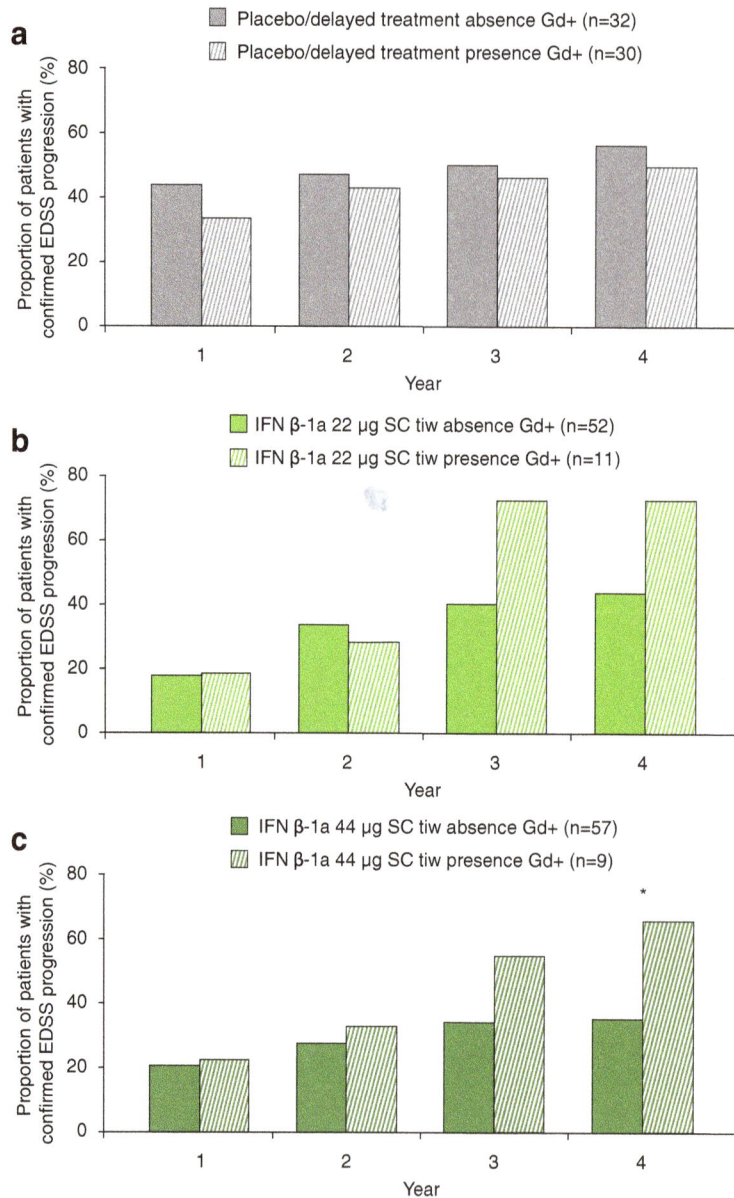

Fig. 4 Proportion with EDSS progression at each year by T1 Gd + lesions at 6 months. **a** Placebo/delayed treatment group; **b** IFN β-1a 22 μg SC tiw group; **c** IFN β-1a 44 μg SC tiw group. There was a significant difference in the number of patients who had T1 Gd + lesions at 6 months and who experienced confirmed disability progression at 4 years in the IFN β-1a 44 μg SC tiw group, albeit in a small number of patients ($n = 9$). No statistically significant differences were seen in the placebo/delayed treatment or IFN β-1a 22 μg SC tiw groups. Values were based on logistic regression model adjusting for number of relapses within the previous 2 years, age, baseline EDSS score, and baseline T1 Gd + lesions. p values were calculated for the predictive effect of T1 Gd + lesions. *$p < 0.05$. EDSS: Expanded Disability Status Scale; Gd+: gadolinium-enhancing; IFN β-1a: interferon beta-1a; SC: subcutaneously; tiw: three times weekly

over 4 years in each group (Fig. 6). Within the IFN β-1a 44 μg SC tiw group, the numeric difference in proportion with progression between those with ≥4 versus 0 lesions grew more pronounced with each year. The predictive value of active T2 lesions at Month 12 for EDSS progression is shown in Table S1(a) [see Additional file 3]. The presence of ≥2 versus 0–1 active T2 lesions at Month 12 predicted EDSS progression in the IFN β-1a 44 μg SC tiw group over Years 3 and 4 (Figure S5 shows this in more detail [see Additional file 6]).

The presence of ≥4 versus 0 active T2 lesions at 12 months was associated with numeric trends toward reduced time to first EDSS progression in each treatment group (HR: 1.215 [95% confidence interval

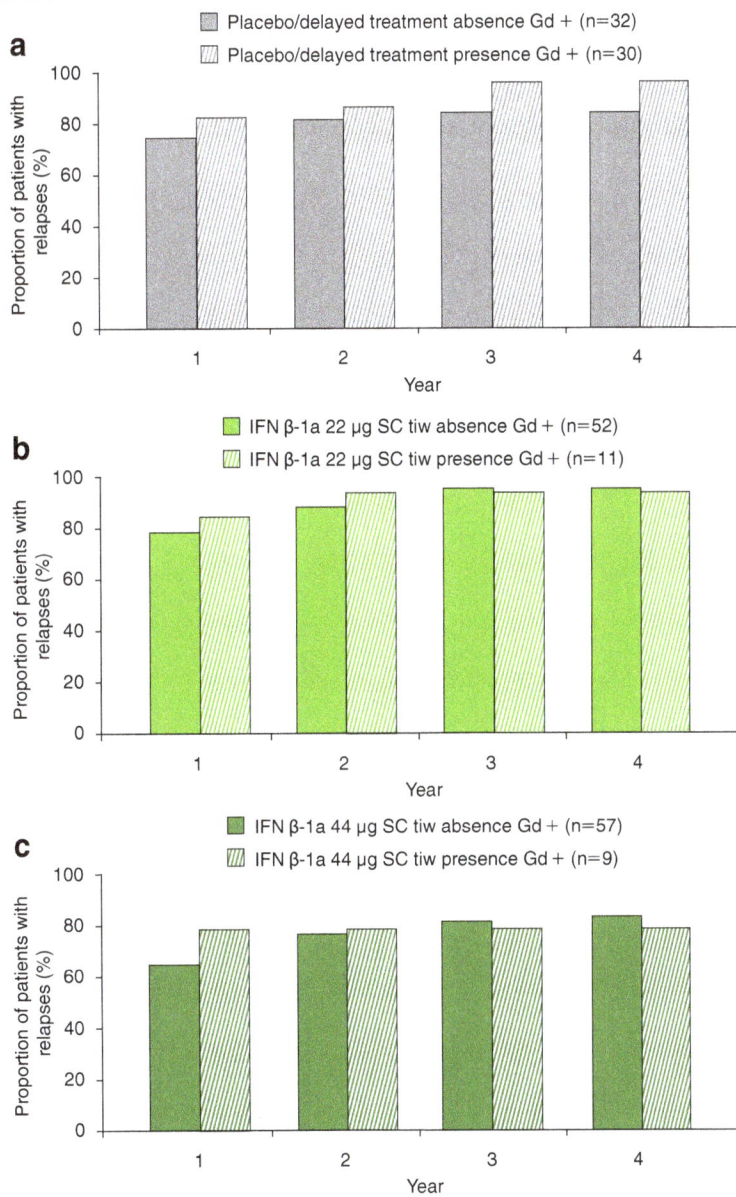

Fig. 5 Proportion relapsed at each year by T1 Gd + lesions at 6 months. **a** Placebo/delayed treatment group; **b** IFN β-1a 22 μg SC tiw group; **c** IFN β-1a 44 μg SC tiw group. No statistically significant differences were seen in any of the treatment groups. Values were based on logistic regression model adjusting for number of relapses within the previous 2 years, age, baseline EDSS score, and baseline T1 Gd + lesions. *p* values were calculated for the predictive effect of T1 Gd + lesions. EDSS: Expanded Disability Status Scale; Gd+: gadolinium-enhancing; IFN β-1a: interferon beta-1a; SC: subcutaneously; tiw: three times weekly

(CI): 0.634, 2.327], 1.358 [0.707, 2.608], and 1.817 [0. 851, 3.879] for placebo/delayed treatment, IFN β-1a 22 μg SC tiw, and IFN β-1a 44 μg SC tiw groups, respectively [*p* > 0.05]). For patients with ≥2 versus 0–1 active T2 lesions, significant reductions in time to EDSS progression were seen in the IFN β-1a 44 μg SC tiw group (HR: 1.970 [95% CI: 1.150, 3.376]; *p* = 0.0136) but not in the placebo/delayed treatment group (*p* = 0.5565) or IFN β-1a 22 μg SC tiw group (*p* = 0.5684).

Relationship between active T2 lesions at 12 months and relapses

Similar to the results seen with lesions at Month 6, the presence of ≥4 versus 0 active T2 lesions at Month 12 predicted relapses in the placebo/delayed treatment group (Years 1–4; Fig. 7), but not in either IFN β-1a SC tiw group. Again, results similar to the effect of lesions at 6 months were seen when patients with ≥2 versus 0–1 active T2 lesions at Month 12 were compared (Figure S6 shows this in more detail [see Additional file 7]).

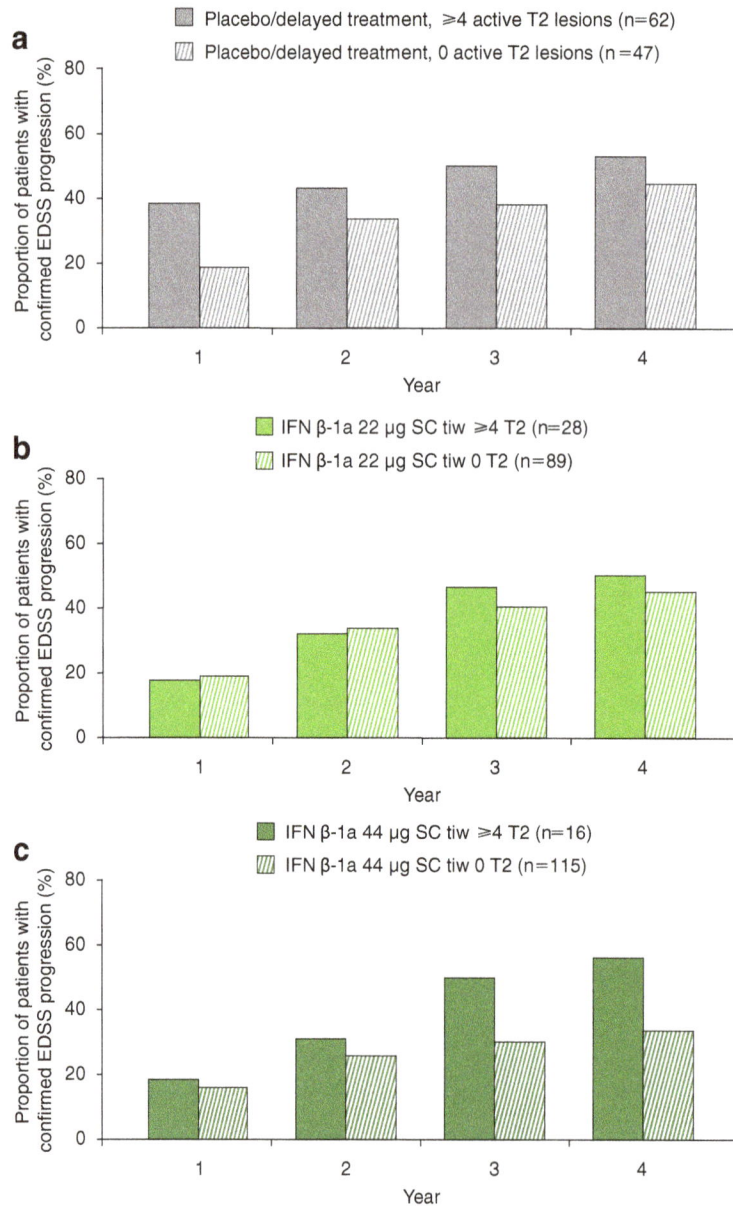

Fig. 6 Proportion progressed at each year by ≥4 versus 0 active T2 lesions at 12 months. **a** Placebo/delayed treatment, ≥4 versus 0 T2 lesions at 12 months; **b** IFN β-1a 22 μg SC tiw, ≥4 versus 0 T2 lesions at 12 months; **c** IFN β-1a 44 μg SC tiw, ≥4 versus 0 T2 lesions at 12 months. No statistically significant differences were seen in any treatment group. Values were calculated with a logistic regression model with predictor (≥4 vs 0 T2 lesions) as a fixed effect; number of relapses within the previous 2 years, age, baseline EDSS score, and baseline burden of disease were independent variables, and p-values were calculated for the predictive effect of T2 lesion subgroups. EDSS: Expanded Disability Status Scale; IFN β-1a: interferon beta-1a; SC: subcutaneously; tiw: three times weekly

Discussion

These exploratory analyses demonstrate that active T2 lesions at Month 6 were not predictive of longer term clinical disease activity in the IFN β-1a 44 μg SC tiw group in PRISMS, and were predictive in the placebo/delayed treatment (EDSS progression and relapses) and IFN β-1a 22 μg SC tiw groups (EDSS progression only). Our data both challenge and extend the previous studies that linked the presence of active T2 lesions to suboptimal treatment responses and clinical outcomes [7, 10, 13, 15]. The results of such previous studies led to suggestions that active lesions identified during treatment with IFN β-1a or other DMDs signify treatment failure and should trigger consideration of treatment changes [7, 15]. Our findings instead indicate that early (6 months) active T2 lesions are not predictive of long-term outcomes with high-dose IFN SC tiw, while T1 Gd + lesions at 6 months may be relevant to future clinical

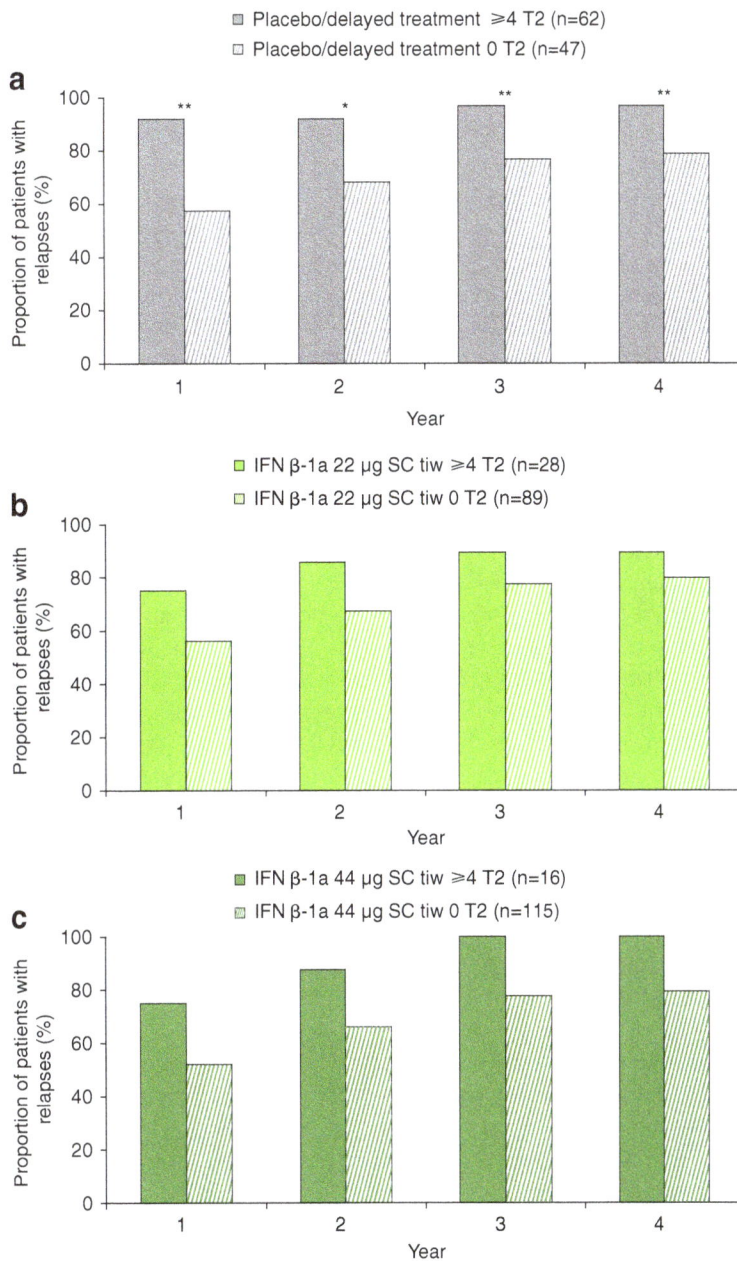

Fig. 7 Proportion relapsed at each year: ≥4 versus 0 active T2 lesions at 12 months. **a** Placebo/delayed treatment group; **b** IFN β-1a 22 μg SC tiw group; **c** IFN β-1a 44 μg SC tiw group. p-values indicate differences between patients with differing lesion loads at 12 months within the treatment group. No statistically significant differences were seen in the IFN β-1a SC tiw groups. Values were calculated with a logistic regression model; number of relapses within previous 2 years, age, baseline EDSS score, and baseline burden of disease were independent variables, and p-values were calculated for the predictive effect of T2-lesion subgroups. *$p < 0.05$; **$p < 0.01$. EDSS: Expanded Disability Status Scale; IFN β-1a: interferon beta-1a; SC: subcutaneously; tiw: three times weekly

outcomes. Additionally, the presence of continued T2 activity after 1 year of treatment suggests that response to treatment is lacking.

Our findings provide new data suggesting that the predictive strength of early on-treatment T2 lesions may be modified by treatment factors. In this historical cohort of patients with RMS, active T2 lesions at 6 months were predictive of clinical outcomes in the placebo/delayed treatment and IFN β-1a 22 μg SC tiw groups, but not in the IFN β-1a 44 μg SC tiw group, suggesting that the predictive strength of early on-treatment MRI lesions may depend on IFN β-1a SC tiw dose. Notably, EDSS progression in the IFN β-1a 44 μg SC tiw group, irrespective of 6-month T2 lesion number, occurred at a rate similar to that in patients in the placebo/delayed treatment group (especially before the treatment switch to IFN β-1a 44 μg SC tiw at the end of Year 2) who had no T2 lesions. Indeed, no trend toward greater likelihood of EDSS progression or relapse was seen in the IFN β-1a SC tiw group, even when patients with ≥4 active T2 lesions at 6 months were compared with patients with no T2 lesions.

Importantly, we also show that on-treatment T1 Gd + lesions at 6 months may be predictive of future disability progression. We propose that the active T2 lesions at 6 months are indicative of accumulated disease activity over the entire period of Months 0–6 when the treatment might not yet be fully effective, while a true lack of treatment response is evident by the T1 Gd + lesion activity at Month 6.

MAGNIMS Consensus Guidelines consider that using a baseline MRI scan as the reference point for new activity after treatment initiation carries the possibility of misinterpretation, as new activity before treatment was initiated or before drug therapy became effective could be mistakenly identified as representing suboptimal response [16]. For instance, in PRISMS-2, the period between baseline and 6 months would include the first 8 weeks of administration, when the dose of IFN β-1a SC tiw was being titrated up to the full assigned dose. Although reduction in MRI activity in the subgroup undergoing monthly scanning was observed as early as 2 months after N β-1a SC tiw treatment began [17], in recognition of the possibility that the full treatment effect may not be evident by 6 months, we also examined as a predictor the new T2 activity at 12 months (with reference to the 6-month scan). The comparison of ≥4 versus 0 T2 lesions at 12 months was not shown to significantly predict future progression. However, numeric trends suggest that lesions at 12 months may be a more useful means of identifying nonresponders to IFN β-1a SC 44 μg than lesions at 6 months; indeed, comparing ≥2 versus 0–1 active T2 lesions at 12 months predicted future progression in this group. Taken together, these observations suggest that T2 activity over the first 6 months of IFN β-1a SC 44 μg treatment may not indicate treatment failure, while activity after a full year is suggestive of nonresponse. Conversely, as the comparison of ≥2 vs 0–1 T2 lesions at 6 months predicted future progression in both the placebo/delayed treatment and IFN β-1a SC 22 μg groups, the IFN β-1a SC 22 μg dose, while beneficial to many patients, shares some similarity with placebo in that results as early as 6 months may be suggestive of future progression.

Previous studies evaluating treatment response according to MRI results in patients receiving IFN β-1a have assessed differing treatment regimens and utilized varying on-treatment MRI time points (6 months to 2 years after study baseline), assessment types (T1 Gd + or T2 lesions), and thresholds for numbers of lesions [8, 10, 12, 18, 19]. As such, the inconsistent results seen between studies suggest that the predictive value of early MRI lesions may depend on IFN β dose, the timing and type of MRI scans obtained, and the overall study protocol. Importantly, a recent study of accrual of long-term disability in a cohort of patients with RMS showed that emergence of new/enlarging T2 lesions in the first 2 years on study did not predict clinical worsening (as measured by EDSS, the Timed-25 Foot Walk, the 9-Hole Peg Test, or the Paced Serial Auditory Addition Test-3) over 10 years, again suggesting that radiological activity alone may not be predictive of long-term outcomes [20].

As the number of effective DMDs available for RMS treatment grows, some experts have advocated a "zero tolerance" approach to subclinical disease activity, suggesting that even a single MRI lesion is evidence of treatment failure and should trigger a change in therapy [21]. However, the results presented in this analysis suggest the need for a more nuanced approach to the prognostic value of on-treatment MRI activity. The predictive nature of T2 lesions is strongly influenced by whether patients are on high-dose, high-frequency treatment at the time when MRI scans are performed, and the presence of a small number of active T2 lesions on early MRI scans should not automatically warrant treatment changes. On the other hand, patients who continue to have T1 Gd + lesions, or active T2 lesions after a year of therapy, may be true non-responders of IFN β-1a SC tiw treatment and might benefit from alternative therapies.

Limitations of this study include the exploratory nature of the analyses and the primary focus on T2 lesions. T1 Gd + lesions were assessed only over 9 months and in just a subset of patients. Data from other studies have suggested that the presence of early T1 Gd + lesions on MRI scans may also be predictive of subsequent clinical outcomes [18].

Conclusions

The results of this study suggest that although early (6 months) on-treatment active T2 lesions may predict long-term clinical activity in patients receiving placebo or low-dose IFN β-1a SC tiw, this association is not seen in patients treated with high-dose IFN β-1a SC tiw (44 μg). On-treatment T1 Gd + lesions at Month 6, however, may predict subsequent clinical outcomes with IFN β-1a 44 μg SC tiw. Notably, very few patients on treatment have T1 Gd + lesions, indicating that the vast majority of patients respond well to the high-dose IFN β-1a SC tiw treatment. Emergence of active T2 lesions after 6 months of IFN β-1a 44 μg SC tiw treatment in the absence of T1 Gd + lesions should not be cause to consider treatment changes. However, active T2 lesions at 12 months and T1 Gd + lesions at 6 months may be cause to consider nonresponse to treatment. Early MRI results can therefore be successfully integrated into the treatment algorithms that are used to decide whether patients are responding to treatment.

Additional files

Additional file 1: Figure S1. Proportion with EDSS progression at each year by ≥2 versus 0–1 active T2 lesions at 6 months. (a) Placebo/delayed treatment group; (b) IFN β-1a 22 μg SC tiw group; (c) IFN β-1a 44 μg SC tiw group.

Additional file 2: Figure S2. Proportion with EDSS progression at each year in the placebo/delayed treatment and IFN β-1a 44 μg SC tiw groups by ≥4 versus 0 active T2 lesions at 6 months.

Additional file 3: Table S1. (a) Performance of T2 lesions on predicting EDSS progression at Year 2 and Year 4. (b) Performance of T2 lesions on predicting relapse at Year 2 and Year 4.

Additional file 4: Figure S3. Time to sustained EDSS progression by ≥2 versus 0–1 active T2 lesions at 6 months. (a) Placebo/delayed treatment group; (b) IFN β-1a 22 μg SC tiw group; (c) IFN β-1a 44 μg SC tiw group.

Additional file 5: Figure S4. Proportion relapsed at each year by ≥2 versus 0–1 active T2 lesions at 6 months. (a) Placebo/delayed treatment group; (b) IFN β-1a 22 μg SC tiw group; (c) IFN β-1a 44 μg SC tiw group.

Additional file 6: Figure S5. Proportion progressed at each year by ≥2 versus 0–1 active T2 lesions at 12 months. (a) Placebo/delayed treatment, ≥2 versus 0–1 T2 lesions at 12 months; (b) IFN β-1a 22 μg SC tiw, ≥2 versus 0–1 T2 lesions at 12 months; (c) IFN β-1a 44 μg SC tiw, ≥2 versus 0–1 T2 lesions at 12 months.

Additional file 7: Figure S6. Proportion relapsed at each year by ≥2 versus 0–1 active T2 lesions at 12 months. (a) Placebo/delayed treatment group; (b) IFN β-1a 22 μg SC tiw group; (c) IFN β-1a 44 μg SC tiw group.

Abbreviations

CI: Confidence interval; DMD: Disease-modifying drug; EDSS: Expanded Disability Status Scale; Gd + : Gadolinium-enhancing; HR: Hazard ratio; IFN: Interferon; MRI: Magnetic resonance imaging; MS: Multiple sclerosis; PD: Proton density; RMS: Relapsing forms of multiple sclerosis; RRMS: Relapsing–remitting multiple sclerosis; SC: Subcutaneously; SD: Standard deviation; tiw: Three times weekly; Y: Year

Acknowledgements
The authors thank Matthew Thomas, DPhil, of Caudex, Oxford, UK (supported by EMD Serono, Inc., Rockland, MA, USA (a business of Merck KGaA, Darmstadt, Germany) and Pfizer Inc., New York, NY, USA) for editorial assistance in drafting the manuscript, collating the comments of authors, and assembling tables and figures. The authors also thank the University of British Columbia MS/MRI Research Group for analysis and review of the MRI scan data.

Funding
This study and analyses were supported by EMD Serono, Inc., Rockland, MA, USA (a business of Merck KGaA, Darmstadt, Germany) and Pfizer Inc., New York, NY, USA. The sponsor planned the post hoc analyses reported here in cooperation with the authors. Analysis and interpretation was performed by the authors. The authors were involved in all stages of development and finalization of the manuscript and received editorial assistance from an

independent medical-writing-services agency paid by EMD Serono, Inc., Rockland, MA, USA (a business of Merck KGaA, Darmstadt, Germany) and Pfizer Inc., New York, NY, USA.

Authors' contributions
DKBL contributed collection of original data, analysis and interpretation of data, and revision of the manuscript for important intellectual content. JF contributed acquisition and interpretation of post hoc analysis data and revision of the manuscript for important intellectual content. AT, MC, FD, and AM contributed to the analysis and interpretation of the data, and to the writing of the manuscript and/or its revision for important intellectual content. AT, DKBL, MC, JF, FD, and AM read and approved the final manuscript.

Ethics approval and consent to participate
Ethics approval was obtained from appropriate Institutional Ethics Committees/Institutional Review Boards: Royal Melbourne Hospital, Melbourne, Victoria, Australia; Ethics Review Committee, Central Sydney Area Health Service, Camperdown, Australia; Health Sciences Centre, University of Western Ontario, London, Ontario, Canada; Ottawa General Hospital, Ottawa, Ontario, Canada; Office of Research Services, Clinical Screening Committee for Research Involving Human Subjects, University of British Columbia, Vancouver, British Columbia, Canada; Forskningsetikkommittén I Lund/Malmö, Lund University Hospital, Lund, Sweden; Independent Review Board, Amsterdam, Netherlands; Newcastle & North Tyneside Health Authorities, Newcastle upon Tyne, UK; Ethical Committee, University Hospital, Nottingham, UK; United Medical and Dental Schools, Division of Pharmacological Sciences, Department of Clinical Pharmacology, St. Thomas's Hospital, London, UK; Central Oxford Research Ethics Committee, Headington, Oxford, UK; Commissie voor Medische Ethiek/Klinisch Onderzoek, UZ Leuven, Leuven, Belgium; Limburgs Universitair Centrum, Diepenbeek, Belgium; Commission d'Ethique Hospito-Facultaire, Université catholique de Louvain, Louvain-la-Neuve, Belgium; Helsinki University Hospitals Ethical Committee, Helsinki, Finland; Joint Commission on Ethics of the Turku University Central Hospital, Turku University Central Hospital, Turku, Finland; Ethik-Kommission de Medizinischen Fakultät der Universität Würzburg, Würzburg University, Würzburg, Germany; Ethik-Kommission des Departementes für Innere Medizin, Kantonsspital Basel, Basel, Switzerland; Academisch Ziekenhuis Vrije Univeriteit Commissie Voor Medische Ethiek/Klinisch Onderzoek, Leuven, Belgium; Medisch Ethische Commissie, Academisch Ziekenhuis Rotterdam, Rotterdam, Netherlands; St. George's Healthcare NHS Trust, St George's Hospital, London, UK; and Commission d'Ethique du Département de Médicine, Hôpitaux Universitaires de Genève, Geneva, Switzerland. All patients gave written informed consent.

Competing interests
A Traboulsee has acted as a consultant for Biogen, Genzyme, Roche, and Teva, and is Principal Investigator on clinical trials for Biogen, Chugai, Genzyme, and Roche.
D Li is the Director of the University of British Columbia MS/MRI Research Group, which has been contracted to perform central analysis of MRI scans for therapeutic trials with Genzyme, Hoffmann-La Roche, Merck Serono, Nuron, Perspectives, and Sanofi-Aventis. He has acted as a consultant to Vertex Pharmaceuticals; has served on scientific advisory boards for Novartis, Nuron, and Roche; has served on a data and safety advisory board for Opexa; and has received research funding from the Canadian Institute of Health Research and Multiple Sclerosis Society of Canada.
M Cascione has received funding/honoraria for research, consultation, and speakers bureau participation from Acorda, Bayer HealthCare, Biogen, EMD Serono, Inc., Genentech, Genzyme/Sanofi, Novartis, Pfizer, Roche, and Teva Pharmaceuticals.
J Fang was an employee of EMD Serono, Inc., Rockland, MA, USA (a business of Merck KGaA, Darmstadt, Germany) at the time of writing.
F Dangond is an employee of EMD Serono, Inc., Billerica, MA, USA (a business of Merck KGaA, Darmstadt, Germany).

A Miller has received research support from Biogen, Sanofi-Genzyme, Mallinckrodt (Questcor), Novartis, and Roche/Genentech. He has acted as a consultant for Accordant Health Services (Caremark), Acorda Therapeutics, Alkermes, Biogen, EMD Serono, Sanofi Genzyme, GlaxoSmithKline, Mallinckrodt (Questcor), Novartis, and Roche/Genentech. He has served on the speakers bureau for Biogen, Genentech, and Sanofi Genzyme for unbranded disease awareness programs only.

Author details

[1]University of British Columbia, S113-2211 Wesbrook Mall, Vancouver, BC V6T 1Z7, Canada. [2]Tampa Neurology Associates, South Tampa Multiple Sclerosis Center, 2919 W. Swann Avenue, Suite 401, South Tampa, FL 33609, USA. [3]EMD Serono, Inc., One Technology Place, Rockland, MA 02370, USA. [4]EMD Serono, Inc., 45A Middlesex Turnpike, Billerica, MA 01821, USA. [5]Mount Sinai Hospital, 5 East 98th Street, 1st Floor, New York, NY 10029, USA.

References

1. Cohen JA, Barkhof F, Comi G, Hartung HP, Khatri BO, Montalban X, et al. Oral fingolimod or intramuscular interferon for relapsing multiple sclerosis. N Engl J Med. 2010;362:402–15.
2. Coles AJ, Twyman CL, Arnold DL, Cohen JA, Confavreux C, Fox EJ, et al. Alemtuzumab for patients with relapsing multiple sclerosis after disease-modifying therapy: a randomised controlled phase 3 trial. Lancet. 2012;380: 1829–39.
3. PRISMS Study Group. Randomised double-blind placebo-controlled study of interferon beta-1a in relapsing/remitting multiple sclerosis. Lancet. 1998;352: 1498–504.
4. Uitdehaag BM, Barkhof F, Coyle PK, Gardner JD, Jeffery DR, Mikol DD. The changing face of multiple sclerosis clinical trial populations. Curr Med Res Opin. 2011;27:1529–37.
5. Fox RJ, Miller DH, Phillips JT, Hutchinson M, Havrdova E, Kita M, et al. Placebo-controlled phase 3 study of oral BG-12 or glatiramer in multiple sclerosis. N Engl J Med. 2012;367:1087–97.
6. Gold R, Kappos L, Arnold DL, Bar-Or A, Giovannoni G, Selmaj K, et al. Placebo-controlled phase 3 study of oral BG-12 for relapsing multiple sclerosis. N Engl J Med. 2012;367:1098–107.
7. Prosperini L, Gallo V, Petsas N, Borriello G, Pozzilli C, One-year MRI. Scan predicts clinical response to interferon beta in multiple sclerosis. Eur J Neurol. 2009;16:1202–9.
8. Rio J, Comabella M, Montalban X. Predicting responders to therapies for multiple sclerosis. Nat Rev Neurol. 2009;5:553–60.
9. Sormani MP, Bruzzi P. MRI lesions as a surrogate for relapses in multiple sclerosis: a meta-analysis of randomised trials. Lancet Neurol. 2013;12:669–76.
10. Rudick RA, Lee JC, Simon J, Ransohoff RM, Fisher E. Defining interferon beta response status in multiple sclerosis patients. Ann Neurol. 2004;56:548–55.
11. Polman CH, Reingold SC, Banwell B, Clanet M, Cohen JA, Filippi M, et al. Diagnostic criteria for multiple sclerosis: 2010 revisions to the McDonald criteria. Ann Neurol. 2011;69:292–302.
12. Rio J, Rovira A, Tintoré M, Huerga E, Nos C, Tellez N, et al. Relationship between MRI lesion activity and response to IFN-beta in relapsing-remitting multiple sclerosis patients. Mult Scler. 2008;14:479–84.
13. Durelli L, Barbero P, Bergui M, Versino E, Bassano MA, Verdun E, et al. MRI activity and neutralizing antibody as predictors of response to IFN-beta treatment in MS. J Neurol Neurosurg Psychiatry. 2008;79:646–51.
14. PRISMS Study Group, University of British Columbia MS/MRI Analysis Group. PRISMS-4: long-term efficacy of interferon-beta-1a in relapsing MS. Neurology. 2001;56:1628–36.
15. Dobson R, Rudick RA, Turner B, Schmierer K, Giovannoni G. Assessing treatment response to interferon-beta: is there a role for MRI? Neurology. 2014;82:248–54.
16. Wattjes MP, Rovira A, Miller D, Yousry TA, Sormani MP, de Stefano MP, et al. Evidence-based guidelines: MAGNIMS consensus guidelines on the use of
    MRI in multiple sclerosis–establishing disease prognosis and monitoring patients. Nat Rev Neurol. 2015;11:597–606.
17. Li DK, Paty DW, UBC MS/MRI Analysis Research Group, PRISMS Study Group. Magnetic resonance imaging results of the PRISMS trial: a randomized, double-blind, placebo-controlled study of interferon-beta1a in relapsing-remitting multiple sclerosis. Ann Neurol. 1999;46:197–206.
18. Bermel RA, You X, Foulds P, Hyde R, Simon JH, Fisher E, et al. Predictors of long-term outcome in multiple sclerosis patients treated with interferon beta. Ann Neurol. 2013;73:95–103.
19. Sormani MP, Rio J, Tintore M, Signori A, Li D, Cornelisse P, et al. Scoring treatment response in patients with relapsing multiple sclerosis. Mult Scler. 2013;19:605–12.
20. Cree BA, Gourraud PA, Oksenberg JR, Bevan C, Crabtree-Hartman E, Gelfand JM, et al. Long-term evolution of multiple sclerosis disability in the treatment era. Ann Neurol. 2016;80:499–510.
21. Giovannoni G, Turner B, Gnanapavan S, Offiah C, Schmierer K, Marta M. Is it time to target no evident disease activity (NEDA) in multiple sclerosis? Multiple Sclerosis Related Disorders. 2015;4:329–33.

21

Environmental exposures and the risk of multiple sclerosis in Saudi Arabia

Osama Al Wutayd[1,2], Ashri Gad Mohamed[3], Jameelah Saeedi[4], Hessa Al Otaibi[5] and Mohammed Al Jumah[6*]

Abstract

Background: Multiple sclerosis (MS) is the most common non-traumatic condition that leads to disability among young individuals. It is associated with demyelination, inflammation, and neurodegeneration within the central nervous system. Information on risk factors of multiple sclerosis is crucial for the prevention and control of the disease. The aim of this study was to determine risk factors of MS among adults in Saudi Arabia.

Methods: A matched multicenter case-control study, including 307 MS patients and 307 healthy controls, was conducted in MS clinics and wards in 3 main cities of Saudi Arabia. Age, gender, and hospital were matched. Information on demographics, family history of MS, past medical and family history, sun exposure at different age periods, tobacco use, diet, consanguinity, and coffee consumption was obtained from self-administered questionnaires. ORs and 95% confidence intervals (CIs) were calculated. A conditional logistic regression model was used to control for potential confounding factors.

Results: The conditional logistic regression adjusted for age and gender showed that being the first child in the family (Adjusted Odds Ratio (AOR) 1.68, 95% CI: 1.03–2.74), having a family history of MS (AOR 5.83, 95% CI: 2.83–12), eating fast food ≥5 times weekly (AOR 2.05, 95% CI: 1.03–4.08), and having had measles (AOR 3.77, 95% CI: 2.05–6.96), were independently associated with an increased risk of MS.
In contrast, eating ≥5 servings of fruit per week (AOR 0.25, 95% CI: 0.16–0.38), drinking coffee daily (AOR 0.46, 95% CI: 0.31–0.68), and having a high level of sun exposure at the primary school level and university level (AOR 0.57, 95% CI: 0.38–0.85 and AOR 0.48, 95% CI: 0.30–0.76, respectively) were independently associated with a decreased risk of MS.

Conclusions: Our study suggested that high levels of sun exposure during primary school and university, consumption of fruits and drinking coffee protect against MS. In contrast, eating fast food was associated with an increased risk of the disease. Encouraging outdoor activity and healthy diets in school, especially for females, is highly recommended.

Keywords: Multiple sclerosis, Case-control studies, Environmental risk factors, Sun exposure, Fast food, Coffee

Background

Multiple sclerosis (MS) is the most common non-traumatic condition that leads to disability among young individuals, and is associated with demyelination, inflammation, and neurodegeneration within the central nervous system [1]. It is commonly diagnosed between 18 and 40 years of age [2]. MS leads to sensory, motor, and cognitive dysfunctions, which may be progressive, temporary, or permanent. Therefore, multiple sclerosis may have adverse effects on relationships, employment, general well-being and the overall quality of life [3]. The prevalence of MS in the Middle East ranges from low to high. These ranges are dependent on the study setting and the particular population under study [4]. Previously, the Gulf region was thought to have a low prevalence of MS, but recent reports have revealed an increase in the disease prevalence and rate of incidence. However, there are still no registries for MS in the Gulf region [5]. In Saudi Arabia, the studies that are available are mostly hospital-based and there is still no regional or national study that has investigated the prevalence of MS, although some investigators have estimated the prevalence at 30 cases of MS per 100,000 individuals in 2009 [6]. It has been estimated that the prevalence in Saudi Arabia was 40/100,000 in 2008 [7]. The etiology of multiple sclerosis is not yet fully understood,

* Correspondence: jumahm@gmail.com
[6]King Fahad Medical City, MOH, KAIMRC/KSAU-HS, Riyadh, Saudi Arabia
Full list of author information is available at the end of the article

but a single causative event is unlikely. Converging evidence shows that MS is normally the result of autoimmune reactions in genetically susceptible persons following exposure to specific environmental factors [8]. The prevalence of MS is high in the Arabian Gulf region and Saudi Arabia. The risk factors that may be associated with MS in Saudi Arabia remain unclear, while the prevalence of MS is increasing. Thus, this study will provide more knowledge about the determinants of MS in Saudi Arabia.

Methods

A total of 307 MS patients and 307 healthy controls matched for gender and age (± 3 years) were selected from 3 main cities of Saudi Arabia, namely, Riyadh (King Fahad Medical City, King Saud Medical City, and King Fahad National Guard Hospital), Jeddah (King Fahad General Hospital), and Dammam (Dammam Central Hospital). MS patients were recruited from neurological clinics and hospital wards. Controls were healthy companions of patients from medical, surgical, and pediatric clinics and wards. The inclusion criteria for MS patients were those who had clinically definite MS that was diagnosed not more than 4 years from first symptoms and who attended MS clinics or were admitted to the hospital, were aged ≥18 years old, and were able to understand the questionnaire and give informed consent. Exclusion criteria for MS patients were those with clinically definite MS that was diagnosed more than 4 years from symptom onset, aged < 18 years old, and patients with current or concomitant illness that would interfere with the individual's ability to complete the study (e.g., cognitive impairment). Exclusion criteria for controls were history of MS, aged < 18 years old, and unable to understand the questionnaire and give informed consent. We adopted a structured questionnaire for this study. It included several sections that addressed demographics, family history of MS, sun exposure, current diet, history of breastfeeding, coffee consumption, medical history and family history, tobacco use, obesity, parental consanguinity, and age of onset of menstruation in the case of female patients. With respect to sun exposure, we used the frequency of participants' outdoor activities at different ages. To ensure the questionnaire's validity, a pilot study was conducted with 30 patients at the King Khalid University Hospital. This study was used to validate the logistics of data collection, and the clarity of the data collection tool and to estimate the time required to collect the data. The questionnaire took 6 to 12 min to complete. Some questions were modified according to the results of the pilot study. To assure the questionnaire's content validity, epidemiologists and Consultant Neurologists reviewed it and it was corrected according to their recommendations. The questionnaire was pretested on 30 participants to assess reliability through tests retests on different questionnaire items and Spearman correlations ranged from 0.62 to 1. These pretested groups were not included in the study. Then, data were collected from participants using the self- administered questionnaire. Trained data collectors were responsible for distributing the questionnaire to the participants and collecting them once finished. They were also responsible for the questionnaires' completeness. Participants filled out the questionnaire but, were supervised closely to address any inquiries they might have and assess whether they left any questions unanswered. The data collectors helped any participants who were unable to fill out the questionnaires by themselves.

SPSS V.21 was used for data entry, management and analysis. The frequencies and percentage of all variables were calculated. The Chi-squared test, Fisher's exact test, and Student's t-test were used to test the association between categorical and continuous variables, respectively. The odds ratio associated with each potential risk factor and its 95% confidence interval (CI) was also calculated. To control for confounding variables, conditional logistic regression analysis adjusted for age and gender was applied in various models using MS vs. controls as the dependent variable and other variables as the independent ones. All variables associated with MS status with a p value < 0.10 were entered into the model. A p value ≤0.05 was considered statistically significant.

Results

Out of the 336 MS patients requested to participate, 307 (91%) agreed, and of 340 matched controls, 307 (90%) agreed, resulting in response rates of 91 and 90% for MS patients and controls, respectively. These rates are similar, are considered satisfactory rates, and not statistically significant. Table 1 shows that the majority of subjects (230; 75%) were females, and (77, 25%) were males. The mean age was 32.91 ± 8.82 years for MS patients and 32.89 ± 8.64 years for controls. Forty-two percent of subjects were 18–29 years old. There was no statistically significant difference between MS patients and controls with respect to their level of education ($P = 0.30$). Further, the primary work status over the past 12 months did not significantly differ between patients and controls ($P = 0.13$). The same was true for average household earnings ($P = 0.19$). Among MS patients with a family history of MS, the median difference in age of diagnosis compared to the age of their relatives with MS is 5 years.

Univariate analyses showed that the risk of having MS among first-born children was increased compared to the ≥2nd child in the family ($P = 0.001$), and MS patients were more likely to have a family history of MS ($P < 0.001$). The risk of having MS among those with

Table 1 Baseline characteristics of MS patients and their healthy controls

Baseline characteristics	MS patients (n = 307)	Controls (n = 307)	P value
	n (%)	n (%)	
Female	230 (75)	230 (75)	1
Male	77 (25)	77 (25)	
Age, mean (SD)	32.91 (±8.82)	32.89 (±8.64)	
18–29	128 (41.7)	128 (42)	0.94
30–39	106 (35)	111 (36)	
40–49	56 (18)	50 (16)	
50–59	16 (5)	16 (5)	
60–69	1 (0.3)	2 (1)	
Level of education			
Less than university	142 (46)	158 (52)	0.30
University	149 (49)	130 (42)	
Postgraduate	16 (5)	19 (6)	
Main work status over the last 12 months			
Employed	158 (52)	186 (61)	0.127
Unemployed	23 (8)	15 (5)	
Student	37 (12)	32 (10)	
Housewife	89 (29)	74 (24)	
Average earnings of the household[a]			
< 7500	87 (33)	87 (31)	0.19
7500–12,499	101 (38)	114 (40)	
≥ 12,500	80 (30)	83 (29)	

[a]62 total missing. (most of them did not know), 39 MS patients and 23 controls

high sun exposure was decreased compared to those with low sun exposure during primary, intermediate, and secondary schools and university ($P < 0.001$).

We found that MS patients consumed less fruit ($P < 0.001$) and vegetables ($P = 0.001$), more fast food ($P < 0.001$) and dairy products ($P = 0.03$), and less coffee ($P = 0.001$) than controls. MS patients were more likely to have a history of measles ($P < 0.001$) and fewer incidences of thyroid disorder ($P = 0.04$), as well as less parental consanguinity with a first cousin ($P = 0.03$) compared to controls (Table 2).

The following exposures were not found to be significantly associated with MS. These included breastfeeding, age of menstruation, and BMI. With respect to diet, the following were not significant: consumption of dates, red meat, and milk. With respect to family or medical history, the following factors showed no significant association with MS: chicken pox, appendectomy, tonsillectomy, medical history of type I diabetes mellitus, migraine, systematic lupus erythematosus, rheumatoid arthritis, Crohn's disease, ulcerative colitis, psoriasis, and family

history of type I diabetes mellitus, migraine, systematic lupus erythematosus, and rheumatoid arthritis. Tobacco use (cigarette and water pipe) and passive smoking during childhood were not associated with MS (Table S1 shows this in more detail [see Additional file 1]).

A total of 604 participants were included in the conditional logistic regression adjusted for age and gender (Table 3). The rest (10) had incomplete data and were excluded from the model.

This showed that being the first child in the family (Adjusted OR 1.68, 95% CI: 1.03–2.74), having a family history of MS (AOR 5.83, 95% CI: 2.83–12), eating fast food ≥5 times weekly (AOR 2.05, 95% CI: 1.03–4.08), and having had measles (AOR 3.77, 95% CI: 2.05–6.96) were independently associated with an increased risk of MS.

Eating ≥5 servings of fruit per week (AOR 0.25, 95% CI: 0.16–0.38), drinking coffee (AOR 0.46, 95% CI: 0.31–0.68), and having a high level of sun exposure at the primary school level (AOR 0.57, 95% CI: 0.38–0.85) and university (AOR 0.48, 95% CI: 0.30–0.76) were independently associated with a decreased risk of MS.

Discussion

Birth order is believed to influence the risk of MS. In our study, the risk of MS among first children in the family was increased 1.7-fold compared to those born 2nd or later. We also compared second- and third-born children to first-born children as a reference category and found a protective effect for those born later. Siblings born late in the birth order are exposed to infection earlier than those born earlier and experience greater challenges to their immune systems. The hygiene hypothesis, which states that exposure to infection early in life provides protection from infection, could mean that younger siblings are at decreased risk for developing MS because they have early contact with microorganisms via older siblings. This is consistent with a study that showed that high levels of exposure to infections in younger infant siblings protected against MS [9]. However, other studies have found inconsistent results [10, 11].

The MS risk was 5.8 times greater when there was family history of MS, and this finding was statistically significant, indicating a strong aggregation in MS cases. We calculated the time difference between age at diagnosis for MS patients and their relatives with MS to establish whether this was attributable to shared exposure to environmental factors or to the genes that are responsible for familial aggregation of MS. We believe both genetic and environmental factors play a role in the development of MS. This is unlikely to be due to chance or recall bias, as the clinical features of MS are obvious, and patients and controls would remember them well. This finding is

Table 2 Bivariate analysis of variables associated with risk of Multiple Sclerosis

Environmental exposures	Exposed cases/Exposed controls ($n = 307/307$)	Crude OR	95% CI	P value
First child in family, yes/no	76/264	2.02	1.34–3.06	0.001
Family history of MS, yes/no	57/294	5.16	2.76–9.64	< 0.001
Sun exposure during primary school, high/low	139/122	0.55	0.40–0.75	< 0.001
Sun exposure during intermediate school, high/low	94/169	0.54	0.39–0.75	< 0.001
Sun exposure during secondary school, high/low	65/192	0.45	0.31–0.64	< 0.001
Sun exposure during university school, high/low[a]	54/184	0.33	0.23 – 0.49	< 0.001
Breastfeeding, yes/no[b]	203/37			
≥ 5 Servings of fruits / week, yes/no	77/145	0.30	0.21–0.42	< 0.001
≥ 5 Servings of vegetables / week, yes/no	145/120	0.57	0.42–0.79	0.001
≥ 5 dates times / week, yes/no	156/146	0.94	0.68–1.29	0.69
≥ 5 red meat times / week, yes/no	38/268	0.97	0.60–1.57	0.90
≥ 5 milk times / week, yes/no	84/239	1.32	0.92–1.91	0.14
≥ 5 Fast food times/week, yes/no	46/291	3.21	1.77–5.80	< 0.001
≥ 5 Dairy products times / week, yes/no	162/172	1.42	1.04–1.96	0.03
Daily coffee intake, yes/no	112/147	0.53	0.38–0.73	< 0.001
Illness or surgical interventions:				
History of measles infection, yes/no	63/283	3.05	1.85–5.02	< 0.001
History of chicken pox infection, yes/no	167/132	0.90	0.65–1.24	0.57
Appendectomy, yes/no	29/268	0.72	0.43–1.19	0.25
Tonsillectomy, yes/no	52/264	1.25	0.81–1.94	0.37
Medical history:				
Type I diabetes mellitus, yes/no	15/285	0.67	0.34–1.31	0.235
Migraine, yes/no	35/269	0.91	0.56–1.49	0.71
Systematic lupus erythematosus, yes/no	1/302	0.19	0.02–1.69	0.22
Rheumatoid arthritis, yes/no	17/289	0.94	0.48–1.86	0.86
Thyroid disorder, yes/no	19/274	0.55	0.30–0.99	0.04
Crohn's disease, yes/no	1/306	1	0.06–16.06	1
Ulcerative colitis, yes/no	18/294	1.41	0.68–2.93	0.36
Psoriasis, yes/no	7/303	1.77	0.51–6.10	0.361
Family history of medical conditions:				
Type I diabetes mellitus, yes/no	154/154	1.01	0.74–1.39	0.94
Migraine, yes/no	53/249	0.90	0.59–1.35	0.60
Systematic lupus erythematosus, yes/no	10/291	0.61	0.27–1.37	0.23
Rheumatoid arthritis, yes/no	69/239	1.02	0.70–1.49	0.92
≥ 13-year age of menarche, yes/no	98/138	1.11	0.77–1.61	0.57
Tobacco use:				
Current tobacco use, cases/controls	58/52	1.16	0.77–1.76	0.47
Ex-smoker, cases/controls	19/15	1.32	0.84–1.56	0.43
Never smoker, cases/controls	230/240	Ref.		
Passive smoking in childhood, yes/no	113/194	1	0.72–1.39	1
BMI:				
≥ 30, cases/controls	76/74	0.92	0.62–1.37	0.67
25–29.99, cases/controls	90/107	0.75	0.52–1.09	0.13

Table 2 Bivariate analysis of variables associated with risk of Multiple Sclerosis *(Continued)*

Environmental exposures	Exposed cases/Exposed controls (*n* = 307/307)	Crude OR	95% CI	*P* value
≤ 24.99, cases/controls	141/126	Ref.		
Parental consanguinity (first cousin), yes/no	63/222	0.67	0.46–0.98	0.03

[a]Not applicable (5 MS cases and 3 controls)
[b]Not know (58 cases and 52 controls)

consistent with many studies of MS, such as one conducted in Saudi Arabia that reported that approximately 20% of MS patients have a family history of MS [12]. Two additional studies conducted in Kuwait reported that a larger number of patients had a family history of MS compared to controls [11, 13]. However, in this study, there was no significant difference between first-, second-, and third-degree relatives.

With respect to the frequency of eating fast food, MS patients ate fast food 2 times more often than healthy controls. This result is consistent with a study of MS patients in which sodium consumption was estimated from sodium excretion in urine samples and showed that increased sodium consumption is associated with increased clinical and radiological activity in MS patients [14]. A diet high in salt (sodium chloride) has been found to increase the stimulation of the Th17 lymphocyte both in human and animal models. The Th17 cells produced by a high salt diet seem to be extremely pathogenic and connected to pro-inflammatory cytokines [15]. However, our study is inconsistent with a recent prospective study (NHS) that showed no association between high dietary sodium intake and the risk of MS [16].

Studies in the literature have been inconclusive with respect to the association between measles and MS. A study prospectively collected serum samples from MS patients and revealed no association between MS and measles [17]. Our study revealed that a history of measles in MS patients was 3.8-folds more frequent than in healthy controls. This study is consistent with a matched case-control study of serology among German children

with MS [18]. In addition, a study reported that MS patients had measles at an older age compared to controls [19]. A possible explanation for this is delayed exposure to common infectious agents. Thus, infection early in life may protect against MS, while conversely, later infections when the immune system has matured may increase the risk. This is consistent with the inverse relationship between MS risk and birth order. However, in this study, the age of getting the measles infection was not determined, and we suggest the need for further study to assess the association between measles and MS taking into consideration the age of infection.

Fruits and vegetables are rich in numerous vitamins and minerals. Vitamins, in particular, contain antioxidants that have been suggested to play a protective role in the prevention of MS [20]. A case-control study conducted in Serbia showed that the frequency of consumption of fruits and vegetables was increased in healthy individuals compared to MS patients [21]. In this study, healthy controls consumed more fruits and vegetables than MS patients, and the association was found to be significant in a bivariate analysis. Although the frequency of consumption of vegetables in healthy controls was greater than that in MS patients, this association was not significant in the conditional logistic regression. This finding was similar to a case-control study among the Iranian population that reported that consumption of fruit has a protective role against MS, but vegetable consumption was insignificant in a multivariate analysis [22].

In this study, coffee intake among healthy controls was increased compared to MS patients. In the conditional

Table 3 Conditional logistic regression model of environmental exposures with multiple sclerosis risk

Environmental exposures	AOR[a]	95% CI	*P* value
First child in family	1.68	1.03–2.74	0.038
Family history of MS	5.83	2.83–12	< 0.001
≥ 5 Fast food times/week, yes/no	2.05	1.03–4.08	0.042
History of measles infection, yes/no	3.77	2.05–6.96	< 0.001
≥ 5 Servings of fruits / week, yes/no	0.25	0.16–0.38	< 0.001
Daily coffee intake, yes/no	0.46	0.31–0.68	< 0.001
Sun exposure during primary school, high/low	0.57	0.38–0.85	0.006
Sun exposure during university school, high/low	0.48	0.30–0.76	0.002

[a]*AOR* Adjusted odds ratio, included variables in the model are age and gender

logistic regression, coffee consumption had a protective effect among healthy controls compared to MS patients and this is consistent with a recently published case-control study in Sweden and the U.S. that reported that those who drank four cups of coffee or more each day demonstrated a protective effect [23]. However, one prospective study (NHS) found no association between coffee intake and MS risk and this may be because it was conducted only in females [24]. Several mechanisms have proposed that caffeine appears to decrease the generation of pro-inflammatory cytokines, and has neuroprotective qualities, credited to phosphodiesterase inhibition and non- specific antagonism of adenosine receptors [25, 26].

The comparison of those with low or high sun exposure during different levels of education was used rather than age groups to increase recall of sun exposure Nevertheless, primary, intermediate, secondary school, and university correspond to the age groups, 7 to 12, 13 to 15, 16 to 18, and 19 to 22 years, respectively. Sun exposure in primary school was associated with reduced risk of MS. This finding is consistent with several studies, such as one conducted in Tasmania that found that increased sun exposure during childhood and early adolescence was associated with a decreased risk of MS [27]. Another study that found an association between sun exposure in childhood and the risk of monozygotic twins with MS reported similar results [28]. Moreover, sun exposure during university was associated with a reduced risk of MS. The mechanism of sun exposure can be explained by Vitamin D, which has been proposed to be the main mediator of this protective effect [29]. Vitamin D receptors bind thousands of genomic sites in immune systems in lymphoblastoid cells, and there is a direct correlation between vitamin D levels and vitamin D receptor binding sites, which bind to fewer sites in primary CD4+ T cells in individuals with low vitamin D levels compared to individuals with normal vitamin D levels [30, 31]. Nevertheless, a population-based case-control study endorses the theory that UVR exposure contributes to reducing MS risk independently of its consequences on vitamin D levels [32]. Moreover, research in Australia recommended that both solar emission and vitamin D have individual protective effects on MS development [33]. There are several pathways through which UVR may influence immune reactions that are independent of vitamin D production, for example, UVB contact influences universal immune responses and assuages systemic autoimmunity through the introduction of regulatory T cells and skin- derived tolerogenic dendritic cells [34].

In this study, current smokers were found more often in the MS cases than in healthy controls; however, this was not statistically significant. This may be due to fact that the majority of MS patients in our study were women and that smoking is more common among men than women in our community. A recent meta-analysis including 10 studies showed that cigarette smoking appeared to increase the risk of MS to a greater extent in men than in women. Additionally, the majority of cigarette smokers were not heavy smokers. We consider that this may be related to MS patients quitting smoking after being diagnosed with the disease. However, this may be unlikely especially in cases of ex-smokers, where differences were not statistically significant between MS patients and controls. On the other hand, tobacco use in our region may have little influence on the development of MS, and this finding is consistent with two studies reported from Kuwait [11, 35].

In our study, as in all case-control studies, there are several limitations. Case control studies are subject to recall bias which is a potential threat to the validity of the results. In the present study, we recruit only MS cases who were within 4 years of diagnosis to minimize the risk for misclassified answers.

Information was obtained retrospectively, with some of the exposures referring to years long before the study, and thus, this study may have exposure misclassification. However, for example, we used school level rather than age period to increase the recall of MS patients and controls regarding sun exposure. Additionally, we asked about viral infections with obvious clinical features, such as measles and chicken pox, which participants could recall easily. Other epidemiological studies need to be carried out to know others that were not assessed in the present study such as Epstein-Barr virus, since this is a major risk factor in other populations. Diet assessment is one limitation in this study, since participants could have changed their current diet since diagnosis. Selection bias is a threat if controls are not representative of the population from which the cases arose. In this particular study, controls were specifically selected from the same hospital as the MS cases. Additionally, selection bias could be considered since controls may have MS as there is a relatively long latency period. However, this is unlikely since MS is not common in the general population. The matched analysis helped to control for these design characteristics.

Conclusions

Our study suggested that high levels of sun exposure during primary school and university, consumption of fruits and drinking coffee protect against MS. In contrast, eating fast food was associated with increased risk of the disease. Encouraging outdoor activity and healthy diets in school, especially for females, is highly recommended.

Abbreviations

AOR: Adjusted odds ratio; CI: Confidence interval; MS: Multiple sclerosis; NHS: Nurses' health study; ORs : Odd ratios; Th17: T helper type 17 lymphocyte; US: United States; UVB: Ultraviolet B; UVR: Ultraviolet radiation

Acknowledgments

We would like to thank all members of arfa MS society which is a group of MS patients in Saudi Arabia for encourage us to conduct this study and Dr. Samah Ishak, and Dr. Ayah Al Jawhary for help with distribution of the questionnaires. Finally, we would like to thank the patients who kindly consented to participate in this study.

Funding

This publication Environmental Exposures and the Risk of Multiple Sclerosis in Saudi Arabia, was made possible in part by a grant from MENACTRIMS, funded by SANOFI – AVENTIS GROUPE (DMCC Branch), representative office of Sanofi – Aventis Groupe SA. The funding body did not have a role in the design of the study and collection, analysis, and interpretation of data and in writing the manuscript.

Authors' contributions

OW and MJ made contributions to review of literature, study design, data management, and analysis, and manuscript writing. AGM made contributions for supervision of the sampling and development of manuscript. JS and HO made contributions to supervision in data collection and management and revising the manuscript. All authors read and approved the final manuscript.

Competing interests

This publication Environmental Exposures and the Risk of Multiple Sclerosis in Saudi Arabia, was made possible in part by a grant from MENACTRIMS, funded by SANOFI – AVENTIS GROUPE (DMCC Branch), representative office of Sanofi – Aventis Groupe SA. The funding body did not have a role in the design of the study a nd collection, analysis, and interpretation of data and in writing the manuscript.

Author details

[1]Unaizah College of Medicine, Qassim University, Qassim, Saudi Arabia. [2]Unaizah College of Medicine and Medical Sciences – Qassim University, Unaizah, Qassim, Saudi Arabia. [3]King Khalid University Hospital, Riyadh, Saudi Arabia. [4]Princess Norah Bint Abdulrahman University, Riyadh, Saudi Arabia. [5]King Fahad General Hospital, Ministry of Health, Jedda, Saudi Arabia. [6]King Fahad Medical City, MOH, KAIMRC/KSAU-HS, Riyadh, Saudi Arabia.

References

1. Compston A, Coles A. Multiple sclerosis. Lancet. 2002;359(9313):1221–31.
2. Compston A. McAlpine's multiple sclerosis, vol. Vol 3. London; Edinburgh; New York: Churchill Livingstone; 1998.
3. Nortvedt MW, Riise T, Myhr KM, Nyland HI. Quality of life in multiple sclerosis: measuring the disease effects more broadly. Neurology. 1999; 53(5):1098–103.
4. Al-Hashel J, Besterman AD, Wolfson C. The prevalence of multiple sclerosis in the Middle East. Neuroepidemiology. 2008;31(2):129–37.
5. Alroughani RA, Al-Jumah MA. The need for a multiple sclerosis registry in the Gulf region. Neurosciences (Riyadh, Saudi Arabia). 2014;19(2):85–6.
6. Al-deeb S. Epidemiology of MS in Saudi Arabia; in 25th Congress of the European Committee for Treatment and Research in Multiple Sclerosis. Dusseldorf; 2009.
7. Bohlega S, Inshasi J, Al Tahan AR, Madani AB, Qahtani H, Rieckmann P. Multiple sclerosis in the Arabian gulf countries: a consensus statement. J Neurol. 2013;260(12):2959–63.
8. Steele SU, Mowry EM. Etiology. Multiple sclerosis and CNS inflammatory disorders. Wiley; 2014. p. 1–9. Retrieved from https://www.wiley.com/en-sa/Multiple+Sclerosis+and+CNS+Inflammatory+Disorders-p-9780470673881. ISBN: 978-0-470-67388-1.
9. Ponsonby AL, van der Mei I, Dwyer T, Blizzard L, Taylor B, Kemp A. Birth order, infection in early life, and multiple sclerosis. Lancet Neurol. 2005;4(12): 793–4. author reply 5
10. Sadovnick AD, Yee IM, Ebers GC. Multiple sclerosis and birth order: a longitudinal cohort study. Lancet Neurol. 2005;4:611–7.
11. Al-Afasy HH, Al-Obaidan MA, Al-Ansari YA, Al-Yatama SA, Al-Rukaibi MS, Makki NI, et al. Risk factors for multiple sclerosis in Kuwait: a population-based case-control study. Neuroepidemiology. 2013;40(1):30–5.
12. Al Jumah M, Kojan S, Al Khathaami A, Al Abdulkaream I, Al Blawi M, Jawhary A. Familial multiple sclerosis: does consanguinity have a role? Mult Scler (Houndmills, Basingstoke, England). 2011;17(4):487–9.
13. Al-Shammri SN, Hanna MG, Chattopadhyay A, Akanji AO. Sociocultural and demographic risk factors for the development of multiple sclerosis in Kuwait: a case-control study. PLoS One. 2015;10(7):e0132106.
14. Farez MF, Fiol MP, Gaitan MI, Quintana FJ, Correale J. Sodium intake is associated with increased disease activity in multiple sclerosis. J Neurol Neurosurg Psychiatry. 2015;86(1):26–31.
15. Kleinewietfeld M, Manzel A, Titze J, Kvakan H, Yosef N, Linker RA, et al. Sodium chloride drives autoimmune disease by the induction of pathogenic TH17 cells. Nature. 2013;496(7446):518–22.
16. Cortese M, Yuan C, Chitnis T, Ascherio A, Munger KL. No association between dietary sodium intake and the risk of multiple sclerosis. Neurology. 2017;89(13):1322–9.
17. Sundstrom P, Juto P, Wadell G, Hallmans G, Svenningsson A, Nystrom L, et al. An altered immune response to Epstein-Barr virus in multiple sclerosis: a prospective study. Neurology. 2004;62(12):2277–82.
18. Krone B, Pohl D, Rostasy K, Kahler E, Brunner E, Oeffner F, et al. Common infectious agents in multiple sclerosis: a case-control study in children. Mult Scler. 2008;14(1):136–9.
19. Bachmann S, Kesselring J. Multiple sclerosis and infectious childhood diseases. Neuroepidemiology. 1998;17(3):154–60.
20. Ghadirian P, Jain M, Ducic S, Shatenstein B, Morisset R. Nutritional factors in the aetiology of multiple sclerosis: a case-control study in Montreal, Canada. Int J Epidemiol. 1998;27(5):845–52.
21. Pekmezovic T, Tepavcevic D, Mesaros S. Food and dietary patterns and multiple sclerosis: a case-control study in Belgrade (Serbia). Ital J Publ Health 2009;6:81–7.
22. Bagheri M, Maghsoudi Z, Fayazi S, Elahi N, Tabesh H, Majdinasab N. Several food items and multiple sclerosis: a case-control study in Ahvaz (Iran). Iran J Nurs Midwifery Res. 2014;19(6):659–65.
23. Hedstrom AK, Mowry EM, Gianfrancesco MA, Shao X, Schaefer CA, Shen L, et al. High consumption of coffee is associated with decreased multiple sclerosis risk; results from two independent studies. J Neurol Neurosurg Psychiatry. 2016;87(5):454–60.
24. Massa J, O'Reilly EJ, Munger KL, Ascherio A. Caffeine and alcohol intakes have no association with risk of multiple sclerosis. Mult Scler (Houndmills, Basingstoke, England). 2013;19(1):53–8.
25. Horrigan LA, Kelly JP, Connor TJ. Caffeine suppresses TNF-alpha production via activation of the cyclic AMP/protein kinase a pathway. Int Immunopharmacol. 2004;4:1409–17.
26. Kalda A, Yu L, Oztas E, Chen JF. Novel neuroprotection by caffeine and adenosine a(2A) receptor antagonists in animal models of Parkinson's disease. J Neurol Sci. 2006;248:9–15.
27. van der Mei IA, Ponsonby AL, Dwyer T, Blizzard L, Simmons R, Taylor BV, et al. Past exposure to sun, skin phenotype, and risk of multiple sclerosis: case-control study. BMJ. 2003;327(7410):316.
28. Islam T, Gauderman WJ, Cozen W, Mack TM. Childhood sun exposure influences risk of multiple sclerosis in monozygotic twins. Neurology. 2007; 69(4):381–8.
29. Smolders J, Damoiseaux J, Menheere P, Hupperts R. Vitamin D as an immune modulator in multiple sclerosis, a review. J Neuroimmunol. 2008; 194(1):7–17.
30. Ramagopalan SV, Heger A, Berlanga AJ, Maugeri NJ, Lincoln MR, Burrell A, et al. A ChIP-seq defined genome-wide map of vitamin D receptor binding: associations with disease and evolution. Genome Res. 2010;20(10):1352–60.

22

Pediatric multiple sclerosis

Raed Alroughani[1*] and Alexey Boyko[2]

Abstract

Background: Pediatric-onset multiple sclerosis (POMS) prevalence and incidence rates are increasing globally. No disease-modifying therapy are approved for MS pediatric population. Hence, we aim to review the literature on POMS to guide treating physicians on the current understanding of diagnosis and management of pediatric MS.

Methods: The authors performed a literature search and reviewed the current understanding on risk factors and disease parameters in order to discuss the challenges in assessing and implementing diagnosis and therapy in clinical practice.

Results: The revised International Pediatric MS group diagnostic criteria improved the accuracy of diagnosis. Identification of red flags and mimickers (e.g. acute disseminated encephalomyelitis and neuromyelitis optica) are vital before establishing a definitive diagnosis. Possible etiology and mechanisms including both environmental and genetic risk factors are highlighted. Pediatric MS patients tend to have active inflammatory disease course with a tendency to have brainstem / cerebellar presentations at onset. Due to efficient repair mechanisms at early life, pediatric MS patients tend to have longer time to reach EDSS 6 but reach it at earlier age. Although no therapeutic randomized clinical trials were conducted in pediatric cohorts, open-label multi-center studies reported efficacy and safety results with beta interferons, glatiramer acetate and natalizumab in similar adult cohorts. Several randomized clinical trials assessing the efficacy and safety of oral disease-modifying therapies are ongoing in pediatric MS patients.

Conclusion: Pediatric MS has been increasingly recognized to have a more inflammatory course with frequent infratentorial presentations at onset, which would have important implications in the future management of pediatric cohorts while awaiting the results of ongoing clinical trials.

Keywords: Pediatric multiple sclerosis, Multiple sclerosis, Clinically isolated syndrome, Acute disseminated encephalomyelitis, Neuromyelitis optics

Background

Multiple Sclerosis (MS), a chronic inflammatory auto-immune disease of the central nervous system (CNS), is most commonly diagnosed in (young) adults, but can also affect children. Pediatric MS, also referred to as pediatric-onset MS (POMS), early-onset MS or juvenile MS, is generally defined as MS with an onset before the age of 16 years (sometimes before the age of 18 years). Between 3 and 10% of patients with MS present under 16 years of age and < 1% under 10 years of age [1]. Pediatric MS has distinctive features and the disease course is different than in adults. Children are less likely to develop primary or secondary progressive MS in childhood. 98% of pediatric MS patients present with a relapsing–remitting (RR) course, compared with 84% of adult patients [2]. Relapses appear to be more frequent in patients with POMS compared with adult-onset MS [3].

Guidelines for pediatric MS recommend that treatment can be started early in the disease course [4, 5]. Disease-modifying therapies (DMTs) for adult patients with MS are also applied in pediatric MS. However, data from large pediatric cohorts are lacking and no large placebo-controlled studies have been published yet. Consequently, level 1 evidence for the appropriate treatment and its timing is still scarce.

Methods

A group of neurologists with expertise in MS met as part of a scientific group (ParadigMS) to address the current understanding of pediatric MS, and to discuss the evolving research and ongoing therapeutic trials in

---
* Correspondence: alroughani@gmail.com
[1]Division of Neurology, Department of Medicine, Amiri Hospital, Arabian Gulf Street, 13041 Sharq, Kuwait
Full list of author information is available at the end of the article

pediatric population. Two MS experts (R.A., A.B.) performed a comprehensive literature search of MEDLINE, EMBASE, and Cochrane databases, systematically reviewing more than 80 published manuscripts from the last two decades that involved pediatric cohorts or any prospective or retrospective studies with at least 10 patients. Case studies with importance to pathology or which have clinical implications, were included as well. The expert panel met again to discuss the topic (pediatric MS) after being extensively reviewed by the authors (R.A., A.B.) and identified the relevant knowledge that needs to be presented in a review article to guide the treating physicians on diagnosis and management of pediatric MS patients.

Results
Clinical features
Children can present with a wide variety of manifestations including optic neuritis (ON), sensory, brainstem-cerebellar, and motor symptoms. The MS course in cases with onset at < 16 years of age is very similar in among populations from Italy, Russia, France, USA, and Kuwait [1–3, 6–10]. The clinical phenotype differs from that of adult patients, in that pediatric MS patients generally experience a more aggressive disease onset with disabling clinical symptoms [11], a polyfocal presentation at disease onset [12] and a higher relapse rate early in the disease course [13]. Though these findings are mostly from the USA and Europe, no were major regional differences in the epidemiological patterns or clinical features, meaning data outside of these regions are scarce. Overall, children tend to have a more favorable outcome after a first clinical event [13]. They also have slower disease progression over time: they take 10 years longer to reach secondary progressive disease phase compared to adults [2]. The relatively slow development of irreversible physical disability in children [14] is believed to result from better plasticity, allowing better recovery from relapses. In pediatric MS time from onset to confirmed disability may be relatively long, but disability milestone is reached at an earlier age.

Axonal damage occurs early in MS and contributes to the degree of clinical disability. In children with MS, there is more pronounced acute axonal damage in inflammatory demyelinating lesions than in adults [15]. Similar heightened axonal damage was observed in a case study of a 12-year-old patient [16]. Evidence was found in a study that was performed on archival biopsy and autopsy tissue of 19 children with demyelinating diseases: MS ($n = 11$) or clinically isolated syndrome (CIS) ($n = 8$). Median age at biopsy/autopsy was 13 years (range 4 – 17 years). The most important outcome was the significant increase, by 50%, of acute axonal damage in early active demyelinating lesions of pediatric

patients (median = 1665 Amyloid Precursor Protein (APP) -positive axons/mm^2) compared to adult patients (median = 1100 APP-positive axons/mm^2, $p = 0.0455$). The numbers of APP-positive axons/mm^2 were significantly higher in the prepubertal age group (< 11 years of age) compared to the pubertal age group (11–17 years, $p = 0.0061$) and adult patients (≥18 years, $p = 0.0044$). Furthermore, significantly more children showed multifocal MRI T2 lesions (71.4% vs 54.5%, $p > 0.05$). Also, the index lesion was larger in pediatric patients (81.8% vs 50% size > 2 cm). There was an increased inflammatory infiltration in pediatric MS lesions, which was shown to be associated with the extent of acute axonal damage in pediatric and adult patients ($r = 0.5381$, $p = 0.0098$).

Besides clinical features that are typical for demyelination, MS is associated with significant cognitive impairment in childhood. In a study in 63 patients, 19 (31%) fulfilled criteria for cognitive impairment [17]. Cognitive outcome in these patients can be heterogeneous, as cognitive performance deteriorated in 42 of 56 cases (75%) after 2 years of follow-up [18]. In a 5-year longitudinal study, cognitive impairment index deterioration was observed in 56% of patients, improvement in 25%, and stability in 18.8% [19].

Prevalence and incidence
One of two methodological approaches to calculate the prevalence and incidence of pediatric MS are usually conducted in scientific publications, which could explain the variation in published data. Subtraction of POMS cases from the total MS cohort, or calculating an age-specific, population-based risk are the common methodological approaches. Other reasons for the variation in the prevalence and incidence are the use of different diagnostic criteria and of a different cut-off age among the studied pediatric cohorts, ranging from 15 to 18 years.

The worldwide prevalence and incidence of pediatric MS is unknown, but data from individual countries and MS centers are available (see Table 1). Several studies indicate that at least 5% of the total population with MS comprises of pediatric patients [6, 7]. Population studies and case-control series show that between 1.7% and 5.6% of the MS population is younger than 18 years of age [2, 6–8]. A recent study showed that incidence and prevalence of pediatric MS in Kuwait in 2013 were 2.1 and 6.0, respectively [20]. Incidence in general is highest in children between the age of 13 and 16.

Risk factors
There is a possible role for Epstein-Barr virus (EBV) in MS pathogenesis. This was suggested by the results of a multinational observational study, which included 137 pediatric MS patients from 17 sites across North- and

Table 1 Incidence and prevalence of pediatric MS: results from various national cohorts

Country	Number	Age range	Syndrome	Diagnostic criteria	Prevalence	Incidence	Reference
Germany	126	≤ 15 years	MS	McDonald 2005		0.64	Reinhardt et al. [45]
Netherlands	86	< 18 years	ADS	Krupp 2007	–	0.66	Ketelsegers et al. [46]
UK	125	1-15 year	ADS	Krupp 2007	–	0.98	Absoud et al. [47]
Italy (Sardinia)	21	0-18 years	MS	Krupp 2013	26.92	2.85	Dell'Avvento et al. [48]
USA	81	0-18 years	ADS MS	Krupp 2007	–	1.66 0.51	Langer-Gould et al. [49]
Brazil	125	0-18 years	MS	Krupp 2007	5.5% of MS population		Fragoso et al. [50]
Iran (Shiraz)	88	1-18 years	ADS	–		0.19	Inaloo et al. [51]
Kuwait	122	< 18 years	MS	Krupp 2013	6.0	2.1	Alroughani et al. [20]

ADS acquired demyelinating syndromes

South-America and Europe [11]. Non-MS controls were matched 1:1 by year of birth with an MS participant enrolled from the same region. The participants underwent standardized assays (ELISA) for IgG antibodies directed against EBV, cytomegalovirus, parvovirus B19, varicella zoster virus, and herpes simplex virus. Over 108 (86%) of children with MS, irrespective of geographical residence, were seropositive for remote EBV infection, compared to only 64% of matched controls ($p = 0.025$). The hazard ratio (HR) to be in the MS group in case of seropositivity for remote EBV was 2.8 (confidence interval (CI): 1.4 − 5.8) ($p = 0.005$). Only anti-EBV nuclear antigen titers were higher in the EBV-positive MS patients compared to EBV-positive non-MS controls ($p = 0.003$).

One of the main risk factors of MS, also confirmed in pediatric MS, is HLA DRB1*1501 [21]. DNA from 56 children with MS (< 16 years of age) was used for HLA-DRB1 typing and compared to healthy controls ($n = 328$), MS patients from the same population ($n = 234$), and 76 parents of 39 pediatric MS patients. Only the frequencies of DR2(15) alleles were higher in both sets of MS patients than in controls. Transmission disequilibrium test (TDT) results showed significant difference in transmission of DR2(15) and non-DR2(15) alleles ($p = 0.00002$).

Natural history
High-quality studies of the natural history of pediatric MS are scarce due to methodological issues. In a comparative study analyzing data collected from two different pediatric cohorts, clinical characteristics and progression of pediatric onset MS (< 16 years) over time were assessed. In the Moscow cohort, 67 cases of newly diagnosed MS were prospectively observed for 2 - 13 years, while the Vancouver cohort consisted of 116 MS cases who were retrospectively observed for 1 - 47 years [1, 9]. The pediatric cohorts were compared with an historical adult cohort to assess the risk of disability progression assessed by expanded disability status scale (EDSS) scores. There were a number of significant differences between pediatric and adult-onset MS [10]. The 50% risks to reach EDSS 3 and 6 were 23 and

28 years after MS onset, compared to 10 and 18 years in the comparator group.

In a longitudinal prospective population-based study the risk of disease progression in POMS was assessed [22]. The interval to second relapse was longer in pediatric patients (5.0 vs 2.6 years, $p = 0.04$) PPMS was less common (0.9% vs 8.5%, $p = 0.003$). Pediatric patients took longer to develop secondary progressive MS (SPMS) (32 vs 18 years, $p = 0.0001$) and to reach disability milestones (EDSS 4.0, 23.8 vs 15.5 years, $p < 0.0001$; EDSS 6.0, 30.8 vs 20.4 years, $p < 0.0001$; EDSS 8.0, 44.7 vs 39 years, $p = 0.02$), but did so between 7.0 and 12 years younger than in adult-onset MS. A high relapse rate predicted faster progression. Complete recovery on the other hand, reduced the risk of progression (reaching EDSS 4) on the long term.

Risk of conversion
Children with initial CIS are more likely to develop MS than those with acute disseminated encephalomyelitis (ADEM) as initial diagnosis. In a study of 123 children (< 18 years of age) with a combined retrospective and prospective follow-up (median 61.5 months), conversion from CIS to MS occurred in 26 of 67 children (38.8%); from ADEM to MS in 4 of 47 children (8.5%) [23]. Female gender, brain stem or hemispheric involvement, and Callen's magnetic resonance imaging criteria [24] were found to predict the diagnosis of MS. Cerebrospinal fluid (CSF) did not prove to be a good indicator for conversion.

A second relapse and initial presentation with brain stem, cerebellar or cerebral dysfunction, or multifocal CIS were strongly associated with the development of MS ($p = 0.002$) in a retrospective study [25]. Sixteen patients (50%) experienced a second demyelinating event, with a mean interval between the first and second episode 21 (± 20) months. 11 (34%) developed pediatric MS after a mean follow-up of 6.1 (± 1.6) years. Asymptomatic brain lesions on MRI and the presence of oligoclonal bands were not predictors of conversion to MS in this study.

MRI parameters

MRI parameters can also be used to predict the risk of MS in children with CIS. In a national prospective inception cohort study at 23 sites in Canada, 284 eligible participants (age < 16 years) were followed up for 3.9 years [26]. Fifty-seven (20%) were diagnosed with MS after a median of 188 days. The presence of either one or more T1-weighted hypointense lesions (HR 20.6) or one or more periventricular lesions (3.34) was associated with an increased likelihood of MS diagnosis. This risk was particularly elevated when both parameters were present (HR 34.27).

A meta-analysis of 14 studies that included children presented with optic neuritis, revealed that older children and those with brain MRI abnormalities at presentation are at greater risk for MS [27]. Data of 223 patients (age range: 2 - 17.8 years) were analyzed. For every 1-year increase in age, the odds of developing MS increased by 32% (odds ratio (OR) = 1.3, $p = 0.005$). The risk of MS was greater in children with abnormal brain MRI scans at presentation compared with normal MRIs (OR = 28.0, $p < 0.001$).

Discussion

Prognosis

In a large cohort from a network of French and Belgian centers, patients with pediatric MS reached secondary-progression and disability milestones at ages approximately 10 years younger than patients with adult-onset disease, despite a slower development of irreversible disability [2]. Among the 17,934 patients, 394 (2.2%) had MS starting at 16 years of age or younger, and 290 (73.6%) of these patients were women. The mean age at onset was 13.7 years. Onset occurred at the age of 14 years or younger in 159 patients (40.4%), and at 10 years or younger in 30 patients (7.6%). The estimated median time between the first two neurologic episodes was 2.0 years.

A more aggressive disease course may be predicted by relapse severity and residual disability in early pediatric MS. In a retrospective study of 105 patients with MS or CIS onset prior to 18 years of age, optic nerve involvement was associated with a severe initial demyelinating event (IDE) (OR 4.30, $p = 0.007$) [28]. A severe initial demyelinating event was associated with incomplete recovery (OR 6.90, $p < 0.001$), with similar trends for second and third events. Incomplete recovery from the first event predicted incomplete second event recovery (OR 3.36, $p = 0.055$).

The importance of presentation at onset for the prognosis is underlined by a study of prognostic indicators of SPMS in a cohort of 127 pediatric MS patients (< 18 years of age) from Kuwait [29]. Twenty patients (15.8%) developed SPMS. At MS onset, brainstem involvement (adjusted HR 5.71; $p = 0.010$) and age at MS onset (adjusted HR 1.38; $p = 0.042$) were significantly associated with the risk of SPMS.

Diagnostic criteria

Many different diagnostic criteria for pediatric MS have been proposed. It is challenging to rule out other disorders that may mimic MS, and to distinguish pediatric MS from various demyelinating syndromes that can occur in childhood. The criteria by the Pediatric International Study Group have been applied in most studies. This is because they have classified the various acquired demyelinating syndromes (ADSs) that may be the first clinical sign of pediatric MS. The classification of ADSs, which dates

Table 2 Diagnostic criteria for pediatric MS [31]

For the diagnosis pediatric CIS, all of the following is required:
- A monofocal or polyfocal, clinical CNS event with presumed inflammatory demyelinating cause.
- Absence of a prior clinical history of CNS demyelinating disease (e.g. absence of past optic neuritis (ON), transverse myelitis (TM) and hemispheric or brain-stem related syndromes).
- No encephalopathy (i.e. no alteration in consciousness or behavior) that cannot be explained by fever.
- The diagnosis of MS based on baseline MRI features (as recently defined) are not met.

For pediatric ADEM, all of the following is required:
- A first polyfocal, clinical CNS event with presumed inflammatory demyelinating cause.
- Encephalopathy that cannot be explained by fever.
- No new clinical and MRI findings emerge 3 months or more after the onset.
- Brain MRI is abnormal during the acute (three-month) phase.
- Typically on a brain MRI:
  • diffuse, poorly demarcated, large (> 1–2 cm) lesions involving predominantly cerebral white matter;
  • deep grey matter lesions (e.g. thalamus or basal ganglia) may be present;
  • T1-hypointense lesions in the white matter are rare.

For pediatric NMO, all of the following are required
- Optic neuritis.
- Acute myelitis.
- At least two of three supportive criteria:
* contiguous spinal cord MRI lesion extending over three vertebral segments;
* brain MRI not meeting diagnostic criteria for MS;
* aquaporin IgG seropositive status.

For pediatric MS, one of the following is required
- ≥ 2 non-encephalopathic, clinical CNS events with presumed inflammatory cause, separated
- by > 30 days and involving more than one CNS area.
- One non-encephalopathic episode typical of MS which is associated with MRI findings consistent with 2010 Revised McDonald criteria for dissemination in space (DIS) and in which a follow-up MRI shows at least one new enhancing or non-enhancing lesion consistent with dissemination in time (DIT) MS criteria.
- One ADEM attack followed by a non-encephalopathic clinical event, three or more months after symptom onset, that is associated with new MRI lesions that fulfill 2010 Revised McDonald DIS criteria.
- A first, single, acute event (e.g. a CIS) that does not meet ADEM criteria and whose MRI findings are consistent with the 2010 revised McDonald Criteria for DIS and DIT (applied only to children ≥12 years old).

from 2007 [30] and has been updated in 2013 [31] is as follows (see Table 2 for diagnostic criteria):

- Pediatric MS
- Optic neuritis (ON)
- Transverse myelitis (TM)
- Clinically isolated syndrome (CIS)
- Neuromyelitis Optics (NMO)
- Acute disseminated encephalomyelitis (ADEM)

There are a number of important changes when comparing the 2007 and 2012 definitions for pediatric acute demyelinating disorders of the CNS [30, 31].

- Arguably the most important change is in the definition of MS (and pediatric MS). "Multiple clinical episodes of CNS demyelination separated in time and space" in the 2007 criteria, has been specified to "≥ 2 non-encephalopathic clinical CNS events with presumed inflammatory cause, separated by > 30 days and involving more than one CNS area".
- Added to the definition of NMO has been the following condition: "Brain MRI not meeting diagnostic criteria for MS".
- Encephalopathy is defined as "An alteration in consciousness (e.g. stupor, lethargy) or behavioral change unexplained by fever, systemic illness or post-ictal symptoms".
- A second event is "The development of new symptoms at least three months after the incident illness irrespective of steroid use".
- Multiphasic ADEM is defined as two episodes consistent with ADEM separated by 3 months but not followed by any further events. The second ADEM event can involve either new or a re-emergence of prior neurologic symptoms, signs and MRI findings.
- Relapsing disease following ADEM that occurs beyond a second encephalopathic event is no longer consistent with multiphasic ADEM, but rather indicates a chronic disorder, most often leading to the diagnosis of MS or NMO.
- Children with MS (under age 12) differ clinically from adolescents with MS. They are more likely than adolescent-onset MS patients to have an ADEM-like first attack, they can have large, ill-defined lesions early in the disease course, and they are less likely to have CSF oligoclonal bands.

Differential diagnosis

As in adults, dissemination in time and space is an essential feature. In general, the more atypical the case and the younger the child, the more consideration is necessary before making a diagnosis of MS [32]. MS must

not only be differentiated from acute ADEM or NMO, but there is also an extensive list of other disorders that can mimic MS which need to be excluded. Examples of such disorders are systemic lupus erythematosus (SLE), neurosarcoidosis, Sjögren syndrome, leukodystrophies, hereditary metabolic disorders, and encephalitic or meningo-encephalitic infectious etiologies.

It is especially challenging to determine whether a child with an initial demyelinating event (IDE) will develop subsequent events that are consistent with MS or not. A list of "red flags" in the differential diagnosis in children presented with their initial demyelinating event have been suggested [32]. It includes encephalopathy and fever, progression from the onset, involvement of the peripheral nervous system or other organs, absence of CSF oligoclonal IgG (40-50% of pediatric MS patients exhibit oligoclonal bands, which is less than in adults) and markedly elevated CSF white blood cells or proteins.

ADEM typically presents as a monophasic demyelinating disease. It may be induced by preceding viral infections or vaccination, e.g. concerning measles or varicella zoster virus (VZV). Seizures or behavioral disorders as common presenting symptoms in ADEM. It can be difficult to differentiate ADEM from the first MS attack based on clinical evaluation. MRI appearance plays a major role in the diagnosis. Two or more periventricular lesions, absence of a diffuse bilateral lesion pattern, and the presence of black holes are frequently seen in MS patients compared to patients with ADEM [33].

The appearance of new lesions in different locations on follow-up MRI strongly suggests MS. Recently it was shown that susceptibility-weight imaging (SWI) may be useful in differentiating initial presentation of pediatric MS from ADEM [34].

Disease-modifying therapies

Studies in adult MS patients suggest significant benefit of early institution of DMTs. The available efficacy data for pediatric MS patients is scarce and mostly based on retrospective studies. An international consensus highlighted the importance of initiating DMT in children and adolescents with MS [35]. A rationale for early institution of DMT in pediatric MS patients was supported by several facts related to natural history data:

- 85-90% has an active relapsing MS course.
- Relapse rate is high in initial phases of the disease and is correlated with a bad prognosis.
- Short duration between relapses and the subsequent accumulation of disability.
- Although progression may be slower than in adults, moderate-to-severe disability is reached at a younger age.

– Brain tissue shows more active inflammation in childhood, so patients may benefit from the anti-inflammatory effects of DMTs.

– Despite the apparent clinical recovery from relapses due to better neuronal plasticity, cognitive impairment is frequent. Postponing treatment may have a negative impact on social activities and school performance.

Evidence of the effectiveness of DMTs in reducing relapse rate and disease progression in pediatric MS patients is exclusively based on observational studies. Four randomized controlled trials are either recruiting or reaching final stages: PARADIGMS (fingolimod), TERI-KIDS (teriflunomide), FOCUS (dimethyl fumarate) and CONNECT (dimethyl fumarate vs. Interferon beta 1a).

First-line treatment

The current first-line treatment of MS in children consists of either interferon beta (IFNB) or glatiramer acetate (GA). The safety profile of IFNB / GA remains favourable in children. No unexpected adverse events and no serious adverse events were documented in 44 pediatric MS patients from 7 countries who were treated with interferon beta-1b [36]. The mean age at the start of therapy was 13 years; 8 patients were ≤ 10 years of age. Most common adverse events included flu-like syndrome (35%), abnormal liver function test (26%), and injection site reaction (21%).

Adult doses of subcutaneous (sc) IFNB-1a (44 and 22 μg, three times weekly) were generally well tolerated by children and adolescents, with no new or unexpected adverse drug reactions, in a large retrospective study, named REPLAY [37]. It is the largest multicenter, multinational review of safety, tolerability, and efficacy outcomes with sc IFNB-1a in pediatric MS patients. Reviewed were records of 307 patients aged between 2 and 17 years, who had received at least 1 injection of sc IFNB-1a for demyelinating events. Despite the lack of a control group, beneficial effects were observed. Annualized relapse rates were 1.79 before and 0.47 during treatment. On the other hand, the experience with glatiramer acetate is very limited. It has roughly the same efficacy as IFNB [38].

Second-line treatment

In children with breakthrough disease (defined as relapses while on first-line therapies), escalation to higher efficacious second-line therapies, such as natalizumab, fingolimod, mitoxantrone, cyclophosphamide, rituximab, and daclizumab may be considered based on the extrapolated data from adult cohorts. However, data on the safety, efficacy, and tolerability of most of these treatments are scarce and have been reported only in small-size retrospective case series [40].

Large observational studies have shown that natalizumab is an effective treatment in children with breakthrough disease, with a good safety and efficacy profile, comparable to those in adult populations [39–44]. A strong suppression of disease activity was observed in all subjects during follow-up in a study of 19 patients (mean age 14.6 +/- 2.2 years) [41]. The mean EDSS score decreased from 2.6 ± 1.0 to 1.9 ± 1.0 ($p < 0.001$). EDSS remained stable in 5 cases, decreased by ≥0.5 point in 6 cases, and decreased by ≥ 1 point in 8 cases. There were no relapses during follow-up ($p < 0.001$), nor new gadolinium-enhanced (Gd+) lesions ($p = 0.008$). A study by the same group of 55 patients showed a dramatic decrease in the number of relapses [42]. The mean number of relapses before treatment was high: 4.4. During follow-up only 3 relapses in all occurred. Mean EDSS scores decreased from 2.7 to 1.9 at the last visit ($p < 0.001$). During follow-up, the majority of patients remained free from MRI activity. Transient and mild clinical adverse events occurred in 20 patients. Anti-JCV antibodies were detected in 20 of 51 tested patients. In a retrospective study of 9 pediatric patients with highly active MS, the use of natalizumab completely halted the inflammatory process [43]. Two patients still had relapses, but they both had neutralizing antibodies against natalizumab. The median EDSS score decreased from 3.0 to 1.0, the median ARR decreased from 3.0 to 0.0. A recent study revealed that treatment with natalizumab was associated with reductions in mean ARR (3.7 vs 0.4; $p < 0.001$), n median EDSS scores (2 vs 1; $p < 0.02$), and in mean number of new T2-lesions per year (7.8 vs 0.5; $p < 0.001$) in children with active relapsing MS.

Conclusion

Pediatric MS has long been an underdiagnosed and undertreated condition. It has distinctive features and the disease course is different than in adult-onset MS. Progression may be slower than in adults due to neuroplasticity, but moderate-to-severe disability is reached at a younger age. It is important to limit the axonal damage secondary to extensive inflammatory changes seen earlier in the disease process by initiating early DMT in these patients and delaying disability accumulation. More prospective, randomized, large cohort studies are needed to assess the safety and efficacy of DMTs in children with MS, especially in those with highly active disease or an aggressive disease course.

Abbreviations

ADEM: Acute disseminated encephalomyelitis; APP: Amyloid Precursor Protein; CFS: Cerebrospinal fluid; CI: Confidence interval; CIS: Clinically isolated syndrome; CNS: Central nervous system; DIS: Dissemination in space; DIT: Dissemination in time; DMT: Disease-modifying therapies; EBV: Epstein-Barr virus; EDSS: Expanded disability status scale; GA: Glatiramer acetate; Gd +: Gadolinium-enhanced; HR: Hazard ratio; IDE: Initial demyelinating event; IFNB: Interferon beta; NMO: Neuromyelitis Optics; MRI: Magnetic resonance imaging; MS: Multiple sclerosis; POMS: Pediatric-onset MS; PPMS: Primary progressive MS; ON: Optic neuritis; OR: Odds ratio; RRMS: Relapse remitting MS; SC: Subcutaneous; SLE: Systemic lupus erythematosus; SPMS: Secondary progressive MS; SWI: Susceptibility-weight imaging; TDT: Transmission disequilibrium test; TM: Transverse myelitis; VZV: Varicella zoster virus

Acknowledgements
The authors write on behalf of the ParadigMS Private Foundation: an independent and non-profit international group of European, Asian and Middle East Multiple Sclerosis experts dedicated to improving Multiple Sclerosis patient care by translating state-of-the-art science into practical education at local level. Board members: Bart Van Wijmeersch, Patrick Vermersch, Bassem Yamout, Celia Oreja-Guevara, Sven Schippling, Nikolaos Grigoriadis, Raed Al Roughani, Mona Alkhawajah, Thomas Berger, Alexey Boyko, Lou Brundin, Andrew Chan, Florian Deisenhammer, Irina Elovaara, Paolo Gallo, Hans-Peter Hartung, Ralf Linker, James Overell, Carlo Pozzilli, Maura Pugliatti, Finn Thorup Sellebjerg, Maria Pia Sormani, Vincent Van Pesch, Tjalf Ziemssen Expert meetings of ParadigMS were supported by Sanofi Genzyme without any involvement of the sponsor in the program and the content. Writing assistance was provided by M. Tent (Montpellier, France), with funding from the ParadigMS Foundation.

Funding
This research did not receive any specific grant from funding agencies in the public, commercial, or not-for-profit sectors.

Authors' contributions
Both authors performed the literature search and reviewed the manuscripts that resulted in the generation of this review article. Both authors contributed equally to the contents and writing of this manuscript. Both authors read and approved the final manuscript.

Competing interests
The authors declare that they have no competing interests.

Author details
[1]Division of Neurology, Department of Medicine, Amiri Hospital, Arabian Gulf Street, 13041 Sharq, Kuwait. [2]Department of Neurology, Neurosurgery and Medical Genetic of the Pirogov's Russian National Research Medical University and MS Clinic at the Usupov's Hospital, Ostrovitianov str. 1, Moscow 117997, Russia.

References
1. Boiko A, Vorobeychik G, Paty D, et al. Early onset multiple sclerosis: a longitudinal study. Neurology. 2002;59(7):1006–10.
2. Renoux C, Vukusic S, Mikaeloff Y, et al. Natural history of multiple sclerosis with childhood onset. N Engl J Med. 2007;356(25):2603–13.
3. Gorman MP, Healy BC, Polgar-Turcsanyi M, et al. Increased relapse rate in pediatric-onset compared with adult-onset multiple sclerosis. Arch Neurol. 2009;66(1):54–9.
4. Pohl D, Waubant E, Banwell B, et al. Treatment of pediatric multiple sclerosis and variants. Neurology. 2007;68(16 Suppl 2):S54–65.
5. Ghezzi A, Banwell B, Boyko A, et al. The management of multiple sclerosis in children: a European view. Mult Scler. 2010;16(10):1258–67.
6. Duquette P, Murray TJ, Pleines J, et al. Multiple sclerosis in childhood: clinical profile in 125 patients. J Pediatr. 1987;111(3):359–63.
7. Ghezzi A, Deplano V, Faroni J, et al. Multiple sclerosis in childhood: clinical features of 149 cases. Mult Scler. 1997;3(1):43–6.
8. Deryck O, Ketelaer P, Dubois B. Clinical characteristics and long term prognosis in early onset multiple sclerosis. J Neurol. 2006;253(6):720–3.
9. Gusev E, Boiko A, Bikova O, et al. The natural history of early onset multiple sclerosis: comparison of data from Moscow and Vancouver. Clin Neurol Neurosurg. 2002;104(3):203–7.
10. Weinshenker BG, Bass B, Rice GP, et al. The natural history of multiple sclerosis: a geographically based study. 2. Predictive value of the early clinical course. Brain. 1989;112(Pt 6):1419–28.
11. Banwell B, Krupp L, Kennedy J, et al. Clinical features and viral serologies in children with multiple sclerosis: a multinational observational study. Lancet Neurol. 2007;6(9):773–81.
12. Gadoth N. Multiple sclerosis in children. Brain and Development. 2003;25(4): 229–32.
13. Yeh EA, Chitnis T, Krupp L, et al. Pediatric multiple sclerosis. Nat Rev Neurol. 2009;5(11):621–31.
14. Chitnis T, Krupp L, Yeh A, et al. Pediatric multiple sclerosis. Neurol Clin. 2011; 29(2):481–505.
15. Pfeifenbring S, Bunyan RF, Metz I, et al. Extensive acute axonal damage in pediatric multiple sclerosis lesions. Ann Neurol. 2015;77(4):655–67.
16. Anderson RC, Connolly ES Jr, Komotar RJ. Clinicopathological review: tumefactive demyelination in a 12-year-old. Neurosurgery. 2005;56(5):1051–7. discussion 1051-7
17. Amato MP, Goretti B, Ghezzi A, et al. Cognitive and psychosocial features of childhood and juvenile MS. Neurology. 2008;70(20):1891–7.
18. Amato MP, Goretti B, Ghezzi A, et al. Cognitive and psychosocial features in childhood and juvenile MS: two-year follow-up. Neurology. 2010;75(13): 1134–40.
19. Amato MP, Goretti B, Ghezzi A, et al. Neuropsychological features in childhood and juvenile multiple sclerosis: five-year follow-up. Neurology. 2014;83(16):1432–8.
20. Alroughani R, Akhtar S, Ahmed SF, et al. Incidence and prevalence of pediatric onset multiple sclerosis in Kuwait: 1994-2013. J Neurol Sci. 2015; 353(1-2):107–10.
21. Boiko AN, Gusev EI, Sudomoina MA, et al. Association and linkage of juvenile MS with HLA-DR2(15) in Russians. Neurology. 2002;58(4):658–60.
22. Harding KE, Liang K, Cossburn MD, et al. Long-term outcome of paediatric-onset multiple sclerosis: a population-based study. J Neurol Neurosurg Psychiatry. 2013;84(2):141–7.
23. Peche SS, Alshekhlee A, Kelly J, et al. A long-term follow-up study using IPMSSG criteria in children with CNS demyelination. Pediatr Neurol. 2013; 49(5):329–34.
24. Callen DJ, Shroff MM, Branson HM, et al. MRI in the diagnosis of pediatric multiple sclerosis. Neurology. 2009;72(11):961–7.
25. Lee CG, Lee B, Lee J, et al. The natural course of clinically isolated syndrome in pediatric patients. Brain and Development. 2015;37(4):432–8.
26. Verhey LH, Branson HM, Shroff MM, et al. MRI parameters for prediction of multiple sclerosis diagnosis in children with acute CNS demyelination: a prospective national cohort study. Lancet Neurol. 2011;10(12):1065–73.
27. Waldman AT, Stull LB, Galetta SL, et al. Pediatric optic neuritis and risk of multiple sclerosis: meta-analysis of observational studies. J AAPOS. 2011; 15(5):441–6.
28. Fay AJ, Mowry EM, Strober J, et al. Relapse severity and recovery in early pediatric multiple sclerosis. Mult Scler. 2012;18(7):1008–12.
29. Akhtar S, Alroughani R, Ahmed SF, et al. Prognostic indicators of secondary progression in a paediatric-onset multiple sclerosis cohort in Kuwait. Mult Scler. 2016;22(8):1086–93.
30. Krupp LB, Banwell B, Tenembaum S. International pediatric MS study group. Consensus definitions proposed for pediatric multiple sclerosis and related disorders. Neurology. 2007;68(suppl 2):S7–S12.
31. Krupp LB, Tardieu M, Amato MP, et al. International pediatric multiple sclerosis study group criteria for pediatric multiple sclerosis and immune-mediated central nervous system demyelinating disorders: revisions to the 2007 definitions. Mult Scler. 2013;19(10):1261–7.
32. Rubin JP, Kuntz NL. Diagnostic criteria for pediatric multiple sclerosis. Curr Neurol Neurosci Rep. 2013;13(6):354.
33. Callen DJ, Shroff MM, Branson HM, et al. Role of MRI in the differentiation of ADEM from MS in children. Neurology. 2009;72(11):968–73.
34. Rubin JP. MRI to discriminate pediatric MS from ADEM. Pediatr Neurol Briefs. 2015;29(2):13.
35. Chitnis T, Tenembaum S, Banwell B, et al. Consensus statement: evaluation of new and existing therapeutics for pediatric multiple sclerosis. Mult Scler. 2012;18(1):116–27.

36. Banwell B, Reder AT, Krupp L, et al. Safety and tolerability of interferon beta-1b in pediatric multiple sclerosis. Neurology. 2006;66(4):472–6.
37. Tenembaum SN, Banwell B, Pohl D, et al. Subcutaneous interferon Beta-1a in pediatric multiple sclerosis: a retrospective study. J Child Neurol. 2013;28(7):849–56.
38. Narula S, Hopkins SE, Banwell B. Treatment of pediatric multiple sclerosis. 39. Curr Treat Options Neurol. 2015;17(3):336.
39. Simone M, Chitnis T. Use of disease-modifying therapies in pediatric MS. Curr Treat Options Neurol. 2016;18(8):36.
40. Yeh EA, Weinstock-Guttman B. Natalizumab in pediatric multiple sclerosis patients. Ther Adv Neurol Disord. 2010;3(5):293–9.
41. Ghezzi A, Pozzilli C, Grimaldi LM, et al. Safety and efficacy of natalizumab in children with multiple sclerosis. Neurology. 2010;75(10):912–7.
42. Ghezzi A, Pozzilli C, Grimaldi LM, et al. Natalizumab in pediatric multiple sclerosis: results of a cohort of 55 cases. Mult Scler. 2013;19(8):1106–12.
43. Arnal-Garcia C, García-Montero MR, Málaga I, et al. Natalizumab use in pediatric patients with relapsing-remitting multiple sclerosis. Eur J Paediatr Neurol. 2013;17(1):50–4.
44. Kornek B, Aboul-Enein F, Rostasy K, et al. Natalizumab therapy for highly active pediatric multiple sclerosis. JAMA Neurol. 2013;70(4):469–75.
45. Reinhardt K, Weiss S, Rosenbauer J, et al. Multiple sclerosis in children and adolescents: incidence and clinical picture - new insights from the nationwide German surveillance (2009-2011). Eur J Neurol 2014;21(4):654-9.
46. Ketelslegers IA, Catsman-Berrevoets CE, Neuteboom RF, et al. Incidence of acquired demyelinating syndromes of the CNS in Dutch children: a nationwide study. J Neurol 2012;259(9):1929-35.
47. Absoud M, Lim MJ, Chong WK, et al. Paediatric acquired demyelinating syndromes: incidence, clinical and magnetic resonance imaging features. Mult Scler 2013;19(1):76-86
48. Dell'Avvento S, Sotgiu MA, Manca S3, et al. Epidemiology of multiple sclerosis in the pediatric population of Sardinia, Italy. Eur J Pediatr 2016;175(1):19-29.
49. Langer-Gould A, Zhang JL, Chung J, et al. Incidence of acquired CNS demyelinating syndromes in a multiethnic cohort of children. Neurology 2011;77(12):1143-8
50. Fragoso YD, Ferreira ML, Morales Nde M, et al. Multiple sclerosis starting before the age of 18 years: the Brazilian experience. Arq Neuropsiquiatr 2013;71(10):783-7
51. Inaloo S, Haghbin S, Moradi M, et al. Acquired CNS Demyelinating Syndrome in Children Referred to ShirazPediatric Neurology Ward. Iran J Child Neurol 2014;8(2):18-23.

Permissions

The contributors of this book come from diverse backgrounds, making this book a truly international effort. This book will bring forth new frontiers with its revolutionizing research information and detailed analysis of the nascent developments around the world.

We would like to thank all the contributing authors for lending their expertise to make the book truly unique. They have played a crucial role in the development of this book. Without their invaluable contributions this book wouldn't have been possible. They have made vital efforts to compile up to date information on the varied aspects of this subject to make this book a valuable addition to the collection of many professionals and students.

This book was conceptualized with the vision of imparting up-to-date information and advanced data in this field. To ensure the same, a matchless editorial board was set up. Every individual on the board went through rigorous rounds of assessment to prove their worth. After which they invested a large part of their time researching and compiling the most relevant data for our readers.

The editorial board has been involved in producing this book since its inception. They have spent rigorous hours researching and exploring the diverse topics which have resulted in the successful publishing of this book. They have passed on their knowledge of decades through this book. To expedite this challenging task, the publisher supported the team at every step. A small team of assistant editors was also appointed to further simplify the editing procedure and attain best results for the readers.

Apart from the editorial board, the designing team has also invested a significant amount of their time in understanding the subject and creating the most relevant covers. They scrutinized every image to scout for the most suitable representation of the subject and create an appropriate cover for the book.

The publishing team has been an ardent support to the editorial, designing and production team. Their endless efforts to recruit the best for this project, has resulted in the accomplishment of this book. They are a veteran in the field of academics and their pool of knowledge is as vast as their experience in printing. Their expertise and guidance has proved useful at every step. Their uncompromising quality standards have made this book an exceptional effort. Their encouragement from time to time has been an inspiration for everyone.

The publisher and the editorial board hope that this book will prove to be a valuable piece of knowledge for researchers, students, practitioners and scholars across the globe.

List of Contributors

Farzin Halabchi and Zahra Alizadeh
Sports and Exercise Medicine, Sports Medicine Research Center, Neuroscience Institute, Tehran University of Medical Sciences, Tehran, Iran

Mohammad Ali Sahraian
Neurology, MS fellowship, MS Research Center, Neuroscience Institute,Tehran University of Medical Sciences, Tehran, Iran

Maryam Abolhasani
Sports and Exercise Medicine, MS Research Center, Neuroscience Institute, Tehran University of Medical Sciences, Tehran, Iran
Sports and Exercise medicine, Sina MS Research Center, Department of Sports Medicine, Sina Hospital, Hassan Abad Square, Tehran, Iran

Danielle Bernardes and Alexandre Leite Rodrigues Oliveira
Department of Structural and Functional Biology, Institute of Biology, University of Campinas, Rua Monteiro Lobato, 255, Campinas, Sao Paulo 13.083-862, Brazil

Meritxell Sabidó-Espin
Frankfurter Str. 250, HPC: F135/201, Darmstadt 64293, Germany

Rick Munschauer
EMD Serono, Rockland, MA, USA

Trygve Holmøy
Department of Neurology, Akershus University Hospital, Lørenskog, Norway
Institute of Clinical Medicine, University of Oslo, Oslo, Norway

Jonas Christoffer Lindstrøm
Institute of Clinical Medicine, University of Oslo, Oslo, Norway
Helse Øst Health Services and Research Centre, Akershus University Hospital, Lørenskog, Norway

Erik Fink Eriksen
Helse Øst Health Services and Research Centre, Akershus University Hospital, Lørenskog, Norway
Department of Endocrinology, Oslo University Hospital, Oslo, Norway

Margitta T. Kampman
Department of Neurology, University Hospital of North Norway, Tromsø, Norway

Linn Hofsøy Steffensen
Department of Neurology, University Hospital of North Norway, Tromsø, Norway
Department of Clinical Medicine, University of Tromsø, Tromsø, Norway

Helena Posová, Václav Čapek and Zdenka Hrušková
Institute of Immunology and Microbiology, First Faculty of Medicine, Charles University and General University Hospital in Prague, Prague, Czech Republic

Dana Horáková, Tomáš Uher and Eva Havrdová
Department of Neurology and Centre of Clinical Neuroscience First Faculty of Medicine, Charles University and General University Hospital in Prague, Prague, Czech Republic

Qi Hao
Institute of Multiple Sclerosis Therapeutics, Nishinokyo-Kasugacho 16-44-409, Nakakyo-ku, Kyoto 604-8453, Japan

Takahiko Saida
Institute of Multiple Sclerosis Therapeutics, Nishinokyo-Kasugacho 16-44-409, Nakakyo-ku, Kyoto 604-8453, Japan
Kyoto Min-Iren-Central Hospital, Kyoto, Japan
Kyoto University Hospital, Kyoto, Japan

Yasuto Itoyama
International University of Health and Welfare, 1-7-4 Momochihama, Sawara, Fukuoka City, Fukuoka 814-0001, Japan

Seiji Kikuchi
Hokkaido Medical Center, National Hospital Organization, 1-1 Yamanote 5-jo 7-chome, Sapporo 063-0005, Japan

Takayoshi Kurosawa, Kengo Ueda and Isao Tsumiyama
Novartis Pharma KK, 1-23-1, Toranomon, Minato-ku, Tokyo 105-6333, Japan

Lixin Zhang Auberson
Novartis Pharma AG, Fabrikstrasse 12, 4002 Basel,
Switzerland

Kazuo Nagato
Mitsubishi Tanabe Pharma Corporation, 17-10,
Nihonbashi-Koamicho, Chuo-ku Tokyo 103 8405,
Japan

Jun-ichi Kira
Department of Neurology, Neurological Institute,
Graduate School of Medical Sciences, Kyushu
University, 3-1-1 Maidashi, Higashi-ku, Fukuoka
812-8582, Japan

Chiara Zecca and Giulio Disanto
Multiple Sclerosis Center, Neurocenter of Southern
Switzerland, Ospedale Regionale di Lugano,
Lugano, Switzerland

Sarah Mühl
Merck (Schweiz) AG, Zug, Switzerland

Claudio Gobbi
Multiple Sclerosis Center, Neurocenter of Southern
Switzerland, Ospedale Regionale di Lugano,
Lugano, Switzerland
Multiple Sclerosis Center, Neurocenter of Southern
Switzerland, Ospedale Regionale di Lugano, Via
Tesserete 46, 6903 Lugano, Switzerland

Michael Munsell, Molly Frean and Joseph Menzin
Boston Health Economics, Inc., 20 Fox Road,
Waltham, MA 02451, USA

Amy L. Phillips
Health Economics & Outcomes Research, EMD
Serono, Inc., One Technology Place, Rockland, MA
02370, USA

**Ilse M. Nauta, Bernard M. J. Uitdehaag and Brigit
A. de Jong**
Department of Neurology, Amsterdam
Neuroscience, MS Center Amsterdam, VU
University Medical Center, Amsterdam, the
Netherlands

Anne E. M. Speckens
Department of Psychiatry, Radboud University
Medical Center, Nijmegen, the Netherlands

Roy P. C. Kessels
Donders Institute for Brain, Cognition and Behaviour,
Radboud University,Nijmegen, the Netherlands

Department of Medical Psychology, Radboud
University Medical Center,Nijmegen, the Netherlands

Jeroen J. G. Geurts
Department of Anatomy and Neurosciences,
Amsterdam Neuroscience, MS Center Amsterdam,
VU University Medical Center, Amsterdam, the
Netherlands

Vincent de Groot
Department of Rehabilitation Medicine, MS Center
Amsterdam, VU University Medical Center,
Amsterdam, the Netherlands

Luciano Fasotti
Donders Institute for Brain, Cognition and
Behaviour, Radboud University,Nijmegen, the
Netherlands
Klimmendaal Rehabilitation Center, Arnhem, the
Netherlands

Nico Arie van der Maas
Institut für Physiotherapieforschung, Lindenweg
48, 2503 Biel, Switzerland

**Theresa Krüger, Anuschka Grobelny and Tanja
Schmitz-Hübsch**
NeuroCure Clinical Research Center,
Clinical Neuroimmunology Group, Charité –
Universitätsmedizin Berlin, Charitéplatz 1, 10117
Berlin, Germany

**Janina R. Behrens, Judith Bellmann-Strobl and
Alexander U. Brandt**
NeuroCure Clinical Research Center,
Clinical Neuroimmunology Group, Charité –
Universitätsmedizin Berlin, Charitéplatz 1, 10117
Berlin, Germany
Department of Neurology, Charité –
Universitätsmedizin Berlin, Charitéplatz 1, 10117
Berlin, Germany

Friedemann Paul
NeuroCure Clinical Research Center,
Clinical Neuroimmunology Group, Charité –
Universitätsmedizin Berlin, Charitéplatz 1, 10117
Berlin, Germany
Department of Neurology, Charité –
Universitätsmedizin Berlin, Charitéplatz 1, 10117
Berlin, Germany
Experimental and Clinical Research Center, Charité
– Universitätsmedizin Berlin and Max Delbrück
Center for Molecular Medicine, Lindenberger Weg
80, 13125 Berlin, Germany

Karen Otte, Sebastian Mansow-Model and Bastian Kayser
Motognosis UG, Schönhauser Allee 177, 10119 Berlin, Germany

Elisabeth Anens, Lena Zetterberg, Charlotte Urell, Margareta Emtner and Karin Hellström
Department of Neuroscience, Section for Physiotherapy, Uppsala University, 751 24 Uppsala, Sweden

Trygve Holmøy
Department of Neurology, Akershus University Hospital, Lørenskog, Norway
Institute of Clinical Medicine, University of Oslo, Oslo, Norway

Hedda von der Lippe
Department of Infectious Diseases, Akershus University Hospital, Lørenskog, Norway

Truls Michael Leegaard
Institute of Clinical Medicine, University of Oslo, Oslo, Norway
Department of Microbiology, Akershus University Hospital, Lørenskog, Norway

Douglas L. Arnold
Montreal Neurological Institute, McGill University, Montreal, QC, Canada
NeuroRx Research, Montreal, QC, Canada

Peter A. Calabresi
Department of Neurology, Johns Hopkins University, Baltimore, MD, USA

Bernd C. Kieseier
Biogen, 225 Binney St, Cambridge, MA, USA
Department of Neurology, Medical Faculty, Heinrich-Heine University, Düsseldorf, Germany

Shifang Liu, Xiaojun You, Damian Fiore and Serena Hung
Biogen, 225 Binney St, Cambridge, MA, USA

Mohammad Ali Sahraian
MS Research Center, Neuroscience Institute, Tehran University of Medical Sciences, Tehran, Iran
MS Research Center, Sina Hospital, Hassan Abad square, Tehran, Iran

Caroline Papeix and Rana Assouad
Neurology Department, GHPS Pitié Salpêtrière, Paris, France

Paolo Ragonese, Paolo Aridon, Giulia Vazzoler, Maria Antonietta Mazzola, Vincenzina Lo Re, Marianna Lo Re, Sabrina Realmuto, Simona Alessi, Marco D'Amelio, Giovanni Savettieri and Giuseppe Salemi
Dipartimento di Biomedicina Sperimentale e Neuroscienze Cliniche (Department of Experimental Biomedicine and Clinical Neurosciences), Università degli Studi di Palermo, Via G. La Loggia, 1, 90129 Palermo, Italy

Marie-Claire Gay and Pierre Vrignaud
Psychology Department, University of Paris West, Nanterre, France

Catherine Bungener
Laboratory of Psychopathology, University of Paris Descartes, Paris, France
Health Psychology, Université Paris Sorbonne Cité, Paris, France

Sarah Thomas, Peter W Thomas and Roger Baker
Clinical Research Unit, Faculty of Health and Social Sciences, Bournemouth University, UK

Sébastien Montel and Michèle Montreuil
Psychology Department, University of Paris 8, St Denis, France

Olivier Heinzlef
Neurology Department, Hospital of Poissy-St-Germain en Laye, Paris, France

Sharareh Eskandarieh
Brain and Spinal Cord Injury Research Center, Neuroscience Institute, Tehran University of Medical Sciences, Tehran, Iran
MS Research Center, Neuroscience Institute, Tehran University of Medical Sciences, Tehran, Iran

Narges Sistany Allahabadi and Malihe Sadeghi
MS Research Center, Neuroscience Institute, Tehran University of Medical Sciences, Tehran, Iran

Hai Qing Li, Bo Yin and Yi Fang Bao
Department of Radiology, Huashan Hospital, Fudan University 12 Wulumuqi Rd. Middle, Shanghai 200040, China

Chao Quan and Hai Yu
Department of Neurology, Huashan Hospital, Fudan University, Shanghai, China

Dao Ying Geng and Yu Xin Li
Department of Radiology, Huashan Hospital, Fudan University 12 Wulumuqi Rd. Middle, Shanghai 200040, China
Institute of Functional and Molecular Medical Imaging, Fudan University, Shanghai, China

Jun Liu
Department of Radiology, The Fifth People's Hospital of Shanghai, Fudan University, 128 Ruili Rd, Shanghai 200240, China

Gulin Sunter, Dilek Ince Gunal and Kadriye Agan
Department of Neurology, Marmara University, Istanbul, Turkey

Ece Oge Enver, Azad Akbarzade, Serap Turan, Abdullah Bereket and Tulay Guran
Department of Paediatric Endocrinology and Diabetes, Marmara University, Fevzi Cakmak Mh. Mimar Sinan Cd.No 41., Ustkaynarca/Pendik, 34899 Istanbul, Turkey

Goncagul Haklaz and Pinar Vatansever
Department of Biochemistry, Marmara University, Istanbul, Turkey

Anthony Traboulsee and David K. B. Li
University of British Columbia, S113-2211 Wesbrook Mall, Vancouver, BC V6T 1Z7, Canada

Mark Cascione
Tampa Neurology Associates, South Tampa Multiple Sclerosis Center, 2919 W. Swann Avenue, Suite 401, South Tampa, FL 33609, USA

Juanzhi Fang
EMD Serono, Inc., One Technology Place, Rockland, MA 02370, USA

Fernando Dangond
EMD Serono, Inc., 45A Middlesex Turnpike, Billerica, MA 01821, USA

Aaron Miller
Mount Sinai Hospital, 5 East 98th Street, 1st Floor, New York, NY 10029, USA

Osama Al Wutayd
Unaizah College of Medicine, Qassim University, Qassim, Saudi Arabia
Unaizah College of Medicine and Medical Sciences – Qassim University, Unaizah, Qassim, Saudi Arabia

Ashri Gad Mohamed
King Khalid University Hospital, Riyadh, Saudi Arabia

Jameelah Saeedi
Princess Norah Bint Abdulrahman University, Riyadh, Saudi Arabia

Hessa Al Otaibi
King Fahad General Hospital, Ministry of Health, Jedda, Saudi Arabia

Mohammed Al Jumah
King Fahad Medical City, MOH, KAIMRC/KSAU-HS, Riyadh, Saudi Arabia

Raed Alroughani
Division of Neurology, Department of Medicine, Amiri Hospital, Arabian Gulf Street, 13041 Sharq, Kuwait

Alexey Boyko
Department of Neurology, Neurosurgery and Medical Genetic of the Pirogov's Russian National Research Medical University and MS Clinic at the Usupov's Hospital, Ostrovitianov str. 1, Moscow 117997, Russia

Index